Management of Communication Needs in People with Learning Disability

Dedication

We dedicate this book to:

Gabriella Tobias who is following her Uncle Sam's footsteps in speech and language therapy

SA

and Evelyn and Graham Hurd, Angela's parents, for all the encouragement and support they have given to her

AH

Management of Communication Needs in People with Learning Disability

Edited by

SAMUEL ABUDARHAM PhD, FRCSLT

and

ANGELA HURD MA, MRCSLT

both of the
University of Central England, Birmingham

W
WHURR PUBLISHERS
LONDON AND PHILADELPHIA

© 2002 Whurr Publishers
First published 2002 by
Whurr Publishers Ltd
19b Compton Terrace, London N1 2UN, England and
325 Chestnut Street, Philadelphia PA 19106, USA

Reprinted 2002

British Library Cataloguing in Publication Data
A catalogue record for this book is available from the British
Library.

ISBN: 1 86156 208 X

Printed and bound in the UK by Athenaeum Press Ltd,
Gateshead, Tyne & Wear

Contents

Preface

'Necessity is the mother of invention' goes the familiar saying. One might say, so is frustration. As academics and practitioners in the field of learning disability (LD), we have for quite some time been struck by the paucity of literature in this field, particularly of text books, written *by* speech and language therapists *for* speech and language therapists (SLTs). On the other hand, there is an abundance of such literature for teachers. There is, of course, no doubt that SLTs can and do learn a lot from the educational world and there are many lessons that can be applied to speech and language therapy. Indeed, SLTs need to familiarise themselves with that body of knowledge and practice, particularly since many work in schools and need to be aware of how their work can contribute to educational requirements such as, in the United Kingdom, the National Curriculum.

This said, however, there are many specialised issues that the educational literature does not address and which are particularly pertinent to the SLT's work. The same can be said about the paucity of literature on speech and language therapy with adolescents and adults with LD. We propose to make some contribution to this 'niche' in the literature. We have included discussion on work with adults, though we acknowledge that we do not pretend to present a perfect balance between discussion of 'paediatric' and 'adult' issues as some of the chapters, such as the one on 'Early Intervention', are on subjects which are entirely aimed at, or more pertinent to, work with children.

This book is primarily aimed at the student and recently qualified speech and language therapist readership. We also address the needs of albeit experienced SLTs who may wish to start work with this client group. The contributors to this book are all SLTs and experienced workers in the area of LD. Many have had their work published in learned and peer-reviewed journals and or have conducted research in the field. We have tried to focus on the practical aspects of the SLT's work, hence the inclusion of case studies anecdotally illustrating clinical issues. Though initially we had planned to allow for more space for this, and provide short reviews of the literature, many of the contributors clearly felt that in order for the practice to make sense, it had to be based on sound theory and so, despite some reiteration of the literature already available, we felt it justified to reconsider the initially proposed balance between theory and practice. The plan for the book was thus to include material which addresses current and central issues in speech and language therapy practice. We do not claim that the coverage is exhaustive in its breadth or depth – space rarely allows this in an edited book. Clearly, as in most publications, the greater the number of topics covered, the less depth there is likely to be. We have attempted to strike a balance to ensure that this book has as much practical value as space allows, without unduly compromising its academic credibility. The choice of topics addressed, the relative emphasis or otherwise, has naturally been left primarily to the contributor though there has, of course, been consultation with the editors from the start of the planning process. We have adopted what seemed to us to be largely a 'chronological' presentation.

One could argue that the success of any speech and language therapy largely depends on the availability of resources and the policies and quality of the service delivery. The first chapter, 'Issues of Service Delivery and Auditing' by Janet Hickman, explores a number of issues related to service delivery and auditing relevant to clients with LD across the infant–adult age range. She makes comparisons across service delivery models. She stresses the need for further evaluation of service delivery, in order to make recommendations for effective management models, and to be able to justify speech and language therapy service provision to the purchaser. Hickman also discusses issues regarding evidence-based practice and current thinking in clinical governance and a number of ways in which intervention outcomes can be measured.

Chapter 2, written by one of the editors, Samuel Abudarham, addresses issues relevant to 'Assessment and Appraisal of Communication Needs'. The chapter is divided into two sections, the first being predominantly related to reviewing the literature and the second to more practical issues. There has traditionally been considerable controversy regarding the assessment of communication skills and needs of individuals with LD and appraisal of such individuals. The major arguments are briefly discussed in this chapter. A holistic approach in the appraisal of both chil-

dren and adults is strongly advocated and a model is proposed. A number
of assessment strategies for both children and adults are discussed. The
major areas of communication skills which should be assessed are
presented with rationales.

In Chapter 3, 'Speech and Language Therapy Management Models',
Della Money argues that the communication strengths and needs of
people with LD are influenced both by their communication partners,
and by their wider communication environments. Communication, she
argues, is the joint responsibility of the focal person, their family and
friends, and the whole multi-disciplinary team and this has implications
for speech and language therapy management and services. Money
presents different examples of management models including direct, indirect, group, individual, and teaching. She also discusses issues related to
location and considers theoretical perspectives i.e. means, reasons and
opportunities.

In Chapter 4, Abudarham discusses issues of 'Early Intervention'.
The nature of early intervention (EI) and its rationale are discussed. He
briefly discusses published programmes such as 'Hanen' and 'The
Picture Exchange Communication System'. Though the focus on effectiveness has been most prevalent in the USA in the last two decades or
so, it has now become very current in the UK. A number of EI
programmes are being evaluated and the British government has started
to fund research into EI programmes such as Sure Start. A slowly
increasing number of SLTs are involved in running and researching into
such programmes.

Chapter 5 by Angela Hurd, the second editor, is entitled 'Development of Pre-symbolic and Pre-linguistic Skills'. Historically, the emphasis
for SLTs has been on the 'precision of the system' (Butterfield, Arthur and
Sigafoos, 1995). However, over recent years there has been a radical shift
towards considering pragmatic aspects and the need for a shared means
of communication. Interactive partners' skills are thus crucial in developing and maintaining communicative exchanges. The more traditional
speech and language therapy approach in developing communicative
competence is, however, critical to success. A five-stage pre-verbal
communication programme based on Bloom and Lahey's (1978) 'form,
content and use' paradigm is proposed which is designed to allow
adequate focus to be placed on the objectives within each stage and also
to consider stage-appropriate activities.

In Chapter 6, Nicola Grove deals with a crucial stage in intervention,
'From First Words to Phrase and from Phrase to Sentence'. She refers to

evidence suggesting that the existence of an intellectual impairment on its own is not necessarily a barrier to the acquisition of language structure. Specific difficulties, however, may be associated with particular syndromes. She discusses a multi-modal developmental perspective for assessment and intervention and a range of approaches to the teaching of sentence structure. She advocates that the guiding principle in speech and language therapy with children with LD should be a search for meaning.

'Augmentative and Alternative Communication (AAC)' is the next topic, discussed in Chapter 7 by Gill Williams. She explores its use and role from the perspective of the individual user and the communicative environment. She presents a description and classification of the different types of AAC and discusses criteria for selecting and introducing different systems, and the roles of individual members of the interdisciplinary team in the assessment and implementation of the AAC system. Williams also advocates a multi-modal approach and discusses the relationship between theoretical models of language acquisition and the development of communicative competence in the non-verbal child. She places a great emphasis on context and how it may affect the child's success at learning and maintaining skills of communication using AAC. Life-cycle issues, relating to the changing needs of the child and family, are discussed.

In Chapter 8, Sue Dobson and Angela Hurd discuss 'Working With Parents, Carers and Related Professions'. They argue that the SLT's work with individual clients is dictated by the differing aspects of the client's assessed communication strengths and needs. However, the style of implementation and the approaches which are acceptable to the significant others in the client's daily living patterns are open to a variety of different creative solutions. The success of these approaches is dependent on the understanding of the partners and the collaboration of the staff and other carers involved with the clients. These approaches involve joint working practices where professional boundaries sometimes become blurred and skills are shared. Such interdisciplinary solutions, therefore, depend on the successful presentation and implementation of a growing therapeutic role, this being the SLT as a resource more than as a practitioner. They also include discussion of speech and language therapy service delivery for whole groups, parents, schools and staff.

'The Management of Challenging Behaviour within a Communication Framework' is the subject addressed by Jill Bradshaw in Chapter 9. She presents an overview of the definitions and prevalence of challenging behaviour, including the ways in which it is defined in practice. In discussing a functional analysis approach, she focuses on the ways in which communication issues are currently addressed. She advocates the consideration of all aspects of communication and considers the communication used by both people in the communication partnership, including examples of the ways in which communication breakdown may lead to challenging behaviour. Bradshaw considers current communication intervention approaches which aim to modify the environment and which are designed to reduce challenging behaviour. Finally, she provides illustrations of, and discusses practical approaches to, developing communication within the partnership.

A growing area of interest is 'Dual Diagnosis', i.e. the co-occurrence of learning disability and mental illness, and this is addressed by Sue Dobson in Chapter 10. She discusses the needs of clients with Dual Diagnosis and how the speech and language therapy service is currently responding to them.

It would be unrealistic to expect that this large and complex subject can be dealt with comprehensively. Currently, research, particularly in the field of early intervention and identification, and work on pre-symbolic and pre-linguistic skills is gathering pace. The progression from the pre-linguistic stage to the first word and beyond has constantly presented a challenge to SLTs. There are palpable signs that much more reflection needs to take place before one selects the most appropriate AAC approach for a client with LD. Rather than a client's having to suit an available AAC strategy, the strategy needs to suit the client and his/her needs. Issues such as the management of challenging behaviour and working with clients with LD and mental illness (Dual Diagnosis) are fast becoming an important consideration in the SLT's intervention. As social and political awareness of the needs of this client group increases and improves, so will the quality of service delivery and innovations in management models. The advent of new programmes such as Hanen, though sometimes criticised for being too prescriptive, obviously meet a need of both SLT and parents/family of the young client.

No doubt, within the near future there will be radical developments in the SLT's role and spectrum of work with clients with LD.

Samuel Abudarham
Angela Hurd
January 2002

Contributors

Samuel Abudarham MSc, PhD, FRCSLT, CertEd (HE), RegMRCSLT, LCST, DipCST. Professor in Speech and Language Therapy, University of Central England, Birmingham.

Angela Hurd MA, BSc(Hons), RegMRCSLT, CertMan, CertEd (HE). Senior Lecturer in Speech and Language Therapy, University of Central England, Birmingham.

Jill Bradshaw BSc(Hons), RegMRCSLT. Lecturer in Learning Disability, Tizard Centre, University of Kent at Canterbury.

Sue Dobson BA(Hons), MA, DipCST, RegMRCSLT. Senior Specialist Speech and Language Therapist, Adult Learning Disabilities, Bradford Community Healthcare Trust.

Nicola Grove BA, MSc, PhD, PGCE, DipCST, RegMRCSLT. Senior Lecturer in Speech and Language Therapy. Department of Language and Communication Science, City University, London.

Janet Hickman BSc(Hons), RegMRCSLT, Advanced Diploma in Dysphagia (MMU). Senior Speech and Language Therapist, Birmingham Specialist Community Health Trust.

Della Bulpitt Money BSc(Hons), PhD, RegMRCSLT. Manager of Speech and Language Therapy Services for Adult Special Needs, Central Nottinghamshire Health Authority.

Gill Williams DipCST, RegMRCSLT. Specialist Speech and Language Therapist, Birmingham Specialist Community NHS Trust.

"If I am slow, I simply have to start earlier"

Robert Lafon

CHAPTER 1

Issues of Service Delivery and Auditing

JANET HICKMAN

Abstract

In the following chapter, issues related to the speech and language therapy service delivery for both children and adults with learning disability (LD) will be discussed. A 'top down' approach has been adopted to explain various perspectives. Firstly, the current philosophical/ideological influences in this area of work such as 'social role valorisation' (SRV), 'inclusion', and 'person centred planning' (PCP), are examined. Discussion follows about the way (British) government papers and initiatives such as *A First Class Service*, *Clinical Governance*, and *Primary Care Groups* are realised in practical terms. The Royal College of Speech and Language Therapists' (RCSLT) requirements concerning competencies are discussed from a professional perspective, as are the effect they will have on speech and language therapists (SLTs).

Finally, the inter-relationships between a number of operational issues, such as models of working, clinical effectiveness, multi-disciplinary team working, prioritisation systems and outcome measures, are explored.

Introduction

The object of this chapter is to present to the SLT student and SLTs entering into this field some of the major themes and influences which will affect service delivery. SLTs are faced with a number of internal and external influences with regard to delivering a service to clients. Beliefs and values derive from several wide-ranging sources, e.g. the World Health Organisation (WHO) health policy, Wolfensberger's explanation of SRV (1983), the concept of PCP, user/consumer empowerment and the movement of 'inclusion', to name but a few.

At a national level in the UK, the National Health Service Executive (NHSE) and social policy makers have acted on British Government White Papers, such as *Our Healthier Nation* (1997), *Partnership in Action* (1998a) and *A First Class Service* (1998b), which outline the way forward for change in the NHS.

Professionally, the RCSLT currently has two major tasks:

- to complete work on SLT assistant (SLTA) and SLT competencies
- to develop evidence-based clinical guidelines so that we have a framework for grading skills, knowledge and expertise in a given clinical area; only the former will be discussed in this chapter.

In addition, UK SLTs are required to meet guidelines laid down in the RCSLT's *Communicating Quality* (1996a), meet local standards and protocols, and document the effectiveness of speech and language therapy services using valid and reliable outcome measures. At a local level, service managers negotiate with health authority purchasers using historical service level agreements. Inevitably, there will be a significant shift in funding arrangements in the next five years as primary care trusts enter the funding picture. Last but not least, the individual SLT must have developed an awareness of models of service delivery and how best to measure clinical effectiveness, be aware of the issues focal to the particular community team working with this client group and service, decide how best, via a prioritisation system, to deliver a particular service to this team, and how to avoid professional isolation. Where possible, how the practical applications of these issues and how they relate to the SLT's practice setting will be illustrated through anecdotal examples.

Influences on service provision of worldwide social policy

From the 1970s onwards, social policy across the western world has moved towards a community-based, person-centred and inclusive way of thinking when providing services. Van der Gaag and Dormandy (1993:109–12) summarised SRV as a philosophy which should embrace all service providers' delivery, regardless of profession or area of work. An American social scientist, Wolfensberger, translated work done in Denmark by Nirje (1969). Nirje and his colleagues had influenced their country's legal system to create a more 'user friendly' environment for the client by statute. This was erroneously translated as 'normalisation'. Wolfensberger (1983) elaborated Nirje's ideas to focus on developing the individual's strengths and interests within society. Wolfensberger (1972, 1983) defined SRV as the most frequently possible use of culturally valued means so as to enable, establish and maintain valued social roles for people. Historically, people with LD were perceived negatively because they had disabilities. The practice before the implementation of the *NHS and Community Care Act* (1990) was to keep them together in hospitals. They were to be 'treated' as if diseased and not to be seen as people who could have normal interests and friends. They were therefore devalued and marginalised from society. Wolfensberger (1983) and his colleagues have endeavoured through their work and training programmes to break down the negative perceptions and attitudes that some carers seemed to have towards their clients. Wolfensberger's aim was to enable people with disabilities to lead more 'normal' lives by effecting the change of society's adverse attitudes to, and pre-conceptions of, disability and people with disability. In this way, carers trained in SRV philosophy could help their clients live more 'normal' lives by creating opportunities to develop clients' skills and thus enable them to integrate successfully into their communities. For example, instead of learning to cook in a day centre, clients would go out on a cookery course for which they would gain certification, qualifications and work where possible; if a client had a particular interest (e.g. landscape gardening, photography, tap dancing or rock climbing) the carer should then aim to exploit the client's strengths via an appropriate activity. The whole philosophy taught service providers and carers to think about 'skilling' clients within the community to enable them to be part of society and not be marginalised. Fundamentally, SRV is a philosophy and underpins good practice in care.

The effect of SRV on the SLT's work

In terms of practice, a SLT needs to attend a SRV workshop, however basic, to absorb its key principles and values. Failing that, the SLT should read the appropriate subject matter, for example in Wolfensberger (1983) and O'Brien and Tyne (1981). The latter are the great exponents of the 'Five Principles':

- choice
- community presence
- respect
- dignity
- relationships.

O'Brien and Tyne (1981) stated that these are the minimum requirements for anyone to live a 'normal' life in society. When a SLT appraises an environment for evidence of these five principles and finds them notably lacking, there is much more work involved than just facilitating the communication opportunities within the environment. Negotiating a contract and joint working with the manager of that environment regarding training with SRV issues as a priority would be a first step in the SLT's management as well as in the assessment of the environment (Woods and Cullen, 1983). If, however, the home/day centre seems to be trying to implement O'Brien and Tyne's five principles, the environment will be more conducive for more specific speech and language therapy input, such as extending clients' options for choice, enabling access to written information and training on the use of assisted communication methods (such as signs, symbols or the role of objects of reference).

Person Centred Planning (PCP)

A number of theoretical perspectives have contributed to the PCP approach. It is primarily a process for 'life-style planning' and a progression from developing clients' skills to enable them to integrate into the community, to developing a desired lifestyle for them. Normally, a care plan would be based on a client's needs. The starting point of the approach involves people working together within a 'circle of friends' in order to actualise the client's 'dream'. Another theoretical perspective influencing PCP derives from 'consumer-directed theory of empowerment' (Kosciulek, 1999). He believed that consumers/clients are experts on what they can do and that choice and control should be introduced into all service delivery. He further held that consumer direction should be available to all, regardless of who the 'payer' might be. Schalock (1996:107) concluded that the ultimate outcome for the consumer is to achieve 'quality of life' (QOL). Kosciulek (1999:197) defined QOL as *'directly related to having individual needs met, control over one's environment, and opportunities to make choices.'* Schalock (1996: 107) believed that in order to be empowered, individuals needed to have some degree of control over their life and all the conditions that affect it; for example, home and community living, school or work. Once empowered, clients can improve the quality of their life. Historically, services were limited by what was available in the day centre attended by the client. If an activity was offered in the centre, it did not happen. If users or clients did not want to spend five days in the day centre, they could express that, but the only option was to stay at home. Ultimately, clients themselves should be able to choose and pay the personnel who care for them using their own finances directly. Currently, health authorities decide if clients have the capacity to spend their money wisely. In time, it may be the 'circle of friends' who administer the direct payment funds for a client.

PCP as a concept has arrived and is established to some degree in social services provision. As its title suggests, PCP is a process of care-planning that has the client/consumer at the centre. All professionals involved are 'back stage technicians' and the clients, their friends and family take centre stage. A facilitator is essential to encourage the exchange of all views and to pull information into a coherent form.

The effect of PCP on the SLT's service delivery

The PCP process moves away from a traditional assessment format in which the professional tests an ability to perform basic functions and tasks, and then records that information in a format which the client/consumer cannot understand. Instead, it involves the people who know the client best in collecting information of that person's strengths and needs in order to form a complete holistic picture. This process is carried out in small groups of people known well to the client and involves the client as much as possible. The model could present some professionals with a number of insoluble challenges in terms of their assessment and intervention model. SLTs, however, tend to describe the client in terms of strengths and needs. The PCP process is not a 'needs-led' approach but more about creating the right conditions to empower clients in their daily life. Regarding care planning, SLTs have tended to write goals agreed with carers in terms of:

'x will be able to do y by such a time, using z.'

The language may change to:

'x wants to do y and needs z to achieve that desired end-point'.

In the future, SLTs may not be deemed relevant by the client's 'circle of friends' because the current assessment or intervention may be perceived as outmoded. Alternatively, SLTs as a profession may be over-whelmed with demands to empower the client in the process.

The following is a summary of a case study conducted by Barclay (1998) of a non-verbal man in his 20s with autistic spectrum disorder. His challenging behaviour excluded him from his day centre and involved regular stays at the local behaviour unit. After a number of bad experiences, he was introduced to PCP by his social worker. The focus of the new plan was on the client's strengths and how carers responded to his anxiety as opposed to the carefully planned structure they had decided for him. Carers also learned not to focus on helping him learn new skills, but on helping him feel safe and in control of what he was familiar with. The outcome of such an approach for this client was more regular sleep patterns and reductions in medication. It was he who determined when he did things and when he saw people. As a result of PCP, four part-time workers were able to provide him with support in a flat near where his parents lived. At the time of writing, this client still exhibited challenging behaviour, but its frequency had diminished considerably.

The PCP approach is not without limitations. For example, gathering an empirical evidence base for research in terms of assessments based on deficits, as suggested earlier, may not be valued by people directly involved with the client, because it may be perceived as a 'deficit' approach. SLTs may therefore not be allowed to carry out formal assessments if this is not seen to help the client achieve their 'dream'. Furthermore, it could in some ways conflict with Wolfensberger's philosophy in that it can focus only on what the client *wants* to do, which may be nothing, and may not help clients become integrated into their community and develop a socially valued role. From a SLT's perspective, the validity of the views of the 'circle of friends' could be called into question as they may be interpreting the views or wants of a non-verbal person who often cannot identify, define or express a 'lifelong' wish, nor appreciate the concept of long-term reward and what is required to achieve it. The role of the independent facilitator is central to an unbiased expression of views to prevent other people's (e.g. carers, professionals, managers) conflicts of interest.

Inclusion

If SRV and PCP are key approaches in working with adults, then 'inclusion' is the main philosophical concern in services for children with LD. Inclusion as a philosophy and a movement is far more advanced in the USA than in the UK. Idol (1997:384) defined inclusion in the following way:

> A student with special education needs attends the general school program and enrols in age appropriate classes . . .

She further stated that

Inclusion is the 100% placement in general education, whereas in 'mainstreaming', a student with special education needs is educated partially in special education programs.

In response to such a fundamental viewpoint, there are groups who advocate the concept and practice of 'responsible inclusion' (see Vaughn and Schumm, 1995: 265) which allows for individual variation in its implementation, includes a graded approach and is appropriate to the needs of the student. Recommendations relevant to 'responsible inclusion' are included in the evaluation of the case study presented below (see later on in this section entitled 'Testing the efficacy of the inclusion model'). Inclusion is rooted, amongst many other disciplines, in 1970s linguistic research. From then on, linguists showed that language was learned more quickly in a naturalistic setting than in a formal clinical one (see Nelson, 1990). The stage was set for SLTs to move into a more participatory and collaborative role. This refers to the extension of the SLT's role, whereby the SLT not only participates in the classroom settings to achieve communication goals, but also plans jointly with the teacher to actualise those goals. In the USA, other movements such as 'regular education initiative' (see Will, 1986) and the inclusion movement itself (see Smith et al., 1995) were challenging traditional classroom methods then current.

In the USA, education was moving on to adopting a more outcomes-based, functional-age-appropriate, curriculum-based learning model (see *America 2000*; US GPO, 1991) and the recommendation proposed 'led to paradigm and naturalistic service delivery models' (*Goals 2000*, 1994). SLTs saw a shift from providing services in isolation to providing them in context (see Nelson, 1990). In 1993, the American Speech and Hearing Association (ASHA) issued a policy statement that recommended 'collaborative consultation' as an appropriate service delivery model for 'some students'. By 1994, a report on inclusion to the US Congress (US Department of Education, 1994) revealed that 80% of students with LD spent some, or all, of their school day in general classes. In the UK, the Green Paper on Special Education Needs, *Excellence for all Children* (DfEE, 1997), appears somewhat more conservative than the American approach. The paper states that, for children to flourish in adult life, they need some experience of being educated alongside their peers. The paper reassures those working in special education that they will still have a vital role to play as they have the specialist resources and expertise, thus advocating a model of 'partial integration'.

There are practical implications of 'inclusion' for SLTs working with children with LD. Before the SLT steps into the classroom, meetings should have taken place between the SLT, special needs co-ordinator and heads of department, to examine the planned schemes of work (as in the example shown below), so that all parties can reinforce curriculum information presented to the students.

The following case study illustrates what might occur in, and the results of, such a meeting. Gill and Ridley (2000) reported on three secondary-age children in the UK, with specific language impairment, but who attended a special school. They were chosen to be integrated into a mainstream school in an inclusive way. In this example, the operational roles of the SLT and the class and support teachers were unclear and overlapped. Areas for the classroom teacher to focus on were highlighted, as were broad means of achieving relevant objectives. These were as follows:

Attention: The children are encouraged to listen, extend their attention span and taught the skills to look as though they are listening.

Comprehension: Complex instructions are broken down into smaller units; ambiguous language is made more concrete; new vocabulary is described and the augmentative sign system (Paget Gorman, 1990) is used to aid comprehension.

Expression: The team's role is to help children to organise their thoughts into coherent sentences and give strategies to produce words.

Organisational skills: Children are reminded to think ideas through during science lessons before acting, and are prompted to record the results of their work.

Social skills: When the child is not sure how to respond pragmatically, the SLT or teacher prompts the child to reply to an adult within the situation as it arises.

Literacy: If the child has difficulty with written information, the teacher/ SLT will have to confirm that the child has understood; if not, more simple language or Paget Gorman Signed Speech (Paget Gorman, 1990) is used.

In this study, the short term aim of the specialist language teacher and the SLT input would be via small groups, to simplify and make less ambiguous the more abstract content of the language required for a particular lesson, such as science, design and technology. Teachers and

SLTs would model and prompt question formation. Such preparation would enable children to realise when they did not understand, and the need to ask for appropriate help.

Evaluation

In this particular study, the three children were selected from the special school to enter mainstream schools on a part-time basis. After a year, the views of all the members of the team were written up. In this case, the exercise was felt to be a positive experience in general. The support teachers and SLT witnessed a change in teaching style of the mainstream teachers, in that it had become more orally driven and with less focus on literacy presentation. One teacher felt encouraged to enter one child for GCSE exams (General Certificate of Secondary Education taken in the UK by pupils aged around 16 years of age). Another teacher changed her scheme of work to adapt to children with special needs. The children themselves appreciated the status of the school and called it a 'proper' school and enjoyed the lessons. They had most difficulty in terms of social interaction and interpreting jokes made. A third child lived outside the borough in which the school was located, so he could not pursue friendships after school. The key to the resultant success of this project was that support teachers and SLTs were available to advise the team, conduct small group work in the classroom and grade the tasks or activities in the worksheets in advance, resulting in a decreased workload for the classroom teacher. In addition, the children were exposed to only a few teachers in the school.

High on the list of recommendations arising from this case study above were the need for:

- annual reviews, especially at the end of Key Stage 3 (National Curriculum, DfEE, 2000c)
- longitudinal studies of the children's progress and attitudes of non-mainstream school peers.

Testing the efficacy of the inclusion model

The sample in the case study above was too small to allow for any generalisations to be made as to whether inclusion is effective or not. The positive effects of inclusion have not been tested on empirical evidence (Vaughn and Schumm, 1995:264), but its face validity is based on a feeling that everyone should have equal opportunities and a right to a mainstream life.

A substantial amount of literature published in the USA from other disciplines would seem to suggest that teachers are responding positively to the more indirect consultative model, that is, one where the SLT advises and recommends appropriate action for the teacher. Cole et al. (1989) selected 61 children to test direct and indirect models of occupational therapy. Tests and re-tests were carried out within 8 months. Testers were blind to the subjects and physical motor tests were carried out. The actual results of the children showed no statistically significant differences between children experiencing direct and indirect intervention methods. The teachers, however, felt they knew the children better by liaising more with the therapists. The same results were found by Elksnin and Capilouto (1994) and Elksnin (1997).

Longitudinal studies may give more detailed, and possibly more reliable data. Components required for successful inclusion are listed by Vaughn and Schumm (1995:267) as follows:

- sufficient time for planning
- being labour intensive in therapy time in terms of planning and adapting the curriculum
- having education and language become integrated in individual education plans (IEPs)
- having collaboration worked at a different level and organically
- having own mission statement on inclusion
- ongoing assessment, monitoring and placement consideration (these being crucial)
- adequate resources in the classroom
- teachers who choose to participate in inclusive classrooms and can give open feedback
- a continuum of services, e.g. not full-time placement if full-time will not work
- staff training and development so they feel they can fully participate
- curriculum designed to meet the needs of all children.

Global and government strategy

Moving away from ideological influences, a brief survey of the influences of global strategy on service delivery will now be conducted. From the 'health' perspective, as far back as 1978, WHO has remained committed to a primary healthcare approach to achieving *Health for All* (see WHO, 1997). The recommendations from the Alma Ata world health conference 'Health For All' were that there should be:

- stronger partnerships between private and public sectors and civic society
- equity oriented policies and strategies

The key themes from this paper were on equity and partnership working, and are echoed in NHSE papers. These themes have not been altogether successful, due to the following:

- insufficient political commitment
- insufficient funding for health
- poverty has increased worldwide, so health has actually worsened in countries that have not been able to secure adequate income levels.

The impact of government policy on service provision and delivery

When the New Labour government came into power in Britain in 1997, its priority was to overhaul the NHS and introduce measures they judged would make a visible impact on the way these services were delivered. A number of papers were published and have now become key references when citing change in the NHS. *Our Healthier Nation* (NHSE, 1997) echoed the WHO message by promising:

- to improve the health of the nation as a whole by increasing the length of people's lives and number of years spent free from illness, and
- to narrow and improve the health gap of the worst off in society.

The Government first set out how it was to deliver better health in the 1998 White Papers *A First Class Service* and *Partnership in Action* (which refer to proposals for England and Wales only).

In the Government's view, quality in the NHS had suffered for four reasons:

- The internal market set up by the former Conservative government was one where general (medical) practitioner (GP) fund-holders were able to offer services more quickly than their non-fund-holding counterparts, and trusts made bids for business in competition against one another. This quickly led to a two-tier health service. Those patients who had a fund-holder GP could access services more quickly as the GP was financially rewarded for being a fund-holder.
- There were no national standards for intervention, so patients did not know what to expect from their services.

- There was patchy appraisal and implementation of best evidence and, therefore, the opportunity for receiving up-to date treatment happened by chance.
- There was no open accountability within trusts so patients did not know how or to whom to express their dissatisfaction.

A First Class Service describes how the NHS intended to create a quality service using a number of frameworks and principles to realise the proposals. Figure 1.1 illustrates the interaction of various frameworks which aim to improve operational aspects of the NHS.

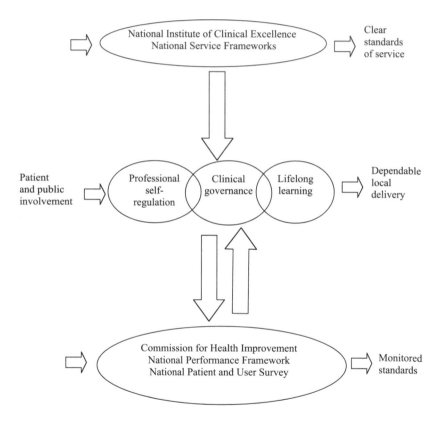

National Service Frameworks will set out common standards across the country for the treatment of particular conditions. The National Institute of Clinical Excellence will act as a nationwide appraisal body for new and existing treatments and disseminate consistent advice on what works and what does not.

Figure 1.1. Setting quality standards.

First, clinical standards are to be established via the National Institute of Clinical Effectiveness (NICE). This body is to act as a type of standards clearing house, evaluating and recommending best medical intervention. Operating alongside NICE are the National Service Frameworks (NSFs). Their purpose is to develop evidence-based frameworks and protocols with the aim of making clear to patients what they can expect in a major disease area or disease groups: cancer, mental health, coronary heart disease and services for older people are currently priority areas. Professional bodies, SLTs and clients will input into the standards setting via lifelong learning, clinical governance (see next section) and involving the client in gaining feedback on services provided. Standards set by NICE and NSFs will be monitored via National Frameworks for Assessing Performance and the Commission for Health Improvement (CHI).

The CHI is an independent body which aims to help avert tragedies similar to those that have happened in the past due to poor internal monitoring of performance by professionals and services. Previously, practice and procedures have been poorly monitored and caused unnecessary loss of life; e.g. babies died in Bristol because a surgeon's poor practice was not monitored; a number of cervical smear results were false negatives; there was also the case of Beverley Allitt, a child murderer who was allowed to practise as a nurse although her superiors knew of her mental health and condition. Inspection visits are made by representatives of CHI, and reports are made to the health authority, trust and government with notes on good or poor practice of the trust concerned.

Clinical governance (CG)

CG is one framework that has had a profound effect on NHS culture. Clinical accountability is a relatively new concept in the UK. An NHS trust chief executive is now both financially and clinically accountable for the trust's actions and will be held ultimately responsible when public enquiries into practice are made. However, because of CG, everyone is now clinically accountable. CG should provide a trust-wide framework for improving quality. It has been defined in *A First Class Service* (NHSE, 1998:33) as

> a framework through which NHS organisations are accountable for continuously improving the quality of their services and safeguarding high standards of care by creating an environment in which excellence in clinical care will flourish.

Among the elements enshrined in the policy are quality improvement, clinical audit, risk management, evidence-based practice, user involvement, clinical supervision, lifelong learning and systems of accountability.

It has been most succinctly defined as 'A framework for continuously improving quality and safeguarding standards of care' (Harvey, 1998:2; also see Table 1.1 for application of CG principles to the work of SLTs).

Outside the National Health Service (England and Wales)

Education strategy

The DfEE set out its strategic framework to the year 2002 in a paper entitled *Learning and Working Together for the Future* (DfEE, 1998c). Many of the aims and terminology have a similar ring to those expressed in *A First Class Service*, mentioned above. The vision in the strategic framework is an inclusive one, whereby each child and adolescent reaches his or her potential, i.e. offering a future to those who have suffered disadvantage. The strategy has three main objectives, with targets and policies, to enable it to become reality:

- to ensure all young people reach 16 with skills, attitudes and personal qualities to help with lifelong learning, work and citizenship
- to develop in everyone a commitment to lifelong learning
- to help people without a job into work.

Targets are set to be measurable, e.g. 65% of 3 year olds will have nursery education. The objectives within the strategy are (1) standards and attainment, (2) innovation and diversity, (3) inclusion, (4) equality of opportunity, access and participation and (5) community focus. Policies and targets have been put in place to ensure the above objectives are actually achieved.

Primary care groups

The creation of primary care groups (PCGs) was first announced in *The New NHS* (NHSE, 1998c). They are groups of GP practices which are sometimes grouped according to electoral constituencies. Their role is ultimately to extend to that of commissioning health services. The rationale was that GPs provided services within a locality and should therefore know what the local health needs are. Once GPs became confident of their local needs, they could move on to a commissioning level to become a primary care trust (e.g. level 4, the status of a primary care group which has become a self governing trust, is allocated monies to care for its population and is able to commission services for their caseloads

Table 1.1. RCSLT clinical governance framework: Birmingham Specialist Community Health (NHS) Trust Learning Disabilities Service clinical governance checklist

Clinical effectiveness	Quality assurance clinical risk management	Staff development
Standardised outcome measures encourage measurable outcome measure	Case file management	Peer supervision – formalise documentation and format
Database for evidence-based practice on specific areas, e.g. challenging behaviour, dysphagia, sensory impairment	Yearly appraisal	Share learning from mistakes – open management style
Access to academic libraries	Ensure standards for dysphagia are met	Develop second opinion protocol
Access to internet, use as for post	Patient's Charter quality data set	Give time to reflect and share learning (create documentation)
Mechanism for courses feedback	Ensure local standards are met, e.g. challenging behaviour, dysphagia	Devise year's programme for clinical governance issues
Develop links with college advisors	Audit clinical practice	Encourage staff to input at the business planning level
Access and feedback to journal club	Check clinical registration	Training programme to enable therapists to input and pull off activity reports
Access to primary care research forums	Check staff competence/knowledge up-to-date	Link in with other SLT teams where appropriate
Standardise therapist assessments	Add to registration information, e.g. appropriate referrals	
	Be aware of PCG agenda	
	Ensure there is cover for all areas	
	Ensure equipment inventory available at all bases	
	Ensure users are involved at every level (work out audit sheet)	
	Use carer/client satisfaction questionnaire – sent out after episode of care by person not involved.	

independently). It is projected in some quarters that community trusts and health authorities will eventually be edged out of the commissioning picture. Specialist community trusts serving people with mental health and learning difficulties are likely to remain as trusts. For SLT managers, the implications are clear. They will now need to address their bids to local GP practices to maintain their teams. Many departments have retained their alignment to GP practices from the fund-holder experience; others have already redefined the local boundaries in anticipation of impending, or likely, change.

Health Action Zones

The concept of health action zones (HAZs) is discussed in full in the paper *Partnership in Action* (NHSE, 1998a). The drive of the British government has been to bring together agencies such as health, education, social services and local councils in England and Wales and to provide the best quality healthcare possible for the consumer. Deprived areas were highlighted and pilot studies initiated across the country to bring together contributions from each government agency in order to make maximum impact on the life of the particular client or consumer. Pre-school services were encouraged to take their services to the community drop-in centre; skill mix strategies were employed to reduce the professional/patient divide, e.g. employing skill mix effectively so that a health professional and an experienced mother could work together, and in different ways to enhance the care of, say, a first-time mother with a child with language delay. The whole approach employs a holistic social model as opposed to the medically oriented disease-intervention model. Over £50m was invested into HAZs in 1998–2000. Future evaluations will indicate whether the initiatives have had an impact on the adverse effects of poverty. The concept of integrated provision will eventually mean that health services will have to pool their budgets with those of social services, housing and leisure to meet a health improvement programme need. Areas of deprivation are likely to attract more financial resource than more affluent ones because of government policy and, therefore, the former will be best served.

Impact of the British speech and language therapy profession on service delivery: the competencies project 2000–2001

Government policy regarding the delivery of quality services, as set out in *The New NHS* (NHSE, 1998c), is starting to make its presence felt across the therapy professions. Currently, two processes are under way, a review of NHS workforce planning and the 'benchmarking' of standards. The results of these will provide a specific overview of what the professions 'do' in the NHS. The competencies project will feed into both these reviews. It appears that the government feels that intervention tasks should be broken down and graded into smaller steps or parts, and that SLTs be rewarded for the complexity of their work, their knowledge and experience. Fish and Coles' work (1998) suggested that there are tensions around the nature of defining professionalism, i.e. is it more science, or is it more craft? The respondents' views in their study indicated that areas such as clinical judgement, decision-making and the ensuing actions cannot so easily be broken down into a discrete task format and graded. Clinical decision-making, in this author's opinion, is refined through an accumulation of clinical practice and is not necessarily task-focused. For example, it informs one's management: to intervene or not, to decide on intensity and style of intervention, when to discharge or not, and so on.

The competencies format

The RCSLT's competencies project leader, Kathleen Williamson, has consulted SLTs across the UK in order to gain a consensus of opinion regarding the area of competencies related to the speech and language therapy profession. The aim ultimately is to develop a professional competencies framework which maps out professional performance objectives in terms of 'knowledge', 'understanding', 'skills' and 'values'. The results of this exercise will enable SLTs to work within the limits of their competency more easily as the relevant guidelines will be published. It will also be easier for developing SLTs to ask for assistance. RCSLT aims to publish the framework by the summer of 2001.

There are three main elements to the competencies exercise:

- defining the care process using a template (Williamson, 2000: 17–18) from referral to discharge; the mapping of the various roles of the SLT; and the decision making process which accompanies each part of the care process
- defining generic qualities of SLTs, e.g. professional attributes, technical skills, knowledge base and emotional skills
- defining workplace performance competencies, which will be different according to the client group and will comprise which level of the care process the SLT is dealing with, e.g. assessment, analysis, intervention, and what specific skills and knowledge and 'critical contextual knowledge and understanding' are required.

Below is a simplified attempt to illustrate some of the competency framework principles and how the competencies are operationalised. The example refers to a SLT working with an adult who has autistic spectrum disorder, and lists likely aims, objectives and competencies required to work with such a client.

Care process

Care diagnosis: Adult with LD with autistic spectrum disorder.

Performance aim: Enabling care (maximises use of existing skills in achieving self care/autonomy through effecting environmental modifications).

Objective: To enable client to develop functional communication skills within his or her own environment.

The SLT is required to possess the following competencies (this list is by no means exhaustive):

Competencies

- *core professional and technical skills* – for example, time management skills, reflective thinking, drawing from an up-to-date evidence base
- *specific underpinning knowledge and skills* – current theories about, and intervention used with, autism; application of theory of language development into an adult context; low-tech methods of assisted and augmentative communication (AAC); knowledge of various symbol systems, in order to assess communication level; knowledge of challenging behaviour and how to manage it within a multi-disciplinary team
- *contextual knowledge base* – SLTs must know the context of the service in which they are working (residential, social care, social services, family situation, dynamics, etc.); have familiarity with the concept of social role valorisation and its relevance and implementation, person centred planning, vulnerable adults policy, appreciates the roles of their multi-disciplinary team
- *professional values and attitudes* – exhibit professional accountability for their actions, adhere to the professional standards
- *emotional skills* – for example, show adeptness in relationships, regulate self, be empathic to carers and clients.

Service delivery issues when working within a speech and language therapy department (children and adults)

Regarding day-to-day work in the practice setting, there are a number of caseload management issues relevant to LD, such as:

- how one delivers the service, e.g. which model and package(s) of care to use, how to employ skill mix, prioritisation procedures, etc.
- liaising with the multi-disciplinary team
- application of outcome measures.

Models of care/service delivery

Historically, not a great deal of information on 'models of care' has been provided at an undergraduate level. Some courses offer professional studies, but service managers report that there is not enough emphasis in undergraduate courses on imparting skills of negotiating, enabling, facilitating and training, all of which are important when undertaking the consultative role effectively. What became apparent in the 1980s was that using the direct client management model only would not sustain an ideal or desired intervention outcome. Training carers in principles of communication and opportunity planning and gaining management support of the communication programme for the client were considered essential to maximise carry-over (Woods and Cullen, 1983). Money (2000:10 and Chapter 3 in this book) refers to models of care as 'the manner in which one delivers the service.' She refers to five 'styles' of intervention:

- direct (individual)
- direct (group)
- indirect (individual)
- indirect (group)
- both indirect and direct (i.e. combined)

and general teaching, i.e. providing training for carer groups away from the client's environment. Money's (1997:462) study of the efficacy of each of these approaches indicated that a combination approach, i.e. using direct and indirect training, provided the best results.

Packages of care

In an attempt to cost therapeutic time, the terms 'packages of care' and 'episodes of care' have become widely used. Thus, a 'package of care' refers to the process and the amount of time required to achieve the intervention goals specified. For example, the package of care for a client with challenging behaviour may be focusing on assessment, delivering a report and making recommendations to the behaviour team. This may take 8–10 sessions (a session generally being a half day) over a period of

2–3 months, including time for observations, report writing, attending reviews, monitoring of recommendations and delivery of training if necessary. A client with complex AAC needs may well require 6–18 months, if not longer, of intensive input using an assistant working 1:1 on a weekly basis and a SLT to plan and monitor the programme. A client who requires the environment to match their communication needs may require 12 weeks' SLT input from assessment to discharge and involve the therapist assessing, informing carers with written recommendations for the environment, modelling of its application, agreeing the symbol system monitoring and placing on review. Factors such as the size of a caseload, the readiness of the environment and the availability of an assistant often determine how many different models one can practise in reality. If one has a large caseload one may have to work in a consultant role only, in order to manage numbers. If one has the resource of an assistant, one can plan for the assistant to carry out treatments more intensively, and for the therapist to monitor, or the therapist can model the intervention, hand over to the assistant and have the assistant report back progress.

Skill mix issues (adults and children)

The newly qualified SLT needs to ask what proportion of time is most effectively spent in direct, hands-on work, indirect advice-giving and monitoring, and with which client needs group. Use of speech and language therapy assistants (SLTAs) is an essential feature of working with children and adults. There are over 500 SLTAs in the UK, making up 10% of the SLT workforce (RCSLT, 1996b). The assistant and SLT collaborate with both the classroom teacher and the classroom assistant to create an adequate IEP. The skills and competencies required of a SLTA vary throughout the country. This is because hardly any two job descriptions are the same, as there does not seem to be a consensus for relevant competencies and, as yet, nothing has been published. More often than not, SLTAs are not allowed to assess, but many are allowed to screen. They have a key role in preparing equipment, working through a programme with a carer, giving feedback to the SLT and developing good relations with care staff in the care setting they work. The majority of a SLTA's work should have clinical focus as opposed to being administration related. As a result of their case study, Atherton et al. (1999) made a number of recommendations for a SLTA's optimal working:

- the focus of the assistant's work should be supporting intervention and management

- assistants provide invaluable help with home visits, assessment, videoing and group work and monitoring progress
- assistants should be encouraged to develop as communicators
- the best training is on the job, supplemented by structured, practical courses of study
- planned time together is essential to exchange views, promote collaboration and confidence
- an agreed focus and caseload gives job satisfaction
- the supervising SLT needs to be mature, confident in how he/she approaches the work and be able to plan work for others (this, of course, takes time and practice)
- planned contact with other SLTAs is supportive (for example, via special interest groups, college courses and in-house training).

The present author's experience suggests a number of advantages and disadvantages of working with assistants.

Advantages

- Continuity of client care when the SLT is absent.
- More intensive and individualised quality of service is possible via the SLTA when the SLT is managing a large caseload.
- More time for planning is allowed as the SLTA completes equipment requests.
- Potentially more face-to-face contacts can be achieved, but this can be disputed as the SLT spends time planning for the clients the SLTA sees.

Disadvantages

- The SLT has to devote clinical time to planning and not face-to-face contacts; this may give cause for less job satisfaction for some SLTs.
- Time has to be devoted to training and supervision of the SLTA (this can be labour intensive for the SLT in the first 6 months, but the benefits should become manifest thereafter).

Prioritisation issues

When one is working often as the 'lone SLT', the potential caseload in any one NHS trust may be over 200 clients. Those referred will often attend a day centre and live in a parental, private or public sector funded home. They will often be assessed and placed on review, or on a waiting list, for further assessment or therapy. The SLT will often have to assess and appraise at least two communication environments, in some cases more, and there will often be 10 or more carers to approach in terms of skills and awareness raising. It may therefore be hard to gain an overview of the client's needs.

Van der Gaag and Dormandy (1993:109–12) recommended the following priorities:

- intervention with people with communication difficulties and challenging behaviour
- intervention with individuals who have an awareness of their communication difficulty and who have expressed a desire for change
- where staff and managers are motivated, to collaborate with the SLT on a contractual basis.

If members of the team involved with the client are not motivated, van der Gaag and Dormandy (1994) suggested setting up training to raise awareness of communication issues.

Using the above criteria, we would have very small caseloads because:

- there are not that many people with 'challenging behaviour' as defined by Emerson et al. (1987a)
- few clients have an awareness of their communication difficulties
- often carers and managers need persuading that they need to support the SLT in the communication programme by building in mechanisms to ensure opportunities are created.

However, what often happens when one sets up a community-based service is that one is inundated with referrals by health and social service professionals in the first year or two, and less frequently thereafter. One can thus develop a feel for the client group and its needs, as the group is often static and re-referral is frequent. The next stage of caseload management, the most difficult one, is keeping a tight rein on review and discharge procedures. This requires effective time management, planning and implementation.

Other prioritisation systems

One can use a 'risk (to the client) management' approach. This would fit in neatly with the current CG framework. The following are considerations in such an approach:

- clients with 'challenging behaviour' which jeopardises either themselves or others, and their placements (Emerson et al., 1987a)

- rehabilitating people in health funded residential units back into their normal environments
- clients with dysphagia (if the SLT is trained and has clinical support)
- school leavers where they need to adapt to new environments
- people with degenerative conditions e.g. Alzheimer's
- clients being resettled into the community from hospital
- adult protection referrals from nurses, social workers and the police
- clients who have assisted communication needs and where there appears to be a mismatch between cognitive and communicative ability (not a 'risk' as such, but the client requires more individual input as well as that of the environment).

Woods and Cullen (1983) stressed the importance of fostering working relations with both the management and care staff of day centres and homes for the successful long-term implementation of programmes. The risk management strategy outlined above needs to be balanced with providing a service to people in everyday communication environments.

When a caseload appears to be getting unmanageable, a few management strategies may include:

- screening the referrals for severity when they first come in, giving out advice sheets and putting on a waiting list for therapy
- employing strict and regular review and caseload management discharge procedures
- applying strict admission criteria, or one can have the whole day centre referred and placed on a waiting list
- assessment-only service.

Advantages in applying such techniques

- The SLT gains an overview of the caseload.
- The Patient's Charter 13-week deadline can be met.
- The caseload is a kept to a certain number that the SLT can feel effective and competent to deal with.

Disadvantages

- Carers can lose faith, as they want the intervention part of the service to follow assessment.
- Resource deficits may be hidden; intervention takes a lot longer than assessment, on the whole.
- Carers prefer treatment to assessment-only.

The multi-disciplinary team

In the UK, SLTs working in a typical LD team may or may not work full-time in that area. The SLT will always liase regarding the client's communication needs with the community nurse, the consultant psychiatrist, psychologist(s), possibly the behaviour team and, if they are fortunate, other community health professionals, as often such resources are not readily available, e.g. the physiotherapist, occupational therapist, dietitian. The social worker is a key team member who will complete the care plan and allocate resources, usually on the advice of the community nurse and other professionals.

In LD teams, as in others for different client groups, certain things become 'hot topics' and one is asked to devote valuable clinical time to such a topic, e.g. developing client-held records. The management team will want a SLT's opinion and input. These are often good opportunities to raise the profile of the service. It can be too easy to strictly adhere to one's prioritisation list. Multi-disciplinary working on projects will ultimately benefit the client. Examples of this are devising a dysphagia pathway, or developing a multi-disciplinary client-held record. Clearly, the SLT has to carefully select in which project to become involved. Working within a LD service, the SLT does need to think more widely than on their own clinical remit in order to maintain a profile within the team. All members of the team need to familiarise themselves with each other's role, expertise and responsibilities.

If a SLT is managed by a SLT manager, it has to be ensured that liaison with the multi-disciplinary team is adequate. If s/he is managed by a LD team, on the other hand, the SLT can risk professional isolation. One therefore needs to ensure that there is access to relevant therapists for advice and sharing experiences. Access to special interest groups (SIGs) is another vital strategy for avoiding professional isolation, maintaining 'continuing professional development' (CPD) and gaining feedback on one's practice via case discussion.

Outcome measures

In the last decade or so, the SLT profession has concerned itself with measuring its clinical effectiveness via the care process (e.g. referral, assessment, case notes, treatment plans, reports) and more recently, by the use of outcomes measure scales. The strengths and weaknesses of some well-known scales used in the UK will now be critically discussed.

Therapy Outcome Measure (TOM)

The most widely known outcome measure in the UK is that of Enderby (1997). She and Alex John were keen to move away from the medical model, which rated 'not dying' as a good outcome! Enderby and John (1999:426) pointed out that the TOM may not be measuring a particular outcome but more 'monitoring of change in patient's performance.' Enderby applied the WHO terminology to the TOM categories and divided the measure into four 'domains' or 'dimensions' (Enderby and John, 1999; John and Enderby, 2000) as follows:

impairment – i.e. the severity of the disorder itself

disability – (renamed 'activity' – Enderby and John, 1999:419), i.e. how the client functions with the impairment, e.g. how much the client can understand and express him- or herself

handicap – (now known as 'social participation'), i.e. how much society's environment is preventing the client from achieving maximum potential, e.g. not providing access or appropriate communication modes

well-being/distress – i.e. how much the disorder distresses both the client and the carer.

Each domain or dimension can be rated on a 6-point scale: from 0 (most severe) to 5 ('normal' population). SLTs have requested a wider rating scale using 0.5 intervals e.g. 3.5, to record more minute change if they feel that the results of the intervention will not reflect a complete transition to the next point in the model.

SLTs working with clients with LD have found the 'impairment' category difficult to rate, especially when it became clear that intervention was not going to affect impairment, i.e. the disorder itself. We could, however, to some degree, influence 'disability' and 'handicap', i.e. 'activity' and 'social participation', and also the sense of 'distress' and 'well-being'. Some of the concerns of British SLTs working in LD who have engaged with TOM are:

- It needs to be applied by equally experienced SLTs, as the amount of practice using the tool affects reliability significantly (John and Enderby, 2000:299).
- SLTs need regular training updates using peers to mark 'unseen clients'; standard presentation of information is an absolute necessity when marking the domains of the measure (John and Enderby, 2000:300).

Advantages

- The tool is quick and easy to apply if one is familiar with the concepts and has appropriate clinical experience.
- The terminology is accessible to the purchaser via the manual.
- '... given sufficient training and practice opportunities ...' SLTs demonstrated '... an acceptable level of reliability when using TOM' (John and Enderby, 2000:301).
- It charts changes/outcomes on a more global level; for example, how much confidence and decision-making one has over one's life, the amount of social integration one manages in one's daily life, as opposed to the specific linguistic goals a SLT would formulate.

Disadvantages

- The tool does not measure what we actually do, i.e. the process, and just measures the change.
- Achieving statistical significance in any change or progress has been questioned with more severely impaired clients as they may only move 0.5 in one domain.
- It is difficult to determine what 0.5 intervals signify as they are not described; for example, it is left to the clinician's judgement to rate the client's disability in domain stage 3, which has a description 'consistently able to make needs known but can occasionally convey more information', or whether to rate 3.5 which has no written description of progress at that point.

TELER outcome measure

Another measure is the 'Therapy Evaluation (by) Le Roux (method)' (TELER – Le Roux, 1999). Again each measure works on a 6-point scale 0–5, and charts either:

- the management process of an episode of care, e.g. referral, access to specialist services, receiving a report, piece of equipment
- the graded effect of therapeutic change on the client, or
- component indicators which list five aspects of recovery that are not clinically related (see Table 1.2 for multi-disciplinary measures for management of dysphagia).

It is used mainly by physiotherapists, occupational therapists, a small number of consultants, and SLTs in rehabilitation. As the tool is copyright, one must purchase a licence from the TELER organisation in order to use the documentation and gain free technical support. The indicators which

Table 1.2. Examples of TELER outcome measure

(a) Hierarchical indicator. The outcomes denoted by the codes occur sequentially
Occupational therapy indicators achieving independent eating and drinking

0. No active participation in eating and drinking process
1. Client assisted hand over hand with no active participation
2. Client participates with physical guidance
3. Client participates with physical guidance and verbal prompting
4. Client participates with minimal verbal prompting
5. Client eats and drinks independently

(b) Component indicator. The outcomes denoted by the codes do not occur sequentially
Multi-disciplinary measures: managing a safe swallow

A. No episodes of respiratory distress
B. Maintains nutritional status
C. Consistent use of prescribed textures to aid safe swallow
D. Achieves suitable positioning and seating
E. Consistent implementation of advice and techniques by clients/care

---

one creates must be sent in to the TELER organisation for approval both by Mr Le Roux and by peers, in order to justify one's clinical experience and knowledge. The TELER outcome measures have been gaining validation by large groups of physiotherapists getting together, and trialling measures relevant to their client group. The West Midlands Collaboration Group (Rosen and Brock, 1998) is a network of physiotherapists who manage their own validation by sharing and trialling indicators by client group.

The following are some key points which need to be borne in mind when using TELER indicators:

- The title of the indicator must reflect the end-point of intervention, e.g. eating independently is the final point of therapy (see Table 1.2).
- The nature of the indicators are explained in greater detail in a handbook of over 150 pages (Le Roux, 1999).
- Only when four or more points in an indicator scale have been achieved can a clinical outcome be said to be 'statistically significant'.

Advantages

TELER's biggest attraction, as reported by therapists who use the system, is its minimalist style of documenting change. In addition:

- There is a reduction in the need for extensive note writing as the significant changes are expressed in the indicator.

- It records changes that are clinically meaningful to the therapist concerned.
- The use of an indicator can be individual and based on the therapist's clinical knowledge.
- A methodology for calculating clinical effectiveness is available (Le Roux, 1999).
- Regular study days are run to demonstrate compliance with the requirements of clinical governance.

Disadvantages

- All changes must follow a five-statement format and this is not always easy or possible to achieve when there are no indicators available and/or there do not seem to be five obvious stages in treatment.
- Achieving statistically significant results (i.e. four points up a scale) in LD is difficult because changes following intervention within this client group are often smaller than moving through 0.5 changes.
- It may only record process and not clinical change. For example, physiotherapists in LD in Birmingham chart the process for wheelchair acquisition from referral to arrival of the wheelchair by using the TELER indicator format. The occupational therapy indicator in Table 1.2 actually records a clinical shift.

East Kent outcomes system (EKOS)

A third outcome measures approach is the one employed in East Kent; it is entitled EKOS. Many SLTs working with people with a LD have become disheartened with the fact that the WHO-Enderby outcome measure scales (TOM) are not sensitive enough to record the clinical changes the client has achieved. The basic premise of EKOS is that 'a good outcome is one where the objectives you set for your client have been met' (Johnson, 1997:476). A 'good' outcome, i.e. as agreed by East Kent SLTs and purchasers, needs to have achieved 70% success rate in reaching objectives set. One can set any number of baselines and objectives defined as end-points of an intervention. Achievement is evaluated at the review date in terms of 'fully' (100%), 'mostly', (70%), 'partially' (50%) or 'not at all' (0%). Success is measured against:

- meeting the objectives
- achieving one or more aims (e.g. the long-term purpose of the intervention, in this case, 'functional communication') and,
- achieving a 'health benefit' gain.

'Health benefits' as a concept have been developed through discussion with Johnson's colleagues in a variety of therapy and nursing disciplines and are referred to by the NHS Executive in their Contract Minimum Data Set (CMDS) care aims for the client (Johnson, 1997:475). Health benefits were defined by the (then) Canterbury and Thanet outcomes project team in 1994 as 'broad categories of healthcare outcome' and the framework attempts to identify and make explicit the general outcome of health professions as a whole, rather than focusing on curative or restorative aspects of the intervention (Johnson, 1997:475). The health benefit set for the adult client in LD is usually 'modification'. This is defined as

> making social or physical modifications to the client's environment to compensate for absence or reduction in normal functioning, when further improvement is unlikely, or gradual over time (Johnson, 1997:473).

With mainstream children or more 'able' LD adults, one would apply the healthcare outcome benefit of 'facilitating development' which is defined as 'facilitating development of new skills where potential exists for improvement in functional ability.' The health benefits cited are among eleven used by EKOS for various client groups.

Case study 1.1

Normally, the following information would be summarised in the EKOS paperwork which is in a boxed format. The following case study illustrates a fairly typical case.
Danny is a man in his late 40s with a cognitive/communication mismatch. He is ambulant, does not take medication and lives at home with his mother; the rest of the family has left home. He has a part-time job three afternoons a week at a local florists, and spends the rest of his time participating in the day centre's gardening business. Danny's comprehension exceeds his expression. He is a keen communicator, speaks in single word utterances, can exchange some news about his home and activities for the most part and supplements his verbal communication with some gesture. He requires the listener to know the topic in order to talk about issues outside the 'here and now'. There are frequent communication breakdowns as Danny uses verbal means and some idiosyncratic gestures to cue people into his chosen topic. The following is an overview of the intervention plan.

Aim: To develop functional communication in a variety of settings
Health benefit: Modification

Baselines	Objectives
1. Danny is understood only by familiar people (Enderby 'disability' 2.0)	He will be understood by some unfamiliar people (Enderby 'disability' 2.5)
2. He cannot transfer information from home to the day centre (Enderby 'disability' 2.0)	He will be able to transfer information home to the day centre (Enderby 'disability' 2.5)
3. Carers do not use signs to assist Danny's communication	Carers will learn 10 functional signs
4. Carers do not use symbols	Carers will use relevant photos to assist communication

The intervention would be supported by treatment targets:

- to assess Danny's needs
- train staff via modelling use of signs and observational techniques
- allocate intensive input twice weekly via SLT and SLTA
- evaluate carer and client satisfaction.

Results of EKOS style intervention

The intervention was carried out for 6 weeks by both the SLT and the SLTA. A review of the objectives set above then took place after 6 weeks. The objectives achieved using the EKOS system after 6 weeks' input were 3 out of 4 (70%, 'mostly'). For example, Danny used symbols to relate news from home when prompted by SLT and SLTA (objective 4 and 2) and was understood by an unfamiliar person, i.e. the SLTA, (objective 1). Staff used only 5 of the 10 signs recommended (objective 3) when observed. The aim of developing Danny's functional communication was realised when supervised by SLT staff only. The application of the Enderby measures helped to give some external objective measure, although it was only used in part to demonstrate change in performance.

Evaluation

This example showed the author's first attempts to grapple with the art of objective-setting using a 'Total Communication' approach. The lessons learnt were to negotiate one's goals more carefully with staff, assess how the client favoured the mode of signing and to set more realistic objectives.

Advantages

Some of the strengths of this approach are:

- As a care planning process, it certainly informs an unfamiliar SLT at a glance what another SLT is doing.
- It is sensitive to the small changes happening to the client.
- Furthermore, health benefits give a broad picture of the type of health gain in terminology which is accessible to the purchaser.
- It *also* allows SLTs to include a range of outcome measures and objective assessments to define one's baseline e.g. Enderby, TELER or scales devised by individual departments.
- The process makes one consider one's goals much more realistically; there can be a wide discrepancy between what one sets and what one achieves, i.e. the therapist is overambitious in objective setting.

Disadvantages

Some of the limitations are:

- EKOS is not an outcome measure system in itself; it is a framework for care planning and evaluating the therapist's input.
- Time and experience are required to learn how to set 'realistic' goals using EKOS.
- People setting up this system outside East Kent with no regular experienced support and feedback run the possible risk of misinterpreting the concepts.
- There is a danger of only setting objectives which one knows can be achieved, and not using an external, or graded measure such as TOM, for example.
- The tendency of making subjective evaluations of one's objectives when using such a system, in turn leads to a less robust evidence base if one wants to move a step on from auditing case notes.
- The TOM measure is static and one has to rate every client using the same terminology in the scale, lending it in theory, greater validity.
- The TOM scale has a more global currency in terms of charting progress. A measure such as TOM can be subjected to rigorous research methodology; this is not the case with EKOS. However, if objectives for specific client groups within LD are set/prescribed as 'packages of care', as is encouraged by East Kent Community Trust, the standardisation of objective-setting draws a little nearer.

Conclusion

The nature of this chapter has been to highlight and discuss internal and external influences on service delivery which affect the SLT working with both children and adults. The role of the SLT working in this field demands a host of competencies, in order to provide for the client maximum opportunities in all environments. The 'consultant' role of the SLT, which has naturally evolved, has made the profession examine how best to deliver the service using skill mix and appropriate models of care. In terms of evaluating clinical effectiveness, the SLT needs to develop and use not only some objective outcome measures and sound documentation, but also have a regular forum for feedback in which to develop either scales or goal setting.

The challenge for the SLT, now and in the future, is to retain the big picture in terms of government, service, and multi-disciplinary demands, while still developing the communication needs of the client.

CHAPTER 2

Assessment and Appraisal of Communication Needs

PART 1
ISSUES AND TRENDS

SAMUEL ABUDARHAM

Abstract

The first section of this chapter includes a brief literature review of issues related to principles of assessment and appraisal of the communication needs of clients with a range of learning disability (LD). We also review and discuss a number of issues related to the nature, assessment and appraisal of their communication skills and needs. The literature on these subjects is extensive but seems to be dominated by the educational, linguistic, social, medical and cognitive perspectives. There is remarkably little literature which has been targeted to the speech and language therapy profession. Until fairly recently, therefore, the profession has had to depend largely on appropriately applying the received wisdom and research findings of related cognate fields. Our contribution in this section is an attempt to harness what can only be considered to be a 'sample' of the knowledge published, and applying it to a proposed holistically client-centred model.

In the second section, we focus more on assessments and appraisal procedures and tools which are relevant to the work of speech and language therapists (SLTs), in the UK in particular, with clients with LD.

Introduction

There are three main purposes for assessment, appraisal and profiling.

- Firstly, the SLT needs to be able to identify the exact nature and severity of the client's impairment (this term is used in this chapter to describe the communication 'disorder' and not in the sense employed by the 1997 WHO–Enderby model which has recently been revised by John and Enderby, 2000). The SLT can also find out, through the client's past records and via a case history, how the impairment developed or was acquired – this information may have management and prognostic implications. A knowledge of causal, contributing and maintaining factors may be acquired via the same methods as just stated and for similar reasons. All this information should contribute to the formulation of a 'differential diagnosis' or as those not wishing to employ terminology related to the 'medical model' might prefer, a 'differential description'.

• Secondly, the results of assessments, appraisals and profiles can also determine the client's strengths and needs including the level at which a client is in the communicative development, what skills are yet to be acquired and which of these should be worked on next. Criteria for the latter may depend on a number of perceived priorities by SLTs and carers which may be developmentally rational, 'functionally' rational, etc. (see Hurd, Chapter 5 in this book).

• Thirdly, the results of repeated (re-)assessment, (re-)appraisal and (re-)profiling can provide evidence for any progress made, the nature and rate of this progress, whether and which learning outcomes have been achieved.

Further, these results should also enable the SLT to test previous hypotheses, reformulate new ones, reflect and 'replan' (Kolb, 1984).

The process resulting in the identification of a LD and its severity is not always successful in determining the existence and nature of such disability. This is an extremely controversial and highly debatable issue. For example, what is the operational definition for the 'severity' of the LD? Is it based on the client's IQ, social criteria, developmental criteria, type and severity of communicative impairment, severity of other disabilities (e.g. physical, sensory, etc.) or is it syndrome-based? It is not within the scope of this chapter to discuss such issues. The reader is referred to published work such as in Grossman (1983), Rondal and Edwards (1997), the *Diagnostic and Statistical Manual of Mental Disorders* (APA, 1994) and discussion of relevant issues in Luckasson et al. (1992), MacMillan et al. (1993), Reiss (1994) and Rondal and Edwards (1997). What is certain is that the debate will not go away. In England and Wales, official policy regarding the identification and assessment of 'special educational needs' (SEN), published in 1994, has been revised in parts and further revisions are imminent.

The terms 'assessment' and 'appraisal' are often used interchangeably and, indeed, they are legitimate synonyms. However, in this chapter, we shall apply them more specifically. The term 'assessment' will be applied to the evaluation of a skill in an individual, for example, a phonological or cognitive skill. The term 'appraisal' will be applied to the evaluation of the 'whole' individual and any factors outside, but related to, the individual, e.g. environment, context. Thus, for example, whereas a grammatical skill is *assessed*, information resulting from a case history is part of the *appraisal* process of the individual. The results of 'assessments' of an individual's skills therefore, contribute to the 'appraisal' process. The proposed distinction between these terms might seem arbitrary, but it is justified on the basis that it introduces a specificity which allows us to consider two complementary and component parts of the evaluation process. A holistic approach to evaluation is essential since we are not dealing with communication impairments and needs 'in' individuals, but 'individuals' with communication impairments and needs. Appraising an individual, in the sense that we have defined it earlier, allows for the consideration of possible causal, maintaining and contributing factors underlying the impairment. It also allows us to consider factors such as the effect or impact that individuals with a communication impairment may have on their environment, and the demands, communicative and otherwise, made on them by factors outside such individuals.

Many SLTs are employing the term communication 'need' rather than 'problems' or 'disorder', i.e. not only those non-verbal, verbal, pragmatic or social skills which the client needs to acquire or develop to become a more effective communicator, but also factors such as environmental or facilitatory strategies that will enable the client to maximise his or her communicative potential. It seems that in the UK we have finally caught up and adopted terms which had been in use in the USA for over a decade (see Haney et al., 1988; Bedrosian and Calculator, 1988).

Appraising any individual with a 'primary' communication impairment (Law, 1996:78–9, Leonard, 1998; Plante, 1998) (i.e. one that is not a result of a learning, physical and/or sensory disability, or structural abnormality) and communicative needs is a complex, often equivocal, process, just as often yielding equally equivocal results. This process becomes all the more complex when the communication impairment is 'secondary' to other factors such as hearing loss, learning or physical disability or maxillo-facial abnormalities. It is further complicated by the fact that one should not use any standardised assessments of communication skills, as we shall see later. Further, there are often many more variables to consider (e.g. cognitive deficits, neurological involvement or environmental barriers to learning) than in individuals who have primary communication impairments and needs, such as a language delay. Individuals with a primary communication impairment are more likely to live, interact and function within a 'normal' environment. For example, a child with a developmental (primary) phonological delay may well attend mainstream school. Some children with mild LD may do so as well, but they are often placed in units or remedial classes with other children with similar disabilities (though see brief discussion on 'inclusion' in the next section of this chapter). In addition, individuals with a LD are more likely to have a multiplicity of problems causing or adversely affecting their communication skills and resulting in other needs, not least communicative. They may have sensory or motor impairment which may or may not be part of a syndrome, or condition. For example, a child with Down's syndrome (DS) may have a hearing loss, which is quite common in individuals with this syndrome, but may have acquired a physical disability (e.g. through peri- or post-natal or acquired brain damage) not commonly associated with the syndrome. These factors may well exacerbate the child's communication impairment.

The political educational context

In order to put the whole issue of the SLT's assessment and appraisal of clients with LD in context, we require a brief overview of the historical and political perspective, mainly relevant to the UK though parallels exist in the USA. SLTs cannot progress through their own assessment and appraisal process without paying due care and attention to the client's social milieu, and particularly in relation to children, their educational and other contexts. The British government's Warnock Report in 1978, and subsequently the 1981 Education Act (Handicapped Children) marked a quantum change in the way that individuals with special needs were perceived, categorised and assessed. Before the Warnock Report, children were categorised as 'handicapped' or 'non-handicapped'. The report recommended that those who were handicapped were to be categorised according to their special need. Four main groups were thus proposed, these being children with:

- specific learning difficulties
- physical/sensory disabilities
- learning difficulties (mild, moderate or severe)
- emotional/behaviour problems.

In 1994, the Department for Education (Welsh Office) published the *Code of Practice on the Identification and Assessment of Special Educational Needs.* The Code recommended that assessment should comprise five stages, as follows:

Stage 1: Class or subject teachers identify or register a child's special educational needs and, consulting the school's Special Educational Needs co-ordinator (SENCO), take initial action.

Stage 2: The school's SENCO takes lead responsibility for gathering information and for co-ordinating the child's special education provision, working with the child's teachers.

Stage 3: Teachers and the SENCO are supported by specialists from outside the school.

Stage 4: The local education authority (LEA) considers the need for a statutory assessment and, if appropriate, makes a multi-disciplinary assessment.

Stage 5: The LEA considers the need for a statement of special educational needs and, if appropriate, makes a statement and arranges, monitors and reviews provision. (DfE, 1994:3).

A 'Statement of Special Needs' is then to be compiled from the assessment results and recommendations for future provision for the child made by a number of relevant professionals such as psychologists and SLTs. A copy of the statement has to be sent by the LEA to the child's parents, and they are entitled to respond to it. They are also entitled to seek further information or query parts of the statement and seek an interview with an appropriate LEA officer. Annual reviews of such statements have to take place. If dissatisfied with any part of the statementing process, or the lack of or quality of the service delivery, parents can put their case to a tribunal and appeal for changes to be made. These requests may or may not be upheld by the tribunal.

Recent British governmental initiatives, following on from the 1998 'programme of action' (DfEE, 1998b), aimed to ensure increased partnerships during a child's education, and the emphasis on life-long learning should help to strengthen transitions. The 'programme of action' also sets out goals on raising the achievements of children with SEN. A SEN update in March 2000 (applying to England and Wales only and not Scotland or Northern Ireland) was entitled *Framework for the Assessment of Children in Need and their Families* (DfEE, 2000a). This framework

provides a systematic way of analysing, understanding and recording what is happening to children and young people within their families and the wider community in which they live. Education professionals working in schools and LEAs who may be asked to contribute to the assessment process will be expected to do so in accordance with the new Framework. In this way, the new Framework offers a unique opportunity to develop a common language and improve communication and collaboration between local agencies.

Issues such as 'multi-agency working' (see also Burke and Cigno, 2000, Chapter 10) and 'inclusion' (i.e. 'the instruction of [special needs] students . . . alongside their non-disabled peers' – Wong, 1998; see also Garcia Pastor, 1999) are also raised in this report. In the USA, inclusive education has been governed by law for some time now. The federal *Individuals with Disabilities Education Act* (IDEA) and its 1997 amendments make it clear that schools have a duty to educate children with disabilities in *general* education classrooms. The British government report requires that inclusive education means that all students in a school, regardless of their strengths or weaknesses in any area, become part of the school community (see Hickman, Chapter 1 in this book). They are included in the feeling of belonging among other students, teachers and support staff. It is not within the scope of this chapter to discuss these proposals in any detail except to state that as a result the demands made on the SLT's assessment and appraisal role are undoubtedly likely to change considerably, in that their involvement in this area is likely to increase (see also Chapter 1 in this book).

The most recent publication from the DfEE, entitled *Special Educational Needs – special edition*, was published in December 2000. It updated developments since the November 1998 report (though other reports have been published since then). It focused on the introduction of the SEN and Disability Bill to Parliament and the responses to the previously conducted consultation draft of the revised *SEN Code of Practice* (DfEE, 1994). It confirmed a positive response from most respondents to the DfEE's recently revised draft of their SEN Code of Practice with the emphasis on several issues including the identification of children's special educational needs as early as possible, and working with parents as partners in their children's education. Some issues of concern were, however, raised by respondents (all members of the teaching profession) regarding matters such as the specifying of provisions in the statements of SEN. The implication for SLT services and individual SLTs of the final recommendations, which it is hoped will become law and come into force for the school year 2001/2002, may be substantial, e.g. each school will be responsible for purchasing SLT services and will prioritise their needs which may or may not include buying in SLT services.

Review of the literature

It is not claimed that the following constitutes an in-depth review of the literature. We shall refer to very focused issues relevant to this particular chapter and oriented towards SLT practice. Other publications, some of which are referred to in this chapter, deal with matters regarding assessment and appraisal in greater detail than we feel is within the scope of this book (see for example, Morse, 1988; Lees and Urwin, 1991; Wolfendale, 1993; van der Gaag and Dormandy, 1993; Beech et al., 1993; Wright, 1993; Wirz, 1995; Fawcus, 1997; Rondal and Edwards, 1997; Wong, 1998; Rondal et al., 1999; Burke and Cigno, 2000). Other chapters in this book also make reference to issues pertinent to assessment, identification and appraisal.

Assessment, appraisal and profiling – conceptual frameworks

Let us first briefly deal with the concepts of assessment, appraisal and profiling. In our introduction to this chapter, we proposed a distinction between assessment and appraisal. The term 'assessment' is the one most used in the literature. Some authors may use both terms 'assessment' and 'appraisal' (e.g. in relation to school 'entry skills' – see Wolfendale, 1992, Chapter 1) without drawing clear distinctions. She used the term 'appraisal' in association with 'reviewing', 'evaluation' and 'accountability' (p. 131). The impression is sometimes given by some authors that the term 'assessment' is employed when referring to the identification and evaluation of skills, both existing and needed, or even other factors such as assessing a 'home environment' as it applies at the time of the assessment exercise. Wong (1998), among other authors, discussed how assessment results form the basis of Individual Educational Plans (IEPs). Morse (1988:116) defined 'assessment' as an attempt 'to determine a client's strength and weakness as a prelude to remediation'. At this point, we would like to argue that the term 'weakness' is counterproductive and carries for us an air of pessimism. It reinforces a type of 'deficit' model which often undermines clients as human beings and frequently leads to an undue focus on what they *cannot/*are *unable* to do, and underplays what they *can* do. We thus prefer to refer to a client's 'needs', as this suggests to us that these clients have needs the same as anyone else in the general population. It therefore behoves society to provide services which will be resourced and geared to meeting such needs.

The term 're-assessment' often refers to the revisiting of such an exercise. On the basis of the re-assessment results, an evaluation can be made about change and how best to respond to it. Assessment and re-assessment are necessary processes, conducted at significant points during the course of remediation and on its completion. Re-assessment is, therefore, one of the strategies employed for evaluating change, short- and long-term aims, and learning and other appropriate outcomes, though much of the re-assessment should take place during the intervention process. However, assessment results of individual *skills* do not on their own provide the total picture, or overview, of the individual's *needs*. The concept of 'profiling' is thus an important one. The definition of profiling often depends on the definer's focus of interest. Crystal (1982) referred to a 'linguistic' profile and defines it as 'a principled description of just those features of a person's use of language which enable him to be identified for a special purpose'. Van der Gaag and Dormandy (1993:48) stated that profiles fall somewhere between standardised tests and naturalistic observations. According to Crystal (1982), profiles are more flexible and comprehensive than tests, and unlike tests which summarise individuals' achievements, they allow for a more subjective evaluation of a whole range of findings. Jeffree (1997:46) attested to the importance of profiling. Referring to developmental profiles in early assessment of children with severe LD, she stated that 'profiles highlight strengths and weaknesses and give an indication of where to start with each individual child.' Of course, the same rationale applies to any client referred for speech and language therapy, including adolescents and adults with LD – mild, moderate or severe.

The concept of 'profiling' is clearly an important one. Here, however, we define 'profiling' more broadly without wishing to suggest that profiling particular skills on their own (e.g. linguistic skills) is not useful. Such a definition would be

> the collection of assessment and appraisal data about an individual, their evaluation and the bringing together of all the resultant information to establish the inter-relationship and interactional effects between different pieces of information, and the determination of how each constituent part is cumulatively responsible for the whole.

So, for example, to consider the severity of the disability on its own without considering compensatory or adversarial factors may result in an inaccurate decision about a client's needs. Individuals with a moderate to severe LD may thrive more than individuals with a mild disability (severe = IQ 20–25 to 35–40, moderate = 35–40 to 50–55, mild= 50–55 to approximately 70 – see Grossman, 1983) because the former may have a more supportive and facilitatory environment which helps them to make fuller use of their potentials than individuals with the mild disability. In this case, the interactional effects between the severity of the LD and the supportiveness of the environment can have prognostic and management implications. It is also possible for some clients with, say, a severe hearing loss, to function as though their hearing was almost normal, possibly because they find other sensory modalities or ways to compensate. We can offer a further rationale for profiling which is very pertinent to the SLT's work, as follows. To profile linguistic abilities without considering communication-related factors such as cognitive skills, environmental needs and demands or the client's affect can easily lead to viewing 'a problem in a client' as opposed to 'a client with a need'. Similar examples can be illustrated by studying and using the holistic model presented later on in this chapter. To put it in popular parlance, to assess and appraise but not to profile is to miss the plot!

An important and widely accepted principle of the SLT's assessment of communicative effectiveness and needs of any client is that the client should be assessed in every relevant context, regardless of what the communicatively impaired client group might be. This principle perhaps applies even more so for clients who have a LD. Examples of such context, are the home, the daytime settings (e.g. adult training centre, day centre, sheltered workshop), educational setting (e.g. school), social domain, and so on. The population with LD is not a homogeneous one, so we cannot make generalisations about the needs of clients with LD; each client has to be considered as an individual. A wide range of communicative and other skills and needs will be encountered in this client group. These may differ significantly between individuals, depending on factors such as the particular individual's environment and setting, their effect on the individual and how he or she is equipped to deal with them. Unlike many clients with 'primary' communication needs, an individual with LD may not be able to compensate for an inability by employing an existing ability. Thus, individuals with LD may be less able cognitively, socially, pragmatically, linguistically and affectively to cope with a range of environments each presenting different demands and challenges to them (see Rondal and Edwards, 1997, for detailed discussion of these issues).

Holistic approach

The practice of applying the holistic approach to assessment and appraisal is currently much vaunted, and one could be forgiven for believing that the concept is new. In fact the need for a holistic approach was recognised several decades ago. For example, as far back as 1966, H. Gunzburg published his *Progressive Assessment Chart* (PAC) of social and personal development (see also Gunzburg, 1977). The PAC is still used by educational and clinical psychologists working with individuals with LD. This assessment is briefly discussed later in this chapter (see the section entitled 'Assessment of related non-linguistic skills', below). Taking one 'snapshot' for the purposes of assessment and appraisal can only provide a limited perspective of the client's abilities and needs. If such an approach is taken, the model of assessment, and immediately following, intervention can be rather static. It rarely provides a full and in-depth perspective of the client, and it is necessary to continue the appraisal and assessment process throughout the therapy interactions.

A holistic approach requires the involvement of more than one individual. A multi-disciplinary approach is needed during the assessment, appraisal and profiling process. Some assessment tools currently in use do require input from more than one person – see the Communication Assessment Profile (CASP; van der Gaag, 1988) and the Personal Communication Plan (PCP; Hitchings and Spence, 1991), for example, in Table 2.1. However, the number of people involved, even in these assessments, often falls short of the ideal, i.e. everyone in daily or frequent contact with the client, and other professions such as education, medical, those allied to medicine, psychological and social services. Over recent years, much research has focused on the influences of the environment and caregivers on the development of the language and communication of clients with special needs. However, there are currently very few formal tools available that attempt to evaluate the communicative competence during natural interactions of an individual with learning difficulty. Kublin et al. (1998:286) noted that

> development is influenced by a child's ability to produce readable signals, a caregiver's
> ability to respond appropriately to the child's signals and the routinisation of such
> patterns.

It is therefore important to view the caregiver as an essential part of the assessment and appraisal process.

It is also vital to consider the dynamic process of communication. One key consideration is how a child or adult actually initiates communication. For people with autism, for example, this is often a significant and important issue. Those involved with clients with LD need to know if there is a difference between people, environments and settings for any one or group of clients. Wirz (1995:124–28) proposed an assessment designed to record those

> strategies and action cycles identified by the competent communicator during interactive exchanges which contribute to successful communication with the client.

In the first section of Wirz's assessment, observations of strategies which a carer or SLT may use to elicit a response from clients with profound LD are recorded. A second section requires an account to be given regarding such clients' 'listening' and 'visual' skills. 'Pre-linguistic skills' such as the client's ability to anticipate, reciprocate (e.g. turn taking), understand cause and effect, seek attention, imitate, initiate interaction, existence of object permanence, make choices (e.g. between two different toys or drinks) are recorded in the second section. The third section addresses 'areas of communicative skills' (i.e. use of gesture, communication of basic needs, rejection and negation, expressing desire for recurrence of objects/actions, symbolic functioning).

Assessment models

A number of assessment models can be employed in the assessment and appraisal of clients with LD. The major ones are:

- behavioural
- psychological/psycholinguistic ⎫
- neurological/neurolinguistic ⎬ neuropsychological
- social
- educational.

Behavioural model

The behavioural model of assessment focuses on the individual's observable behaviour in a given situation, and over a given period of time. In order to understand and evaluate such behaviour, one needs to consider its antecedent, i.e. what occurred prior to and was likely to result in that behaviour. It is also important to observe the consequence of a client's behaviour. This approach is often referred to as the ABC model (for antecedent, behaviour, consequence) and provides for a functional analysis not only of the behaviour but also what precedes or causes it, and what follows or results from that behaviour. Lister Brook and Bowler (1997:21) argued that

> Functional analysis techniques are not only concerned with identifying overt behaviours but . . . also . . . with the role of cognitions and internal physiological states in the ABC relationship.

Thus, physiologically determined sensitivity to intense stimuli such as sound or vision may result in a particular behaviour by the client such as withdrawal or aggression. Similarly, such behaviour may be triggered by cognitive processes such as the client's understanding or misunderstanding of a situation or something said to them. Such a model depends on information provided by others, client included, observation schedules (checklists and the like) and probing strategies used to determine how a client will respond to another person's non-verbal or verbal behaviour.

Psychological model

The psychological model can include a number of approaches all designed to assess psychological systems and sub-systems. There are similarities between the psychological and the neurological model. The former focuses more on the individual's actual cognitive deficits and skills. Lister Brook and Bowler (1997:23) stated that cognitive assessments

> can be of great value in providing a very individualised assessment of a child's ability to process and organise information available to them in their environment.

The psychological model may also include psychometric testing, such as of IQ. When linguistic behaviour is the focus of the assessment, psycholinguistic models may be employed (e.g. Hewlett, 1990; Stackhouse and Wells, 1997; Groome et al., 1999; Chiat, 2000) as well as neurolinguistic models.

Dockrell and McShane (1993:11) discussed a *cognitive* approach to assessment with children with LD. In Chapter 1 of their book, they presented and discussed a cognitive frame of reference and stressed the need to conduct task analyses, the aim of which is to 'decompose a larger task into a series of smaller tasks'. The concept is an important one as, no matter what skills are being assessed, one needs to be able to explore the level at which a client is succeeding or not by assessing their ability to cope with 'subtasks'. They also highlighted the need to explore the client's 'cognitive system' and the client's cognitive structure required for learning (pp. 20–5). They identified four levels: the client's 'cognitive architecture' (i.e. the inborn organisational structure for processing information), the 'mental representation' (i.e. the structure of information related to the storage of information in the long-term memory), the 'task processes' involved in the ability to 'transform external input to an internal representation' (p. 23) and the 'executive processes' concerned with planning and regulating activities and meta-cognitive knowledge (i.e.

'knowledge about one's own cognitive system and how it functions' p. 24). They also discussed the assessment of 'auditory processing', 'working memory' and 'cognitive processes' (pp. 76–8). Metaphonological and metalinguistic skills also need to be assessed both at a 'receptive' and an 'expressive' level to establish whether the client has an understanding of, and ability to use, phonological and other linguistic rules.

LD and language learning impairments can be due to problems in auditory processing of incoming sound or language. The relationship between poor auditory discrimination and phonological impairment has long been debated. Auditory processing difficulties may result in a degraded signal being available for phonological representation (Dockrell and McShane, 1993:77). Gathercole and Baddeley (1990) concluded, after their research with a group of 7–9 year old children with language difficulties, that compared with age-matched peers without a language difficulty, their subjects were less able to retain material in their phonology working memory and this could affect the development of a stable representation of a new sound sequence in their long-term memory. Poor working memory may also affect the development of other linguistic skills such as vocabulary or syntactic rules. Bishop (1992) discussed the relationship between language difficulties and poor performance in tasks requiring symbolic representation. It is possible that, rather than cognitive deficits being (entirely) responsible for (language) learning difficulties, the latter may impact on the development of the former. The whole story about the cause–effect–cause relationship between language and cognitive difficulties is, therefore, yet to be told unequivocally. Methodological weaknesses in a number of studies exacerbate the search for the 'truth' (as happens in other fields of research too). It must also be borne in mind that there are inter-relationships between different language skills, so that if there is a deficit in one, there may be a deficit in others. However, this is not always the case, as discussed by Rondal and Edwards (1997). This would suggest that a cognitive deficit may adversely affect one language skill (e.g. phonology) and not another (e.g. semantics).

Neurological model

The neurological model will range from the medical-neurological approach to assessing an individual's physical (e.g. cerebral palsy) and sensory skills (e.g. central auditory impairment, visual deficits, etc.) to neuro-psychological assessments which attempt to assess the existence of neurological impairment, including brain dysfunction, and how it may explain other impairments. Montgomery et al. (1991:588–90) discussed neurological correlates of 'speech and language disorders'. Having briefly reviewed some of the literature, they concluded that 'different locations within the central nervous system may show malfunctions in different groups of language-impaired children.

Advocates of *neuro-psychological* assessments of clients with LD will argue that their justification lies with those who view that the disability is due to a central nervous dysfunction (Batchelor and Dean, 1991:311). They argued that

> the diagnosis of learning disorders would require demonstration of achievement deficits concomitant with neurological and neuro-psychological dysfunction.

Rourke and Del Dotto (1994:74) believed that neuro-psychological assessment of clients with LD should be 'comprehensive' in nature. A comprehensive neuropsychological assessment should involve 'the measurement of principal skills and abilities that are thought to be subserved by the brain' (p. 75). They also advocated that

> a fairly broad sampling of tasks involving sensory, perceptual, motor/psychomotor, attentional, mnestic, linguistic, and concept-formation/problem solving/hypothesis-testing would need to be administered (p. 75).

They further recommended that fairly comprehensive personality and behavioural data on the client is available. Analysing the results of a number of neuro-psychological assessments given to several hundred subjects with LD, Batchelor and Dean (1991:323) concluded that

> There would appear to be some common neuro-psychological elements to reading, spelling and arithmetic performance, including auditory attention and short term memory, remote verbal memory and symbolic language integration.

They did, however, acknowledge methodological problems in studies such as theirs and warn that 'a more conservative approach to existing data in this area' should be taken. Further details about neuro-psychological assessment used with children and adolescents with LD can be found in Rourke (1981) and Rourke et al. (1986). The fact that a number of the neuro-psychological assessments available are only open to certain individuals and professionals should not deter SLTs who believe in the usefulness of such assessments from working in collaboration with, say, psychologists who may be trained to conduct and evaluate the results of such assessments.

Social models

Social models predominantly address issues of social constructs of disability. Particularly with adolescent and adult clients with LD, one needs to recognise if, how and to what extent clients' disabilities have been adversely affected over the years by the way society has treated them, oppressed them (Barnes, 1996; Barton, 1996), set up barriers to their quality of life and deprived them of opportunities (see Swain et al., 1993), excluded them or even victimised them. It has been universally acknowledged that people with LD experience negative relationships and fewer social contacts than peers without LD. They also experience rejection and low expectations from society. In the not too distant past, institutionalisation often robbed the client with LD of opportunities of achieving independence, developing skills to make their own decisions or being their own advocates. Despite advances made over the last few decades, clients with LD may still suffer such disadvantages. Others have had a lifetime's negative experience and it often becomes too late or very difficult for them to change so as to improve their quality of life. One needs to determine how a client's particular environment can be enhanced to eradicate, or at least limit, any existing disadvantages. This may be achieved through persuasive dialogue and negotiation with both managers and carers so that the environment and the society within which the client lives can become enabling ones (Hales, 1996). Such conditions may, however, be created within the client's family and must start very early on in life. Inadequate social relationships can sometimes start from birth as a result of parents rejecting their child and failing to develop parent–child bonding. In later years, factors such as 'odd' facial features or behaviour, and poor communication and cognitive skills may lead to different levels of social isolation, lack of friendships and other social needs. The development of learning and communication, particularly pragmatic skills, is dependent on a number of social contingents, the absence of which almost invariably has an adverse effect on the development and maximisation of a client's communicative skills. The social model cannot be considered in isolation but provides a significant contribution to the assessment, appraisal and profile of the communication skills of clients with LD from 'cradle to grave'.

One can develop strategies within a 'social' framework designed to assess the nature of a client's non-verbal and verbal interaction with the social environment. Bradshaw (see Chapter 9 in this book) discusses the relationship between communication impairment and challenging behaviour in clients with LD. She also discusses the relationship of both of these with the client's environment. In the present chapter, we have noted that several assessments consider the client's social interaction with the environment. Bradley (1998:55) presented her assessment and intervention 'model of communicative development' which includes examples of clients' non-verbal and verbal communication skills and needs. A client, for example, may 'respond to her internal feelings such as hunger . . . ' but may 'not try to communicate or change the situation'. Bradley suggested that such a client needs 'a close relationship with key workers . . . have clear routines . . . have a quick response to distress or happiness'. She advocated the use of meetings and interviews with carers (see Bradley, 1991a), observational techniques, schedules to assess communication and multi-disciplinary involvement. These strategies are used to assess and appraise a client's social skills, activities, routines, interests and lifestyle, core signals and signs (employed and understood by the client, for communicating), likes and dislikes, tactile defensiveness, interaction styles, conversational strategies, etc. Ouvry (1998) highlighted the importance of social relationships. She referred to the current attention given to enhancing the quality of life of clients with LD (p. 66) and the importance of relationships and of limitations experienced by many of these clients. Processes such as bonding and forming close relationships for people with profound and multiple learning disability (PMLD) are being addressed in appraisal and intervention. Ouvry (1998) stated that there is little literature on this subject relevant to individuals with PMLD.

Education model

The educational model is probably the most frequently and widely published. This model is predominantly concerned with the assessment and appraisal of any factor which may be relevant to the individual's education. It also focuses on the individual's skills in numeracy, literacy and writing skills, verbal reasoning, and all other skills which are learned in school and are included in the UK National Curriculum. The literature is well served in this area and there is therefore little need to discuss the issue further here. Clearly, a SLT's assessment and appraisal (and intervention) needs to interface with a client's educational needs. The SLT also needs to be able to recognise, and if necessary act upon, the implications of the results of educational assessments, needs and provision for a wide range of clients with LD (see Robson, 1989; Norwich, 1990; Wolfendale, 1992, 1993; Robertson, 1997; Tod, 1997; Marvin, 1998).

The SLT needs information yielded by all these models before effective intervention can be planned. Dependence on one model of assessment and the information it can offer cannot provide the SLT with an overview of the client's needs as the development of communication depends on and affects other needs (e.g. educational, social and so on).

Approaches to assessment

The issue of 'types' of assessment has been addressed extensively. However, we feel that the issue needs to be included, if not reiterated in this chapter as the subject should be considered simultaneously with some of the other chapters in this book.

Assessments can be 'formal' or 'informal'. We define 'formal' assessments as those which generally require the assessor to follow a prescribed procedure and format set by the authors of the assessment. One of the advantages of following a prescribed procedure is that any assessor will follow the same administrative procedures, use the same material, format and evaluation criteria, providing both equability and equity. Inter-assessor and inter-assessment reliability are also enhanced if everyone employs the same procedures. Tests are formal assessments which, in addition, provide quantitative or sometimes qualitative data which may be compared to standardised norms. Other tests, while still providing quantitative or qualitative analysis, do not allow for comparisons with normative data. Tests can be 'screening' or 'diagnostic'. The former are designed to provide a quick and brief overview of a client's skills and needs, but are not meant to provide an in-depth assessment. These tests usually do not take long to complete but can help to identify at-risk individuals who may need further and more detailed assessment before a more accurate conclusion can be made as to their needs. Some tests are said to be 'diagnostic', but we believe that a differential diagnosis can rarely be formulated without a proper profiling of all the client's strengths and needs. Tests may well be part of, and contribute to, such profiling.

Standardised tests have a number of limitations, especially in terms of their usefulness with clients with LD. At this point we invoke the truism that 'a test only tests what it tests'. Tests can usually only 'sample' an individual's skills in a particular area. Furthermore, there are times when comparisons with normative data are inappropriate and this is especially so in the assessment of the needs of clients with LD. The reason for this is that the standardisation of tests is based on the 'normal' population. For this to be permissible, the population must be homogeneous.

The quandary facing the SLT regarding whether to use standardised assessments, especially when non-standardised ones appropriate to a particular client do not seem to be available, has long been recognised. Furthermore, standardised assessments are unlikely to be available for adolescents and adults with LD. Morse (1988) addressed another contra-indication to the use of standardised assessments. He pointed out that such test materials have been designed for use with individuals who do not have LD. The format and presentation of such assessments may thus not be appropriate for clients with LD. For example, many assessment instruments use pictorial material, such as line drawings, with which clients with LD may not be familiar. These clients may be more familiar with photographs, for example, and the lack of familiarity with line drawings, rather than a deficit in the skill being assessed, may cause them to underachieve in such assessments. Morse (1988:110) posed the question often asked:

> How does one adhere to standardised procedures . . . knowing that the adult with mental retardation . . . has receptive or expressive difficulties that are atypical of the established norms?

Morse (1988:110) also asked the rhetorical question 'if one modifies administration procedures or materials, have not the tests lost their signif-icance?' He went on to acknowledge that the dilemma in using standard-ised assessment is especially pertinent when attempting to use them with adults with LD who have 'severely restricted language, lengthy histories of institutionalisation, experiential deprivation, and varying degrees of sensory and motor handicap'. There is an acknowledgement that many professionals may still use standardised tests with clients with LD. Morse (1988) suggested that the 'materials' employed in such tests may under certain circumstances and if appropriate (e.g. mental age/cognitively appropriate) be modified and used so long as the results are not norm-referenced.

As stated before, the population with LD is not homogeneous and indeed is likely to be very heterogeneous, despite the fact that client groups such as those with DS may demonstrate a higher level of homo-geneity than other groups with LD. There is thus a general consensus that standardised assessments are therefore not appropriate for the LD client group. Rondal and Edwards (1997:7) stated that

> There is no good reason to believe that [language] assessment should be basically different from that in MR [mentally retarded] individuals or in other developmental disorders.

It is difficult to know what exactly they mean, as they did not elaborate. However, there is a potential interpretation with which we would take issue. There are similarities between the assessment of the communication needs of clients with LD and those who have communication impairment which is not due to LD. There are also major differences not only in the type and format of the assessment (e.g. as argued before, the use of norm-referenced assessments, especially for diagnostic purposes, is not appropriate with clients with LD) but also in the way and the context in which assessments are conducted. Added to this is the likely need to consider a multiplicity of factors with clients with LD such as poor attention span, sensory deficits or physical impairment (see for instance Rondal and Edwards, 1997; Rondal et al., 1999).

There are a number of strategies and tools available, other than norm-referenced ones, for assessing LD clients, e.g. the CASP (van der Gaag, 1988) and the PCP (Hitchings and Spence, 1991) – see Table 2.1. This type of test is often referred to as a criterion-referenced or content-related test. Such tests commonly aim to identify a client's abilities and needs without the need to compare these to those of other individuals with or without LD.

Informal assessments are generally not restricted to prescribed administrative procedures; any scoring is likely to be arbitrary and exclusive to the assessor conducting such an assessment. There is no doubt that informal assessments have a role to play, particularly in the field of LD and especially when no appropriate, valid or reliable assessment is available for a particular client. However, the validity and reliability ('test–retest' and 'inter-tester') of such assessments are likely to be very low.

One cannot stress enough the value of observation as part of the assessment and appraisal assessment, both formal and informal. Lister Brook and Bowler (1997) stated that the most common assessment procedures used with clients with LD involve direct and indirect observations. Such observations can be 'free range', when the observer just records as much as possible of the client's behaviour across a number of modalities e.g. linguistic, social, cognitive, pragmatic and play skills. Other observation strategies (see Table 2.1) may employ questionnaires, check-lists, rating scales and daily logs. Observations should take place in natural settings. However, observations solely of the client's behaviour, no matter how detailed, need to be considered in perspective. It is important to describe the setting in which the observations have been conducted, the people present and their possible effect on the client's behaviour. Adopting an ABC model allows observations and the recording of the 'antecedents' to each 'behaviour'. This allows the observer to make sense of how the behaviour came about. The 'consequences' of such behaviours also need to be recorded, for similar reasons. There are limitations to assessment via observations: the main one is that observations are vulnerable to observer subjectivity, not only in what is being observed but also in the way that interpretations are made of such observations and their consequence. Other factors that may influence the validity and reliability of observations may be how the observer actually brings about certain behaviours, or even non-behaviours. For example, the client may not be familiar with the observer and may become silent or inactive. Though this is less likely to happen if the observer is well known to the client, or if a participant–observer approach is adopted, other limitations may come into play. For example, as a participant, the observer may find it more difficult to make contemporaneous recordings of observations made and may not recall all observations when attempting to record them after the session. The outcome may also be determined by whether the observer is passive or active, the setting, who else is present, the type of tasks and probes the observer chooses and how appropriate they are, and the subjective judgements used not only in the choice of those but in the evaluation and resultant action following the outcomes. In order to minimise such limitations, Lister Brook and Bowler (1997) suggested that analogue situations can be used within a controlled environment. During such situations, two or more people make and record observations and these can then be discussed and interpreted by the dyad, or group. A 'triangulation' approach may also be employed. This involves receiving assessment data from the use of three different strategies (e.g. observation, informal assessment and formal assessment, or indeed three different sources employing the same or different strategies). Other strategies for assessment have been implemented for some time now. Examples of these are 'ethnographic' and 'ecological' assessments. Falvey et al. (1988:50–2) provided an anecdotal example of an ecological observation session. Van der Gaag and Dormandy (1993:47–8) discussed both in some detail.

Ethnographic approach

An ethnographic approach comprises the assessment of an individual's behaviour and skills in their natural environment. This approach contrasts with the setting up of a contrived, non-natural situation for the purposes of assessment. Ethnographic assessments require a long period of time and resources, and this expectation may be unrealistic. However, if well planned and co-ordinated, several strategies can be employed to achieve this type of assessment. Carers, key and case workers who are in regular, even daily, contact with clients may be trained to contribute to such an assessment. Assessment sessions should be as unobtrusive as possible. Observations via wall-mounted, remote-controlled video cameras may be more reliable so long as technical problems do not interfere. Long or short periods of clients' interactions and other behaviours can be recorded for subsequent study. CCTV cameras are often used for other purposes such as security and, if it is considered ethically appropriate, recordings from these (e.g. clients' behaviour in a playground or workshop) may be used for assessment purposes.

Ecological approach

A type of ethnographically based strategy is the ecological approach. Essentially, this 'requires all the assessments to be carried out in the context of whatever skill is being taught at the time' (van der Gaag and Dormandy, 1993:48). An ecological assessment aims to identify the skill that a non-LD age-matched peer individual needs to have to perform the activity and determine whether the client with LD has this skill. For example, an adult without LD should have a well-developed pragmatic skill such as maintaining a topic of conversation. This skill is then assessed in the adult with LD and if not manifest can be worked on, provided it is thought that the client has a potential for developing it in the near future. An ecological personalised inventory can therefore be created for each client comprising activities to be worked on under different broad skill headings, e.g. physical, communicative and social skills. This approach, argued Falvey et al. (1988), ensures 'the teaching of chronologically age-appropriate and functional skills'. They stated that these inventories and subsequent instruction should take place in 'natural environments i.e. those frequented by non-handicapped peers who live, work, and recreate in the same community as the student with a handicap'. Falvey et al. (1988:50) recommended that skills should be taught in response to 'natural cues and correction procedures, natural consequences and natural materials'.

In this section, general issues regarding assessment, appraisal and profiling of communication needs have been discussed. Theoretical perspectives and models have been briefly reviewed. The following section deals with more practically oriented issues relevant to the assessment and appraisal of communication needs.

PART 2
ASSESSING COMMUNICATION EFFECTIVENESS AND NEEDS

Introduction

Having provided what can only be considered an overview of general issues related to assessment, appraisal and profiling, we now turn to what communicative skills and processes we need to assess, appraise and profile in clients with LD. The answer can be presented simplistically by stating that the SLT needs to collect data not only on a client's communication skills, but also on any other factor related to or required for the communication process (e.g. cognitive, medical or environmental). Clearly, the SLT is not equipped to assess all this, and other professionals and non-professionals, because of their experience and expertise, all form part of the assessment or appraisal team. The SLT needs to understand the role of each member of the team, be able to interpret the results of their assessments, and utilise such data when profiling the client's abilities and needs and when formulating appropriate intervention plans.

The appraisal process is complex and wide-ranging. In this chapter, we can only address some of the communicative factors which need to be assessed and which are discussed in some of the literature. Most individuals with LD will have at least a mild communication impairment. This will present as predominantly articulation, phonological, receptive and expressive language impairment. Many will also present with pragmatic impairment. Often, depending on the causal factors underlying the LD and/or a common feature of a particular syndrome, there may also be voice and fluency impairments. For example, in individuals with DS there is a high incidence of dysfluency and voice disorders (see later). Often there are physiological or (maxillo-facial) structural abnormalities which may be responsible for any of these communication impairments.

As a general rule, the more severe the LD, the more severe the communication impairment. However, many other factors may come into play. For example, as stated earlier, an individual with a 'moderate' LD in a supportive environment may achieve higher levels of communication than a peer with only a 'mild' disability but a non-supportive environment. This is one of the reasons why a holistic model is necessary. Rondal and Edwards (1997) provided a very detailed account of communication impairment in individuals with LD. Non-linguistic impairments such as sensory and cognitive deficits have been discussed by many authors for a number of years, some of the most recent being Marcell

(1995), Rondal and Edwards (1997:153), and Rondal et al. (1999, Chapters 9–13). The communication impairment of an individual with LD is generally secondary to the LD itself. Here, we need to make a distinction between two terms commonly used and, often, just as frequently confused, or at best used interchangeably. We shall adhere to the differentiation currently made by Burke and Cigno (2000:1 and 12–14) between 'learning difficulty' and 'learning disability'. They argued that

> Learning disability implies actual intellectual impairment, and thus more clearly defines our subject group than the all-inclusive term 'learning difficulties', which every person has in relation to some aspect of daily life.

An individual with a LD usually presents with delays in most or all developmental modalities, though not necessarily to the same degree.

Another term, sometimes used synonymously with LD, is 'special needs'. We do not reject the usefulness of this term but believe that it is a generic term embracing all individuals who need extra attention from a range of educational, social and medical service providers. Individuals with LD of whatever age would be included in this category, as well as those with affective disorders, perceptual and sensory difficulties, physical disability (with and without a LD), autism, and so on. We recognise, of course, that the 'terminology' issue may be debatable and may not be as simplistic as we have implied here. However, we do not think it is within the scope of this chapter to present further discussion on this matter as such debate has been expertly presented by other authors (see Wong, 1996, 1998; Rondal and Edwards, 1997).

We now turn to some general issues regarding the assessment of communication effectiveness and needs of the client with LD.

Van der Gaag and Dormandy (1993:17) stated that 'the very existence of communication assessments relies on two tacit assumptions'. These assumptions, they argued, depend on whether optimal communicative proficiency exists and, if so, whether it can be measured. They adopted the term 'communicative efficiency' or 'effectiveness' because they suggested that this involves considering the client's linguistic and non-linguistic skills. However, they recognised that having linguistic skills is not enough. The individual needs to be able to apply what linguistic skills they do have appropriately, e.g. in social situations. They further suggested another term, 'strategic competence', to define the individual's abilities to 'use strategies for making the best use of what one knows about how language works, in order to interpret, express and negotiate mean ing in a given context'.

rehension versus expression

It has not been uncommon in the past for SLTs to focus on the assessment of clients' expressive skills, especially those with moderate and mild LD. As mentioned earlier, some clients with LD may seem to produce quite complex utterances but these may be stereotypical. It is very important to assess their comprehension and other receptive skills as their expressive skills may belie serious comprehension deficit. So often, erroneous judgements are made about clients being stubborn, lazy or badly behaved, as a result of a false expectations based on a misperception of the client's understanding of languages and pragmatic rules (see Haney et al., 1988; Reichle et al., 1988; Kelly, 1997; Bradshaw, Chapter 9 in this book). Phonological skills are often predominantly assessed at the expressive level. It is important, however, to assess a client's meta-phonological abilities as well as more general meta-linguistic skills. Thus, every level of communication – non-verbal and verbal – must be assessed at both a receptive and an expressive level (see also Stackhouse and Wells, 1997). Meaningful expressive communication can rarely develop in the absence of comprehension.

Pre-linguistic and pre-symbolic needs

Not until the last quarter of the last century were the importance and significance of the pre-symbolic, pre-linguistic, and non-verbal communication skills in clients with LD, especially during their early development, widely recognised in the SLT profession. Some individuals with severe and profound LD are unlikely to be able to communicate verbally, or even by using perceptible gestures. However, they may be able to communicate via other means, such as what has been referred to as 'referential gaze' (for example, see Fischer, 1983). Gaze patterns have been found to be different in children with DS. Jones (1977:394) described one example of referential gaze used by a DS child who glanced upwards to make some reference to his activity. In doing so, there is a transfer of attention from the activity itself to the interlocutor (often the child's mother). After this referential gaze, the child will look at the interlocutor's face and then resume the previous activity. Wooton (1989) stated that the vocal initiation rate of children with DS when interacting with their parents is less than in 'normal' children. Fischer (1983) found that about 24% of DS children (language age 13 months) initiated vocally compared to 52% of normal children with the same language age. So parents of children should respond even more than those of normal peers. Perhaps DS children use referential gaze in lieu of vocal initiation. Parents must be aware of this and respond appropriately, in order to encourage communicative behaviour. These forms of communication can easily be missed and thus, ignored. One of the dangers of ignoring non-verbal communicative behaviour is that the individual does not get a positive response to the behaviour and it may be 'extinguished', thus possibly preventing future communicative attempts. Opportunities for responding to the client's attempt to communicate may thus be missed, with an added consequence that, if not rewarded with appropriate responses, the client may not be encouraged or motivated to continue trying to communicate in this way (see Abudarham, Chapter 4 in this book).

Dunst et al. (1990) noted that one of the most important variables to assess is 'readability'. It is vital to establish how the client communicates and the response that this engenders in the caregiver. Various aspects need to be considered, particularly with clients with profound and multiple LD. These include

- how eye gaze and facial expression are used to influence interaction and indicate emotion
- range of the client's communication functions
- the client's means of communication and how mature these are
- frequency and rate of imitation response
- repair strategies
- symbolisation skills, e.g. language comprehension, production, play, and so on.

These aspects may also be relevant to the notion of 'opportunity' provided by the caregiver and also the use of the 'scaffolding', i.e. building on the client's existing abilities, by the communicative partner, as well as the communicative partner's interaction style (see Reason, 1993:73–74).

The assessment and appraisal exercise also aims to identify behaviours not demonstrated by a client either because they have not developed them, or because they cannot, or will not, exhibit them. One example of such a behaviour is 'joint attention', defined as attending jointly and simultaneously with another person (Jeffree, 1997:56). Many assessment, appraisal and intervention activities may not be possible without this skill. Jeffree (1997) stated that it is often difficult to get such attention of young people with learning difficulties. She warned that 'Direct confrontation may have a bad effect' (Jeffree, 1997:56) and advised that ignoring such a behaviour may achieve the client's attention; that is, of course, if the client is able to attend jointly. Attention levels are cognition related and may be varied in clients with LD. Cooper et al. (1978) discussed different levels of attention, and it is important to assess these in clients with LD. For example, a client who has only a one-channelled attention is unlikely to be able to attend to more than one channel input – say, visual and auditory. Knowledge of a client's attention level may thus determine the type of, and the manner in which, activities should be presented, whether during the assessment or intervention phase.

Despite general agreement about the importance for later development, the early signalling and interaction behaviour of infants with LD has received only minimal attention. Concepts such as the 'proto-conversation/proto-dialogue' ('primitive' or 'initial' conversation or dialogue) are regarded as important precursors of language and must be related to the development of pragmatic skills. Smiling, laughing, showing and pointing have all been studied as early forms of social and communicative sharing. Research in the 1970s indicated that even 'crying' is seen as contributing to later language development (Dore, 1975; Rheingold and Adams, 1980). A study by Jones (1977) of pre-linguistic non-LD children and infants with DS found that at 8–18 months the average rate per minute of interactional exchanges for mother–child pairs is about the same for normally developing and children with DS. But children with DS tend to vocalise in continuous strings, or repeat vocalisation with less than 0.5 seconds left for dialogue – lapses in interactive turn-taking. Jones (1977) reported a high frequency of 'vocal clashes' between children with DS and their mothers, as compared to normally developing children of corresponding age and their mothers. Several studies report delayed smiling in infants with DS, at 5–9 weeks. The amount of time they spend smiling is also less than in infants with no LD.

Owens and Rogerson (1988:206–8) provided tacit guidance for the assessment of pre-symbolic skills, albeit of adult clients with LD. These guidelines can also be applied, however, to the younger client (see Hurd, Chapter 5 in this book, who discusses pre-symbolic skills in children). Owens and Rogerson (1988) listed the following targets for pre-symbolic training: responding, motor initiation, object permanence, turn-taking, functional use of objects, means–ends, communicative gestures, receptive language and sound initiation. The assessment tools they listed (p. 208) are based on direct assessment, interviews, observations or questionnaires filled in by caregivers. Rondal and Edwards (1997:142–52) discuss issues relevant to pre-linguistic development in some detail. They reviewed the literature regarding sensori-motor development, sound discrimination and different aspects of babbling, including symbolic babbling.

Phonology

There is a consensus in the literature that in individuals with LD there is a high incidence of phonological and meta-phonological impairments (see

Menn and Stoel-Gammon, 1995; Stoel-Gammon, 1997). Much of the literature seems to be related to those with DS (see Stoel-Gammon, 1980, 1981; Borghi, 1990) but these impairments have also been found in non-DS individuals with LD. Having comparatively reviewed a number of studies, Rondal and Edwards (1997:135) concluded that

> phonological development is not complete in most DS adolescents' etc. and the speech levels reached by . . . older subjects do not differ markedly from those of . . . children, even if some improvement may occur with age.

A client's phonology can be analysed by using assessments such as the *Phonological Analysis of Children's Speech* (PACS) (Grunwell, 1985). Although this assessment is designed mainly for children, the phonology of an adult client with LD can be qualitatively analysed by comparing it with the expected non-LD adult's phonology as indicated in the PACS. Similarly, the assessment section of the *Metaphon Resource Pack* (Dean et al., 1990) may be used if appropriate for the client; the pack has a section suggesting intervention which includes the development of the client's phonology through the development of meta-linguistic awareness. Psycholinguistic approaches to the assessment of phonology can also be used (see for example, Stackhouse and Wells, 1993, 1997).

Pragmatic skills and needs

As a general rule, both child and adult clients with LD are likely to have very poor pragmatic skills, e.g. eye contact (see referential gaze, earlier), initiation, turn-taking, interaction, sharing, requesting and responding. The severity of impairment may depend on a range of factors, ranging from mental age or IQ to the quantity and quality of opportunities presented to them to develop such skills. Burke (1990) defined pragmatics as the function of a behaviour and the effect that this has in regulating the behaviour of a listener. Pragmatic behaviour can be subdivided into two main areas: 'needs and wants', and 'social interactions'. 'Needs and wants' can include variables such as 'feelings' and 'affection'. Examples of these are those messages given by the client to express their wishes, requests for help, rejection, choice and simple messages such as 'yes' and 'no'. All of these may be expressed verbally or non-verbally, and even by the use of 'eye gaze'. Behaviours that help to regulate social interaction may include 'displaying attention', 'acknowledging', 'turn-taking', 'responding to questions', 'requesting information', 'responding to name' and 'greetings'. Many young and adult clients, though they may have some language, might not have reached the stage when they are able to learn or use pragmatic skills. Of course, pragmatic skills do not need to depend on there being language. For example, profoundly deaf individuals may be able to use appropriate pragmatic skills through sign. The adult with profound LD may also not have acquired, or be able to use, certain pragmatic skills. Particularly in the older client with LD, poor pragmatic skills may affect their communicative effectiveness, attempts at living independently, social development, advocacy ability and opportunities for empowerment. For example, they may find a shopping experience challenging or confusing, especially on occasions when they may need to assert themselves, as they might not have the skills required to request or complain in a socially accepted way. In the societal domain, they may find similar difficulties even if they spend most of their day in protected environments. They are often not able to maintain topics during conversation or apply other social rules such as turn-taking.

One approach to assessing whether a client has such skills is via careful, detailed observation, especially in natural settings, during key events and times in the client's daily life. Such assessments can be conducted either by the SLT or by caregivers and key workers who usually spend more time with clients and are likely to be more familiar with them, their likes and dislikes, when they are likely to be most responsive, their daily routines, and so on. Analysis of these events and times also ensures that caregivers are responsive to even the most subtle of signals from the client. One can, of course, use well-established questionnaire/observation type schedules, or behavioural checklists to assess pragmatic (and other) skills. An example of such a schedule is the *Pragmatics Profile of Everyday Communication Skills in Children* (Dewart and Summers, 1997). Dewart and Summers (1997) also developed an assessment for adults, the *Pragmatics Profile for Everyday Communication Skills in Adults*. In a personal communication (2001) Summers stated that the Profile had been used with clients with special needs such as Asperger's. In addition, Dewart and Summers (1996:24) stated that 'It is intended that the questions in the Profile should be applicable to a whole range of severity of learning disability'.

Butterfield et al. (1995) noted that three essential elements of the communication process need to be considered. These comprise the integrated 'quality of interaction' model. It is therefore important to consider the following:

- context – i.e. partners, activities, preferences
- skills – abilities, forms, functions
- partner skills – chances, opportunities, routines, expectations.

Articulation

As mentioned earlier, an articulation impairment could be due to some organic aetiology. This could be neurological, physiological or structural (anatomical). Neurological involvement of the articulators is more common in clients with severe LD, but it may also present in individuals with a less severe disability. Individuals with DS may have a 'floppy' or hypotonic tongue (Rasore-Quartino, 1999). Though it is generally accepted that this is due to a neurological impairment, Brinkworth (personal communication, 1983) hypothesised that it could be due to the fact that these individuals often have very narrow external nares and consequently, they have to breathe through their mouths. In addition, their oral cavity is commonly less deep than in non-DS individuals, and during early development, they find it difficult to keep their tongue inside their mouth, and this produces a flaccidity in the tongue. It used to be thought that individuals with DS had an oversized tongue (macroglossia). However, it is now accepted that the tongue is only 'relatively' large because the buccal cavity of these individuals is too small to accommodate what is considered to be a 'normal'-sized tongue found in the non-LD population (see Rondal and Edwards, 1997:152–63 for more details about the speech of individuals with LD and DS). A weak velum may also be found in DS individuals and this may be responsible for an incompetent velo-pharyngeal sphincter which can result in hypernasal speech (see Rondal and Edwards, 1997; Buckley, 1999).

These abnormalities of the articulators may be responsible for, or contribute to, an articulatory impairment. Individuals with LD may also present with other neurological impairments such as dysarthria and dyspraxia. They may also suffer other structural abnormalities such as a high palatal arch, or a cleft palate, which may affect their articulation. Rondal (1999:144) identified 'articulatory and co-articulatory difficulties particularly with the more delicate phonemes' in persons with DS. It is thus important to conduct an oral assessment when a speech impairment is suspected. The size, structure, position at rest and the mobility of the articulators, and the strength and speed at which they move, for both speech and non-speech activities, should be studied. Evidence for or against neurological involvement should be sought. The client's phonetic inventory should be established through appropriate quantitative and qualitative assessment. It is important to establish whether the client can 'articulate' speech sounds, in isolation, clusters, blends, word initially and word finally. This can be established through assessing which sounds the client actually uses, albeit inappropriately, and whether they can imitate sounds.

Although articulatory breakdown may not be apparent at the single sound or word level, it may manifest itself when a more complex articulatory behaviour is necessary, such as in continuous speech. Breakdown of speech at this level is not necessarily diagnostic of a *phonological* impairment, though of course it may be due to a combination of both an articulatory and phonological impairment.

Eating and swallowing

Clients with LD may also have eating, drinking and swallowing problems. It is interesting that this is not a subject which is widely discussed in the literature. During research with very young DS children, Brinkworth and Abudarham (1984) identified several subjects who had needed help with feeding for some time, partly because of hypotonic musculature in the muscles used for sucking, chewing and swallowing. Some clients with LD, with and without DS, may remain for quite a long time at a stage when they can only take in fluids or semi-solids, so the transition to solids may be severely delayed. It is therefore important to conduct a detailed eating and swallowing assessment, especially for infant clients, so that appropriate and practical advice can be given to carers. As can be expected, parents can become very distressed when they find that their child is not able to eat or swallow properly, and they need advice (see case study in Chapter 4 of this book). Assessment of eating and swallowing is best conducted informally, though formal assessment allows for a more focused approach in enabling the study of the client's ability to drink, eat and swallow particular types of food and drink. It is possible that some clients are kept on certain foods, e.g. soft or liquid, for longer than necessary. Formal assessment can provide evidence for moving on to more appropriate food and drink. The informal assessment should take place during a client's natural feeding times as the client will be feeding in the way that is natural to them. There are other aspects which can be assessed during such times, e.g. carer–client interaction, manual motor and dexterity skills, social skills, and so on.

Language needs

Abudarham (Brinkworth and Abudarham, 1984) studied the communicative development of 15 children with DS from age 3 months to 5 years. These children's LD ranged from mild to moderate. Abudarham and Brinkworth's findings confirmed what other research had shown, that speech and language development in these children progresses in a developmentally rational way from the qualitative point of view but that it is delayed in all areas. Much of the later research does not contradict these findings. Issues related to communication development and functionality (Rondal and Edwards, 1997, Chapter 5) and related issues (e.g. IQ) are discussed at some length by Rondal and Edwards (1997:41–5; see also Rondal, in Rondal et al., 1999, Chapter 13). They concluded that, regarding 'language development and functioning', there are no good reasons for postulating 'qualitatively different language organisations in mildly, severely and profoundly MR [mentally retarded] persons.' They asserted that 'there is fundamental continuity in language at the various psychometric levels of mental retardation'. They conceded, however, that

> Of course, the language problems of moderately and severely MR people are more pervasive and more important than those of mildly MR subjects, particularly in some areas. (p. 35)

Examples of such areas are given as articulation, morpho-syntax and written language.

Clients with LD may have deficits across all linguistic parameters, i.e. vocabulary, semantics, grammar, syntax. It is important during the assessment process to distinguish between vocabulary and semantics. Some clients may seem to have a comparatively large vocabulary which they use without much meaning, thus giving the impression that they are communicatively competent and effective. Often they use stereotypical words or phrases which they have heard and learned but cannot always use appropriately. They may also learn formulaic expressions which they feel allow them to take part in social interaction. However, they may use words and expressions without really understanding their (semantic) meaning. Further in-depth discussion on lexical and semantic skills can be found in Rondal and Edwards (1997). Grove (Chapter 6 in this book) also discusses assessment of linguistic skills such as lexicon, semantics, syntax, morphology and pragmatics. She, like others before her (see Rondal and Edwards, 1997), advocates a multi-modal approach to assessment. Component parts of language, e.g. vocabulary, phonology and grammar, cannot be considered individually and independently as they interact with and relate to each other to form the 'whole' (see Rondal and Edwards, 1997, Chapter 4). Furthermore, one component of language may be more advanced developmentally than another. In addition, an impairment in one, for example phonology, can affect grammar e.g. a client who cannot use an 's' sound may not signal plurals. Rondal and Edwards (1997) also discussed evidence of exceptionality in individuals with LD when they demonstrate a skill in language which is higher than expected, supposedly in relation to IQ. The validity of this conclusion will obviously depend on factors such as whether whatever the expectation was related to, e.g. IQ, was reliably measured.

Writing and reading

It is fair to say that most of the research published about reading and writing skills in individuals with LD, certainly in the UK, has been about children with DS. One of the British authorities on the subject is Sue Buckley. She reported (1999:104) that her research over a period of two decades had indicated that with early reading instruction children with DS have achieved

> functional levels of reading and writing abilities i.e. above eight year reading ages, and spelling abilities with good comprehension.

More recently, Appleton et al. (2000) found that 3 year old children with DS were able to learn sight words at the same speed as pre-schoolers matched for age. They further found that a large number of their 6 year old subjects with DS were at the same reading level (including comprehension reading) as measured by standardised tests, after 1 year in school, as 'typically' developing peers matched for age.

There seem to be very few publications regarding reading and writing in clients with LD but with no DS (see Conners, 1992). Many questions are currently being asked regarding the relationship between a number of cognitive and psycholinguistic skills and the development of reading and writing. Among these are the 'phonological awareness' required to be able to segment phonemes, morphemes and syllables. Can 'reading with meaning' be achieved in the absence of these cognitive skills? If not, can an individual with LD learn to read orally, with or without some level of understanding? Can only those with a mild LD ever expect to learn to read at whatever level? Brinkworth (personal communication, 1983), for example, taught his daughter who had DS how to type. Her standard was good enough for her to be able to successfully achieve some paid employment.

Much more research is needed into the skills required to achieve different levels in literacy skills. We need to research into the role of factors such as auditory and visual memory, attention levels, auditory/visual sequencing, speech and 'verbal' language skills, figure–ground awareness and symbolic understanding, which are relevant to individuals with LD. Until these questions are answered, it is difficult to develop any valid and reliable assessments which will identify the skills required for individuals with LD to read or write.

Voice and fluency

There is a high incidence of voice and fluency impairment in clients with LD, particularly in clients with DS. Voice problems in clients with DS may be the result of congenital, neurological, anatomical and physiological abnormalities in the vocal folds, or frequent upper respiratory tract infections which may be responsible for attacks of laryngitis (see Rondal and Edwards, 1997:154–5 for further discussion). Vocal function should be assessed using current methods of assessment, through either observation or electronic instrumentation or both.

Fluency disorders may be of the 'stuttering' type; again, quite common in clients with DS. However, non-fluent speech resulting from difficulties in encoding language and executing articulatory or phonological processes may present as pauses, hesitations, repetitions, prolongations, and sometimes even forms of struggle behaviour during the articulatory attempt. Whether this dysfluency is of the type seen in stutterers is difficult to establish. Lebrun and Van Borsch (1991) reported on an adolescent client with DS who had 'stuttering symptoms'. It is difficult to state with certainty, but the dysfluency may be due to cognitive or pragmatic difficulties, neurological impairment, language processing impairments, slow patterns of thinking or other difficulties in 'central' (cortical) abilities. When assessing the fluency of a client with LD, one has to consider whether the assessment strategies employed for stutterers or clutterers are appropriate. Observation can be made regarding the nature and severity of a client's dysfluency, such as atypical hesitations, pauses, fillers, repetitions, prolongation, blocks and concomitant behaviour. The effect of the non-fluency/dysfluency on the client and his/her environment must be explored in order to determine how it affects their communicative effectiveness and needs.

From a management point of view, voice and fluency disorders may not be the first focus of attention when the client may benefit from work on developing non-verbal communication, language or pragmatic skills. However, they need to be assessed and monitored as they can be major contributors to unintelligibility and ineffective communication. Voice and fluency disorders can also make clients more conspicuous and add to the negative responses they may get from society.

A holistic model

Let us, be more precise about what we do or do not mean by the term 'holistic'. Our experience has all too often indicated that some students, and even some colleagues, perceive holism as the consideration of all aspects of a client's communication *impairment*. Such an approach would suggest that if one explores, say during assessment, all aspects of communication skills, for example, speech, both receptive and expressive language skills, voice, phonology, pragmatics, fluency, and so on, the holistic approach has been fulfilled. Others, ourselves included, believe that although this is part of the holistic approach, it does not fully fulfil the required brief. The development and acquisition of communication depends on many factors, e.g. hereditary, organic (neurological – sensori-motor, physiological, structural), cognitive, environmental, and affective (emotional). An impairment at any of these levels may have an adverse effect on the acquisition of communication skills.

Communication does not take place in a vacuum. It is an essential part of the general learning process, social and educational development, social and communicative interactions, and indeed, one's well-being may well be determined by an ability to communicate one's ideas, wishes or desires to others. A communicative environment can have an effect on an individual if it transcends their ability to understand. Similarly, individuals' own abilities to communicate may allow people in their environment to understand or not understand them. For this and other reasons, we need to consider all these factors during our appraisal of an individual's communication needs.

In Figure 2.1 we illustrate a possible approach to a holistic model. On the right of the model appear all those variables related to communication itself. At the top of the model are represented aspects of communication. These are generally the component parts of human communication and where communication could break down or not develop. Below this appears a variable which is often ignored, especially during the appraisal stage, although we feel that information about this has diagnostic and prognostic value. This is the need to explore the course and development of the communication impairment.

At the bottom of this side of the model is another set of variables we consider to be important, which should be considered during the appraisal stage, this being the exploration of causal, maintaining and contributing factors. The fact that it is not always possible to accurately determine the diagnostic and management significance of the course and development of the communication impairment, or the causal, maintaining and contributing factors, does not mean that one should neglect exploration of issues which can provide crucial insights into the appraisal, diagnostic and management exercise. On the left-hand side of the model appear issues regarding environmental factors which need to be

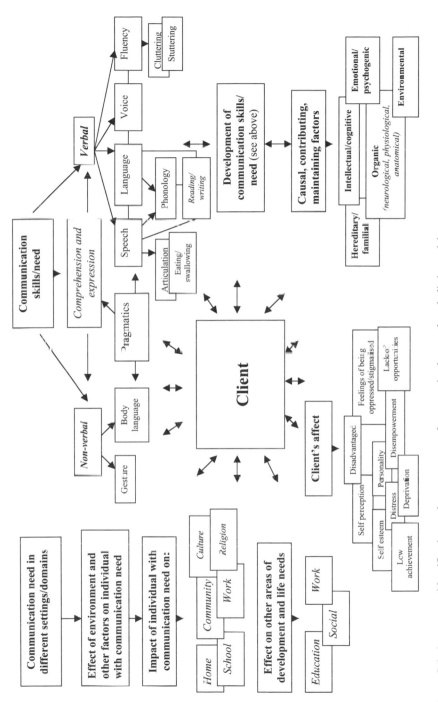

Figure 2.1. Assessment, identification and management of communication need – a holistic model.

considered and which have to do with the client's communication needs. Examples of these factors are the settings or domains in which communication may take place, the communicative and other demands that these domains may make on an individual, the communication skills needed to be able to communicate in these domains and the effect that individuals with LD may have on these settings. One cannot omit consideration of the client's affect, often adversely determined by negative social or cultural attitudes and stigmatisation (and sometimes those engendered by religious law and dogma). Similarly, a client may be disadvantaged because of underprovision of adequate and appropriate services, as a result of the social, educational and health policies of local and central government.

It cannot have escaped the reader's notice that we place the 'client' in the core of the model. The arrows emanating from the client are bidirectional, to illustrate that each factor is two-way, potentially impinging on the client and arising from, or inherent in, the client. Thus, a particular setting may make certain demands on the client (e.g. linguistic, emotional, practical), but a client may also have an effect on the environment.

Assessment, appraisal and profiling

General principles

In our introduction, we made the point that a distinction between 'assessment' and 'appraisal' has value. Essentially, we suggested that the term 'assessment' can be applied to the assessment of skills, whereas 'appraisal' is a term which can be applied to the whole individual. Thus, assessments are part of the appraisal of the individual. However, collecting information from the assessment and the appraisal process does not provide the full picture of an individual's needs, and as discussed before, the total picture of a client's communication skills, communication needs and related skills and needs can only be obtained by an accurate and detailed profiling exercise.

Nature of the communication impairment

The main aspects of communication have been discussed earlier. Other chapters in this book deal with some of them in more detail (see Chapters 4 and 6). One of the hotly debated issues has been the usefulness of the terms 'delay' versus 'disorder' or 'deviance', in relation to speech and language impairment (see Law, 1992a:31–2; Donaldson, 1995; Law and Elias, 1996:79–81; Rondal and Edwards, 1997). One of the arguments has been that when speech (including phonology) or language is delayed, it presents in a developmentally rational manner. The delay is thus indicated 'quantitatively' but not 'qualitatively'. Although clients with a delay may demonstrate 'less' speech and language than their non-LD peers, the particular communicative skill belongs to an earlier developmental stage. A 10 year old with LD may thus not have the rich vocabulary of a peer with no LD, or may not be able to use simple sentences, but the language level can be related to an earlier biological age, often though not always commensurate with their 'mental' age or IQ. Articulatory or phonological errors in 'deviant' or 'disordered' speech may not be associated with earlier phonology or with the phonology of the client's language. Some will argue that, given that in 'normal' development the discrepancy between comprehension and expression is usually not more than 9–12 months, a client with a demonstrable greater discrepancy could be said to have a language 'deviance' or 'disorder'. A similar argument applies when a client demonstrates a greater competence in 'expressive' than 'receptive' language, since receptive language precedes and exceeds 'meaningful' expressive language. Kamhi and Masterson (1989:83, and reiterated in the 1997 edition) stated that 'it is time to move beyond the delay and difference controversy and ask different and more appropriate questions', an example of which is the LD client's cognitive abilities, environmental and affective determiners and their relationship to language.

Despite their hope that the issue is never revisited, Rondal and Edwards (1997:105–108) addressed it in their book. Clearly it is not one that will go away easily. The likelihood is that at a management level, the difference may be fatuous because the developmental model is employed extensively during intervention. However, we shall desist from pursuing this matter. What is probably more relevant is to be able to differentiate between and identify different stages and levels of linguistic acquisition, different types of impairment (e.g. dysarthrias, dyspraxias, etc.) and the severity of the impairment. In a holistic approach it is the client and everything about them that comes first, not just their linguistic impairment, as has already been argued.

The case history

The case history is an important element in the process of documenting and subsequently evaluating a client's developmental, social or educational antecedents. We believe that the practice (sometimes encouraged) of focusing only on a client's present and future and ignoring their past is misguided and results in much previous information about the client being missed. The client's current needs must be considered in the context of relevant history which will include information about earlier needs, how they were or were not assessed or managed, social and residential history and so on.

Assessment of communication skills and needs

We have argued before that standardised tests have severe limitations, especially when used with clients with LD. We have also declared our preference for criterion referenced, or content related, assessments. However, it seems to be quite common practice by some educationalists and SLTs to use standardised tests for clients with LD. If the practice is to use the materials of such tests, so long as they are appropriate to the client's level (e.g. linguistic, cognitive, social, etc.) the practice may provide some useful information about the client's skills. However, what is not appropriate or acceptable is for the client's performance to be scored and statements made which are based on information drawn from derived scores (e.g. standard scores, standard deviations, age equivalents).

Kersner (1992) provided an overview of a range of tests employed in SLT. We shall briefly mention at this point some of those more commonly used with this client group and include some which are specially designed for clients with LD.

Informal assessment

Despite the fact that informal assessment typically suffers from the assessor's subjectivity, it is a strategy that is frequently employed and often justified. For example, the approach is appropriate with very young clients especially when there are no 'formal assessments' designed for them. Informal assessment can also be employed with older clients, including adults. When assessing informally, it is important to do so in naturalistic environments. There is much to be gained from conducting these assessments with parents and carers who spend a large part of the day with the client, as they can often furnish the SLT with much valuable information and insights into the client's skills and needs. The use of video and audio recordings can be of great benefit as one can study the client's behaviour in greater detail and depth. Observation during informal assessment can be related to a developmental framework if appropriate; for example, to establish where in the developmental continuum the client is operating. Once this is known, one can again use the developmental framework to determine what the developmentally rational 'next step' can be expected to be. For example, observations may indicate that a young client with LD has enough vocabulary and appropriate cognitive skills to move on to two-word utterances, or even phrase level. Informal assessment may also be driven by more immediate and functional needs. For example, can an adult client with LD make requests when perhaps the environment does not require them to do so, because everything is done for them?

Probe methods can also be used as part of one's informal assessment to explore the client's ability to deal with a particular 'challenge'. Tasks can be presented to clients to see how they cope. For example, without needing to resort to formal assessments which may include a particular task, one can present a client with a number of objects in the client's environment – a brush, say – assess the client's symbolic understanding, whether they can relate the object to its function, and so on. Other skills such as social and pragmatic skills, parent/carer–child/adult interaction, attention span, sensory skills (such as ability to scan visually) can sometimes be assessed more effectively via informal means that do not restrict the SLT to a prescribed set of assessment instructions nor constrain the therapist to assessing, as in the case of a formal assessment, or studying only what the assessment aims for. As mentioned earlier, informal assessments are likely to suffer from subjectivity. It is therefore important, particularly when conducting the informal assessment jointly with a parent or carer, that the assessment session is preceded by discussion about each participant's role and a list of shared objectives is arrived at. It is not only professionals who use jargon, and it is important that key terms are defined. For example, when asked whether her child had a word in her vocabulary, a mother replied in the affirmative. She was then asked to say what the word was. 'She says "mamamama" when she wants food' was the reply. Furthermore, one needs to establish whether a client 'correctly' responds to language, or is the response due to an ability to guess because of contextual clues?

Formal assessments

Most of the formal assessments available for this client group are of the criterion-referenced type, but some use developmental criteria. Several formal assessments have already been described (Kersner, 1992) and discussed in other publications (Lees and Urwin, 1991; Beech et al., 1993; van der Gaag and Dormandy, 1993; Wirz, 1995). Most of these assessments are still in current use. There is little point in discussing these here, but Table 2.1 provides some key information on a selection of the formal assessments available and used with this client group.

Table 2.1. Selection of formal assessment used with clients with learning disability

Name	Reference	Client group	Format	Aims
Affective Communication Assessment (ACA)	Coupe et al. (2000) David Fulton Publishers	Children at early stage of sensori-motor development; severe LD	Observation schedule	Pre-intentional communication skills and communicative behaviour
Communication Assessment Profile for Adults with a Mental Handicap (CASP)*	van der Gaag (1988) Speech Profiles/ Winslow Press.	Adults with severe to mild LD	Assessments by: Section 1- Carer (Questionnaire) Section 2 – Therapist (assesses 'event knowledge', 'auditory skills', 'vocabulary', 'comprehension', expression, 'communicative functions' – also 'concepts', 'articulation', 'gesture imitation', 'oro-muscular skills' Section 3 – Joint (includes client's own views, profile summary, communication, environment rating scale)	Examines communicative abilities within client's communication environment and in everyday situations
Derbyshire Language Scheme*	Knowles and Masidlover (1982) Masidlover Derbyshire Education Authority	For children at all levels of learning difficulties. Also available is a screening test for adults with LD	Uses both toys (not included) and pictures	Language Comprehension and Expression (in terms of information carrying words – ICW)

Table 2.1. (contd)

Name	Reference	Client group	Format	Aims
INTECOM*	Jones (1990) NFER-Nelson.	Adults with LD	Communication checklist	Aims to INTegrate carers into the client's assessment and development of COMunication skills – deals with communication environment, relationships, and opportunities for day-to-day communication
Personal Communication Plan (PCP)*	Hitchings and Spence (1991) NFER-Nelson.	Adolescents – Adults (age 14 and above) with mild-severe LD	Involves as many carers in the client's everyday environment as possible via a checklist and using a 'normalisation' framework, elicits background information, assesses speech, language, social communication skills and environment	Assess functional (expressed) communication skills and environmental opportunities
Phonological Assessment of Children's Speech (PACS)	Grunwell (1985) NFER-Nelson.	Children (but if adult-related qualitative analysis required, can be employed with adults)	Employs contrastive analysis and phonological process analysis. Comparisons can be made with expected adult phonology and also with that expected of children at the same developmental stage.	Aims to provide a detailed phonological analysis of children's speech

(contd)

Table 2.1. (contd)

Name	Reference	Client group	Format	Aims
PIP Development Charts	Jeffree and McConkey (1976) Hodder & Stoughton Educational.	Aimed for assessing 5 areas of development in children with severe LD (covers first 5 years of 'normal' development – can be used with children without LD	Employs developmental charts. Provides a developmental profile in: (a) physical (b) social (c) eye–hand (d) play (e) language	Provision of a basis for facilitating a client's development
Portage Early Education Programme*	Cameron and White (1987) NFER-Nelson.	Children with developmental delay	Checklists	Examines developmental achievement in 6 areas: (a) infant stimulation (b) self help (c) motor (d) socialisation (e) cognitive (f) language
Pragmatics Profile of Early Communication Skills in Children* (There is also a version for adults by the same authors)	Dewart and Summers (1996, 1997) NFER-Nelson.	Predominantly children with no LD from 9 months–5 years but can be used with children with severe LD	Structured but informal interview with carer results in a pragmatic skills profile	Assesses the following: (a) communicative intent (b) response to communication (c) interaction and conversation (in a wide range of communicative settings) (d) contextual variations

(contd)

Table 2.1. (contd)

Name	Reference	Client group	Format	Aims
Pre-verbal Communication Schedule (PVCS).*	Kiernan and Reid (1987) NFER-Nelson.	Children and adults with severe LD and others	Checklist observation schedule Four sections: (a) pre-communicative (b) informal communication skills (c) formal communication skills (d) receptive skills	Assesses communication skills of non-speaking clients or those with very little expressive language – words, signs and symbols, pre-communicative, communicative and receptive skills
Symbolic Play Test	Lowe and Costello (1988) NFER-Nelson.	Predominantly children with no LD from 1–3 years of age. Sometimes used with client with LD with suspected mental age of below 3	Miniature toys	To assess the level of representational functioning without using language; assesses early concept formation and ability to recognise and manipulate symbols

*Also provides comments and suggestions for intervention.

Assessment of related non-linguistic skills

There are many factors that are both directly and indirectly relevant to the development of communication and the client's learning needs which the SLT is not equipped to assess and appraise. The obvious ones are those which need medical expertise. Others such as cognitive skills can be assessed via means other than IQ tests. For example, much can be gleaned through observing the client's play behaviour, such as object permanence, ability to recognise relationships such as 'in-ness' (e.g. if when presented with a spoon and a cup, the child puts the spoon in the cup without being prompted; this may indicate that they possesses the concept of 'in-ness'), symbolic understanding, attention levels (see Cooper et al., 1978), joint attention, verbal and non-verbal functions, numeracy, etc. These are precursors to the development of corresponding verbal behaviour. Jeffree (1997) discussed issues related to the observation of play behaviour as a means of early assessment of children with severe LD. However, there are tests which are 'closed' to SLTs and may only be ('legitimately') conducted by qualified and trained psychologists. Many clients with LD may have visual problems needing assessment by optometrists, opticians or even ophthalmologists. Similarly, auditory problems may require assessment by audiometricians, audiologists, and even ENT specialists. The SLT must recognise when these assessments are required and make the appropriate referrals. SLTs also need to know how to interpret and evaluate the resulting reports and identify their implications for the SLT assessment, appraisal, differential diagnostic and management.

Our holistic model would require the assessment and appraisal of skills and needs related to linguistic ones. Examples of the former are cognitive skills (including 'attention levels' – see Cooper et al., 1978) and sensory skills (see Chapter 4 in this book). Social skills are often lacking or underdeveloped in clients with LD. This can undermine effective social interaction in any number of domains, from relationships with peers, to those between children with LD and adults with and without. The lack of appropriate social skills can affect the progress of a child with LD through school and into adolescence and adulthood. Not infrequently, communicative impairments may result in, or be associated with, a social skills deficit. Kelly (1997) discussed this matter at some length and described non-verbal behaviour such as body language (e.g. eye contact, facial expression, posture and personal appearance) and paralinguistic skills, or vocal cues (e.g. volume, rate of speech, clarity, intonation and fluency) as elements of social skills. She described verbal behaviour in terms of conversational skills (e.g. listening, initiating a conversation, asking and answering questions, relevancy, turn-taking, repair and ending a conversation) and assertive behaviour (e.g. expressing feelings, disagreeing, complaining, apologising, requesting explanations). Kelly (1997) stated that all these were important skills in maintaining and developing social relations and interactions. Clearly, many of these are pragmatic skills as well (e.g. 'turn-taking', 'requesting explanations'). There is thus a very close relationship between social and pragmatic skills. Examples of assessments of social skills currently used in the UK are Rinaldi's (1992) *Social Use of Language Programme*, Kelly's (1996) *Talkabout* and the social skills section of the *Personal Communication Plan* (Hitchings and Spence, 1991).

Clients' affect, motivation and personality may all play their part in determining the level of progress in communication skills. Strengths in these areas can have a positive impact on a client's prognosis for change. Often, the results of such assessments and appraisals are considered in the 'prioritisation' process and will determine if and when a client will be seen, how frequently, in what context, and the most appropriate provisions and service delivery. Information about a client's cognitive skills, environment, affect, and so on can also suggest causal, maintaining and contributing factors. Knowledge of these may equally contribute to issues related to prioritisation, IEPs, resources needed for such clients (e.g. audiology services or consideration of residential facilities) and rationales for speech and language therapy intervention strategies.

Gunzburg's (1977) PACS, mentioned earlier, is perhaps not entirely holistic as it is predominantly skills-based and does not include items to do with possible causes, but it does comprise four major areas of development: self-help, communication, socialisation and occupation. The subcategories under each of these and the skills assessed under them differ according to the client group being appraised. There are thus versions for individuals with DS (Chart 1 – see Gunzburg, 1977) and adults with severe LD (Chart 2). General skills such as manual activities, cleaning, social awareness, shopping, language, reading and writing, numeracy, play activities, mobility, dexterity, agility, table habits, etc., are assessed via a questionnaire-based approach. The results of the assessment are recorded on to a chart comprising a circle divided into the four main areas of assessment. Within each quarter are further small sections representing specific skills. Shading the skills achieved provides an overview of the individual's skills and developmental profile.

Lastly but by no means least, a careful appraisal of the client's environment (home, day setting, etc.) needs to be conducted. One cannot just assess the 'means' (Kiernan et al., 1987; see also Money, Chapter 3 in this book) for communication but also the 'functions' and 'reasons' for communicating (Kiernan et al., 1987) and 'opportunities' (Money, Chapter 3). The existence, or lack, of reasons and opportunities for communication are mostly triggered and provided by the client's environment. It is thus important to observe clients' in their natural settings, including home, school or workplace. The particular type of service delivery (see Hickman, Chapter 1, and Money, Chapter 3 both in this book) and provision, the expertise, motivation, co-operation and collaboration of significant people in the client's environment may hold back or enhance a client's development of communication skills and wish to communicate.

Case studies

In presenting these case studies, we aim to illustrate several issues related to assessment and appraisal and particularly make implicit reference to the holistic model presented earlier.

Case study 2.1

This case provides a brief illustration of a number of factors. The potential 'bilingual' status of the child exacerbated matters. However, the differential diagnosis was between a second language (L2) problem and a specific language impairment (SLI). His home background and communication needs there and at school also had to be assessed, as did a number of cultural issues (e.g. social stigma).

Bashir was an 8 year old Asian child attending a school for children with LD. Because he came from a non-English background and English was not spoken at home, a teacher of English as a Second Language (TESL) was asked to see him. This teacher had minimal experience in teaching children with LD. An approach from her to a SLT indicated that she was experiencing substantial frustration at not being able to help the child develop his knowledge and use of English. She was surprised that, having worked for quite some time on certain basic grammatical rules, the child was only able to use them in the context taught (stereotypically) and was not able to generalise them. The SLT assessed the child and concluded that he had an articulatory dyspraxia which no doubt contributed to his language difficulties. There being no bilingual co-workers available, a postgraduate special needs student was asked for help in the assessment.

It was quite obvious from observations and the class teacher's reports that the child's English was extremely poor. One needed to know whether he had a L2 learning problem or a specific language learning impairment, or SLI (Abudarham, 1998). Before embarking on any assessment, the first issue that had to be addressed was what language he used at home. This was predominantly Punjabi, though the home lexicon included vocabulary from other dialects. Once the names given at home for certain familiar objects, actions and concepts were established, we were able to devise an information assessment based on these. As a result, it became evident that the child had a severe language disorder, with extremely poor receptive and expressive vocabulary and no language structure. His poor language skills were well below what might have been expected for his IQ as reported by the school's educational psychologist. However, his non-verbal communication was more functional, as were his pragmatic skills. His parents could not understand or speak English and seemed to be embarrassed by their child's problems. Following assessment and appraisal, a summary of which has been presented, it was possible to identify the child's communicative abilities and needs and formulate an action plan with the class teacher. It was agreed that TESL intervention was not appropriate at that point. The SLT took an advisory role in the language programme but worked on the child's dyspraxia.

Case study 2.2

The following case study illustrates how it is important to consider factors which may impinge on a client's communicative development. It also demonstrates the teamwork that is needed between the SLT and client's carer, and between both these and other professionals. Furthermore, this was one of many typical cases which, as referred to constantly in the literature (see Guralnick, 1999:52–5), suffered from many of the stressors which can affect a family and child, and adversely affect the child's development.

Christiana was referred to speech and language therapy at the age of 6 months. She was born with DS. Initially, her parents were advised by the consultant paediatrician that it was unlikely that she would live to see her first birthday because of a congenital heart condition. Christiana had an older sister who was 'normal'. Both parents were educated professionals. Initially, they both rejected Christiana. However, her 35 year old mother changed her mind and decided to take her home when she left the hospital but her father was not able to conceal or cope with his feelings of rejection. Because they had been told that Christiana's health prognosis was so poor, they decided to try for another child, despite the risk of having another child with DS. Halfway through the third pregnancy, Christiana's father left the family for a female colleague. His wife was naturally very bitter and developed a distrust for many of the professionals and services associated with her daughter. This, however, seemed to reinforce her determination to do the best for Christiana so that she could make the most of her predicted short life. The mother was therefore quite happy to co-operate with the SLT whom she also used as a sounding board and counsellor. Despite this, she was not prepared to accept any advice without rigorously questioning the rationale, and challenging the SLT as she felt appropriate. The SLT's response was positive and enabling throughout. As her carer, the mother's focus in life was Christiana's every need, sometimes seemingly to the detriment of the older sibling. However, the mother was able to provide detailed information about Christiana's strengths and needs. She was encouraged by the SLT to keep a diary of Christiana's development of communication skills, both verbal and non-verbal. The SLT, who saw them every 6 weeks for an hour and a half, was able to confirm the mother's reported observations of Christiana's communicative and related development, and inform and guide her about the range of behaviours and events (e.g. medical experiences) which were relevant to Christiana's communication needs. Though primarily Christiana was part of a research group of 15 children with DS (see Brinkworth and Abudarham, 1984), our ethical imperative resulted in including providing advice and some intervention work once the research requirements (i.e. collection of data on communication and related development) had been fulfilled for a particular session. Inherent in the research was the need to train parents in observation skills and enable them to become aware of developmental issues, e.g. communication-related terminology, identification of stages in communicative development, non-verbal communication, such as pre-symbolic stage, holophrastic stage, emergence of two-word utterances, concepts of 'pivot' and 'open class', etc.

Over the four and a half years of contact, the mother learned about and was able to observe, and sometimes anticipate, the emergence of Christiana's pre-linguistic and linguistic skills, from eye contact, to the communicative role of referential gaze, the acquisition of object permanence, the communicative importance of objects of reference, the emergence and recognition of the first 'word' and eventually, two-word utterances. By the age of 3, Christiana was placed in a play group which she attended every weekday morning. The very welcoming staff initially had little idea of what to expect or do. However, both her mother and the SLT were able to assess the environment and resources available (including equipment and staff's skills) and advise staff how best to meet Christiana's needs.

Sadly, Christiana died after her fifth birthday, having outlived all medical prognoses of a more premature death.

Conclusion

The field of assessment, appraisal and profiling is large. In the two sections in this chapter, we have attempted to address a number of major issues, but by no means all. In the second section, we have dealt with the more practical issues, having discussed a number of theoretical ones in the first section. We have stressed the need for a holistic approach and have considered not only the assessment, appraisal and profiling of communication skills and needs but also highlighted the need to consider factors related to such skills and needs.

CHAPTER 3

Speech and Language Therapy Management Models

DELLA MONEY

Abstract

The main models of speech and language therapy management from past to present are presented in this chapter. The research evidence is discussed and some recommendations for future work are suggested. The chapter is divided into five sections. The historical and theoretical perspectives that have influenced speech and language therapy models are briefly presented. A current model of communication is discussed as a proposed basis of all management models. The main models of speech and language therapy management currently in use in the UK are explored, as are the incidence and practical implementation of different management models. The findings of some surveys into management models and a case study example of a combination model are presented. A summary of the limited research evidence available to support different models of management is provided. Finally, recommendations are made for the future development of management models and possible directions for research.

Introduction

The aim of speech and language therapy management with children and adults with learning disabilities (LD) is to maximise their potential communicative competence. The challenge for speech and language therapists (SLTs) is that communication does not occur in a vacuum, and communication breakdown could be the result of the individual's skills, their partner's skills, and/or their environment. Hymes (1974) described a competent communicator as someone who knows when and when not to communicate, what to discuss, with whom, when, where and in what manner. This means that communication and the environment are inter-linked and interdependent, serving to facilitate, or exacerbate, communicative competence. Successful management models of speech and language therapy services need to reflect this.

Review of the literature

Historical and theoretical perspectives

This review starts with a historical and theoretical perspective of management models practised in the UK over the last two decades or so. In the past, the focus of therapy and research was the individual with LD and that individual's communication deficits. It was assumed that communication problems were solely the result of an individual's lack of competence and skill (Leudar, 1981). Although it cannot be ignored that a person with LD may have a specific communication difficulty, communicative competence is necessarily the result of interchange between the skills of the speaker and events in the environment (Halle, 1988). Ultimately, this means that all communication partners have a vital role in promoting a person's communicative competence, and current speech and language therapy models of management have to reflect this. To achieve this, SLTs and relevant staff need a greater understanding of the communication environment, the communication skills of staff, and a shared model of communication.

Communication environment

In the early 1980s, researchers began to explore communication within the context of the whole environment. They found that people with LD can be handicapped as much by the under-expectation of those who live and work with them as by their primary disabilities (Mittler and Berry, 1977). Additionally, communication skills are under-utilised if they are in an environment that does not make sufficient demands on individuals with LD to communicate (van der Gaag, 1989), and increased environmental opportunity correlates highly with improved communication ability (Blackwell et al., 1989). Leudar (1989:296) concluded that 'communication environments for mentally handicapped people are systematically distorted and do not provide the same opportunities as those of average persons'.

As the importance of the role of communication environments in promoting opportunities for communication became highlighted, it was clear that individuals with LD frequently do not have the same opportunities for meaningful interaction. Halle (1988) studied carer interaction and found that carers often unintentionally pre-empted natural occasions for language. Pre-empting could be environmental, whereby the physical environment negates the need for communication; non-verbal, where carers provide objects, events, or activities without requiring any interaction; or verbal, where carers inhibit communication by providing prompts, or using closed questions before the person has had time to initiate speech. Pre-empting at its greatest is exemplified by Ryan and Thomas (1980:35) through an excerpt from Frank Thomas's diary, written while he was working as a nursing assistant and volunteer in various hospitals and schools: 'Tea mixed with milk and sugar to save time, mess and trouble. How many lumps, say when with the milk? You must be joking.'

Although tea may no longer be served from large urns as described by Thomas, it can still too often appear at specified drink or break times already prepared with added milk and sugar, thus pre-empting opportunities for communication. Ultimately, it is staff and carers who have the greatest opportunities to communicate with people with LD, and who play a vital role in creating and maintaining the communication environment (Landesman-Dwyer and Knowles, 1987). Management models of speech and language therapy have to address these environmental needs.

Communication partners

Every communication partner has their own unique contribution to developing communicative competence. A communication partner is a major factor in the success or failure of many communicative interactions (McNaughton and Light, 1989). However, staff working with children and adults with LD often use communication that is limited in terms of its quantity, purpose and form. They may fail to provide appropriate settings of demand, expectation, and opportunity for effective communication (Mittler and Berry, 1977). Money (1997) studied the quality and quantity of staff/carer interaction with adults with LD. Unfortunately, the results are not encouraging.

In her study of interaction between staff and service-users (i.e. clients), Money (1997) analysed 2029 utterances from 20 dyadic 12-minute interactions between staff and service users in day services, from health and social services settings. The vast majority of staff utterances were initiations (93.4%). These were further analysed in terms of both their form and function. Overall, statements were the main form of initiation (37.5%), followed by closed questions (29.7%), and multi-uttered initiations (19%).

Open questions accounted for 10.3% of staff initiations. The use of requests for information (53.8%) and requests for action (31.1%) were the most frequently recorded functions of staff initiations.

Money (1997) found that staff provided 1079 initiations and, therefore, an equal number of opportunities for clients to respond. Over one-third (34.3%) of staff initiations failed to elicit a response. Analyses of staff–client interactions in terms of their use of additional modalities indicated that clients used additional non-verbal modalities over one-third more than staff, and that clients use twice the amount of formal modalities (i.e. signs and symbols) as staff.

These findings are supported by other researchers. McConkey et al. (1999a) summarised four main points about staff communication following their research.

- Clients were presented with few opportunities to engage as equal partners.
- Staff overly relied on verbal communication, even when communicating with predominantly non-verbal clients.
- Staff favoured the use of directives and questions.
- The majority of staff failed to adjust their language to the client's level of understanding.

Similar results have been found with children. Ware (1990) studied staff–pupil interactions and found that interactions occurred once every 12–13 minutes with pupils with profound and multiple LD. Additionally, she found that staff initiations were less likely to expect a response with pupils who had the greatest difficulty.

The results of such research imply that two issues need to be addressed before SLTs can be effective in changing staff communication.

- Why do staff communicate the way they do?
- What is or is not acceptable in terms of the quality and quantity of staff–client interactions, i.e. what dimensions constitute a good communication partner or environment?

McConkey et al. (1999a) suggested two possible reasons for staff communication that need further investigation. Do staff misjudge the communicative competence of their partners and, for example, not use enough simple language or additional modalities, or provide time? Or is it because of the way that staff and/or their employers perceive both their role as paid employees and service users as either peers or patients? This point is illustrated by this excerpt in Frank Thomas's diary (Ryan and Thomas, 1980:56):

> Nursing in full glorious colour! Make a bed and you get praised. Interact socially with a patient and you get accused of loafing.

A shared model of communication

From the research already presented on communication environments and staff communication skills, it is evident that an effective model of speech and language therapy management needs to consider all aspects of communication in terms of the individual with LD, their partner and the environment. Staff and SLTs must work jointly and share a model of communication for assessment and intervention. Communication needs to be considered in the context of how staff and service users communicate (means), why they communicate (reasons), and with whom, where, and when do they communicate (opportunities). A model of means, reasons and opportunities for communication has been evolved by the current author (Bulpitt, 1989) and is illustrated in Figure 3.1.

This model now underpins all models of service delivery in Nottinghamshire for both training and therapy, with children and adults (Money and Thurman, 1994; Money, 1997b; Thurman, 1997; Sutton and Thurman, 1998). Although the models of speech and language therapy management vary, they all reflect means, reasons and opportunities for communication, throughout assessment and management. Therapists use these dimensions of communication to observe and monitor both the person and their communication partners, and the impact and relationship between them. This model ensures that the equal importance of means, reasons and opportunities for communication is reflected in the rationale for the most appropriate management model.

Intervention

Models of speech and language therapy management

From the 1970s, models of management were primarily centred on teaching the client new skills in highly structured situations. The role of the partner and the environment was viewed as secondary. Although some success was recorded in therapy sessions, there was little or no carryover, or generalisation, into everyday communication. From the mid-1980s, approaches to speech and language therapy service delivery developed significantly in terms of both areas and styles of intervention. It

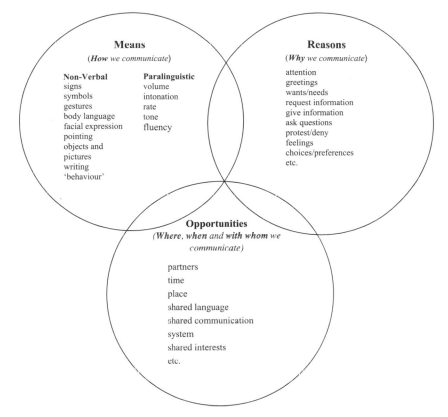

Figure 3.1. Means, reasons and opportunities model.

was clear that there was little justification for planning communication intervention as an isolated activity because communication is the tool that facilitates individuals to function in daily living activities (Calculator, 1988). The emphasis of therapy had shifted to an environmental, or ecological, approach and this had far-reaching implications for speech and language therapy management models.

There are many management models that can be considered valid and successful and they all view the roles of the person, partner and environment as equal in effecting change. *Communicating Quality*, the professional standards published by the Royal College of Speech and Language Therapists (RCSLT, 1996a), recognises that developing improved physical surroundings, personal circumstances and appropriate communication used by carers, will significantly benefit the client's communicative success. It recommends that these should always be the primary focus for intervention. *Communicating Quality* states that the style of speech and language therapy intervention should be direct, indirect or a combination of both.

Direct approach

This style focuses on developing the client's communication abilities, through either:

- individual goal planning integrated into daily one-to-one situations
- individual goal planning integrated into already existing group situations
- the use of specifically planned groups to develop targeted skills.

The rationale for this approach is that direct therapy aims to develop a specific skill, generally in conjunction with significant others. Examples may include assessment of specific language skills, anger management, intensive interaction, facilitating signs and symbols in the classroom or activities, social communication skills, individualised sensory environments and developing parent–child interaction through approaches such as the Hanen Programme (Manolson, 1992).

Case study 3.1

Nick has a high-tech communication aid on loan from the Communication Aids Centre. He needs specific individual direct therapy to teach him how to maintain and use the aid. He needs to learn how to access the vocabulary, how to delete and how to 'speak' the message. At first he needs a lot of practice time to find his way around the aid, explore what it can do for him and enjoy using it. This needs to be overseen by the SLT but also involves all his care staff and his mother. Direct therapy needs to be provided at home, at the day centre and within the community to ensure real and meaningful reasons and opportunities are used.

Indirect approach

This style concentrates on developing opportunities for communication, through one or all of the following:

- training for carers in any aspect of communication pertinent to the client
- a programme to make the physical environment more conducive to good communication for the client
- a programme to amend carer communication to any appropriate style, thus enhancing the client's communication skills
- advice and support to the carers
- referral on to another agency.

The rationale is that indirect therapy aims to develop and influence significant others' communication skills by providing them with information, models and/or experiences that enable them to adapt their communication and/or the communication environment. This adaptation should in turn facilitate the service users' communication skills. Some examples may include specific individualised training, support for using augmentative and alternative communication, facilitating groups for sign/symbol befrienders or peer tutors, jointly developing, reviewing and evaluating care plans, participating in case conferences or providing access to information for individuals.

Case study 3.2

Alison has a hearing impairment. She knows many signs but has not used them for several years. She has recently moved into a residential home and recommenced day services. She can remember her signs but neither the day nor residential staff use signs. Staff in both these settings need to learn signs, but this has to be in conjunction with a joint understanding of the importance of a shared communication system and promoting positive reasons and opportunities for Alison to sign.

Combination approach

Here, intervention is a combination of direct and indirect approaches. There are publications that detail and support this approach, through assessment to management, for example *ENABLE* (Hurst-Brown and Keens, 1990) and the *Personal Communication Plan* (Hitchings and Spence, 1991).

The rationale for this approach is that using one single approach to intervention is rarely appropriate. Therapy needs to be tailored to individuals, and an eclectic approach is necessary. People often have specific needs which require targeting both directly and indirectly, and through a range of management models.

Case study 3.3

Carol is 16 and has left school to go to college. She uses a combination of single words, signs and symbolic noises. Both Carol and the staff need help using signs and symbols within the college curriculum. A combination of working directly within her timetabled activities alongside her staff and peers is provided, together with facilitating a workshop specific to Carol's needs, regular support at review meetings, and being available as a resource for Carol, her family and college to use.

Whichever approach is used, SLTs recognise that all aspects of management models must ensure that people with LD have the right to dignity, respect, choice, community presence and participation and should be valued, as well as the right to achieve their maximum potential (RCSLT, 1996a). This is the principle of normalisation which is a foundation for planning and running services and a vantage point for judging service quality (O'Brien and McTyne, 1981). With the change to environmental approaches, the use of indirect models of management has increased, and many SLTs now feel they predominantly use this approach. Within indirect models, SLTs are moving from the role of an 'expert', whereby they give expert advice, through the model of 'transplanting' knowledge to significant others to enable them to carry out communication care plans, to a 'partnership' where significant others and SLTs work equally together benefiting from each other's skills.

However, working indirectly is not always easy. Indirect approaches involve a transition from a traditional therapy role, requiring a different set of skills, and detailed re-appraisal of the aims and objectives. SLTs often feel that they are ill-prepared in training for the practical implementation of indirect therapy for this client group (Enderby and Davies, 1989). These issues were first raised nearly 20 years ago, as newly qualified SLTs found it difficult to emerge from the 'speech and language therapy room' and to change from direct one-to-one work to become part of a team approach (Stansfield, 1982). However, even in the year 2001 speech and language therapy students and newly qualified SLTs find it challenging to work indirectly with service users, through staff and carers.

Examples of indirect approaches

Three models that exemplify indirect approaches are discussed now: the advisor, the training and the team management models.

Advisor model

This is an example of an 'expert' management model. In order to use speech and language therapy time most effectively, SLTs needed to work with, and through, other people, in an advisory and consultative role. The need to move away from a traditional role, to the specialist role of advisor, staff trainer and team member was described by Stansfield (1982) and Cottam (1986), among others. One conclusion was that SLTs should act as advisors to staff and/or carers on a regular basis, because the level of speech therapy service provision was inadequate to meet the need.

Working through the advisor model is not, however, purely a supply and demand issue about speech and language therapy resources. Many SLTs choose to work within the speciality of LD because of the philosophy that underpins it. Working together with others is a more practical approach to intervention than the traditional medical and developmental models used within speech and language therapy, because people with LD are neither 'ill' nor 'children' (van der Gaag and Dormandy, 1993).

One challenge of the advisor model is the all too common problem of developing the role of care staff. In practice, other agencies generally feel the responsibility for communication still belongs with the speech and language therapy service (Dobson, 1995). For example, SLTs in Somerset reported that staff would send their clients to them to 'do' signing, instead of regarding it as a tool for them to use to help clients communicate better (Jones et al., 1992). In North Tees, instructors and carers did not consider communication skill development as their responsibility, and resented SLTs for putting additional demands on their time (Siddons and Wray, 1995).

These types of comments demonstrate the limitations of the expert role, and the need to move towards transplant and partnership models. However, some examples of when the advisor model may be appropriate include:

- working in schools or colleges, giving advice on the communication curriculum
- working with other professionals in specific working parties developing guidelines for sexuality, abuse, bereavement, etc.
- liaising with primary care staff for hearing assessments, general practitioners (GPs), appointments, parenting skills
- facilitating access to communication through easy language and symbols.

Training model

Training staff is no longer an optional component of the work of a SLT, but an essential, ongoing commitment (van der Gaag and Dormandy, 1993). However, the number of people needing training is as great as the number of people working with clients with LD in the UK health and social services, as well as families, voluntary and private organisations and generic services (Mittler, 1987). Although there are many unpublished local communication training initiatives (for example, six within Trent Regional Health Authority in 1991), there are only a few published workshops, e.g. INTECOM (Jones, 1990), Assessing Communication Together (Bradley, 1991) and Talkabout (Money and Thurman, 1994).

Teaching can be an effective model of service delivery, provided it is flexible, small scale, facilitated by local SLTs, moulded to the needs of the individual staff, practical and straightforward, and supported by management (Cullen 1988; van der Gaag and Dormandy, 1993). However, the style of training provided by SLTs varies from one department or trust to another. Dobson (1990) found that some SLTs ran large intensive workshops, and others ran small regular unit-based training which was less intensive but took place over a much longer period of time. Another option was large single-day workshops for whole staff or professional groups. Dobson found that one main difference was whether SLTs waited to be invited to provide courses, or whether they initiated courses and invited carers to attend.

There are clearly pros and cons to all these variations in styles of training models, and the research evidence supporting training is discussed later on in this chapter. The training model is essentially a transplant role whereby SLTs are transferring information to significant others so they can achieve communication aims. Some examples of use include:

- training specifically tailored to an individual's, or environment's, need
- opportunity for problem-solving
- training for specific techniques or needs e.g. hearing loss, understanding, choices, abuse, challenging needs, signs and symbols
- induction for new staff.

Team model

SLTs work as part of a multi-disciplinary team to provide clients with LD with well co-ordinated packages of care (RCSLT, 1996a). *Communicating Quality* (RCSLT, 1996a) discusses the diverse role of the SLT in this field, which involves working in partnership to meet overall team objectives through:

- raising awareness of the communicative needs of an individual
- advising service purchasers on policy issues as they relate to the communication needs of the individual with a LD
- educating these groups who may include commission teams, GPs, social services, further education funding bodies and care managers
- being a case manager/co-ordinator
- developing protocols, procedures and guidelines to meet identified needs

- participating in support/supervision policies
- developing local standards and local service level agreements for working in a multi-agency team.

Teams must strive together to work towards these goals. SLTs work within the team's framework for assessment and intervention. One example of a 'systemic framework' is used by Eastbourne and County Health-care Intensive Support Team. They aim to achieve high-quality, collaborative inter-disciplinary relationships that can have a powerful positive influence on people's lives. Thurman (1997) described the success of a communication-centred team approach with a commitment to optimum opportunities for fulfilling activities and minimum levels of intrusiveness, within the context of a close-knit team who value the individuals with whom they work. Team models of speech and language therapy management must truly encompass partnerships.

Practical application of management models

There have been three main types of surveys investigating the use of management models in the UK, and these are discussed below.

Surveys of models of management in the UK

Dobson (1990) compared four different models of management across 15 districts in the UK. These were an indirect assessment/advice model, a direct individual model, a direct group model and a training/facilitating model. She found that only one approach, staff training, was identified as used by all districts. A direct approach, combining both individual and group work, was predominantly used by two-thirds of the districts. Most offered a group-based service. An indirect model of service delivery was only exclusively used by four districts (two by choice and two through expediency), and none of the districts surveyed used an exclusively individual model of service delivery.

A variety of models was also found by Enderby et al. (1992) in a survey of therapy services to South West Regional Health Authority (SWRHA). The most frequent intervention approach in all 10 districts covered by SWRHA was staff/carer support and training, but there was variation in the other approaches. Five districts frequently used an environmental modification approach and five frequently used an individual approach. Others frequently used approaches including sensory integration and a multi-disciplinary approach.

Both surveys found that the training model was the only model identified by all districts. However, whereas Dobson (1990) had found that most districts were providing a group approach, Enderby et al. (1992) found that only three districts listed group treatment as a frequent approach, with instead a greater emphasis on environmental approaches.

Money (2000) surveyed speech and language therapy services in Trent Region in England to explore the current models of management in use, and establish the extent of evidence-based practice. Nine NHS trusts responded. SLTs were asked to identify from a choice of five (see Table 3.1) the management models they predominantly used to deliver different areas of intervention.

Table 3.1. Definitions of models of service delivery

Direct (individual) Working directly with an individual, concentrating on developing their communication abilities

Direct (group) Working directly within specifically planned groups, to develop targeted skills of two or more individuals

Indirect (individual) Working indirectly with an individual by working through significant other(s) to develop their communication environment or targeted skills. May include training

Indirect (group) Working indirectly, through the significant other(s) to develop targeted skills of two or more individuals within specifically planned groups

General teaching Teaching that is not specifically planned to meet an individual's need, but to develop overall awareness, communication skills, etc.

Use of the five models of intervention varied up to 25% between both individual SLTs and across trusts. These variations in models reflected differences in caseload size, fixed timetable sessions at one place, differences in local policies on criteria for active vs. review vs. discharged, and/or differing management responsibilities and specialisms (for further details, see Money, 2000).

The survey found that the strengths of an indirect approach were flexibility and being within the context of the environment, delivered at the most appropriate location together with a multi-disciplinary team and staff. This supported Dobson (1990) who found that the strengths were that staff and carers were facilitated and the environment was supportive. However, there can be disadvantages around the implementation of programmes, and the perception of SLTs as being distanced rather than 'hands on'. This is also supported by the Trent Region survey where the constraints of service delivery were around staff morale, motivation and skills mix, and with other agencies with changing policies and agendas.

The least frequent model of intervention for five trusts in the Trent Region was direct groups. There are several constraints to direct groups with problems around carers not always being involved, therapy not being part of daily living, and SLTs becoming exclusively responsible for communication, thus creating dependence, and taking communication out of context (Dobson, 1990). Some areas of intervention were delivered by specific styles. For example, models of management for social communication skills and basic interaction skills predominantly use direct group approaches although half of the service is also provided indirectly. This compares to low-tech alternative and augmentative communication (AAC) which appears to be delivered using all the models of intervention equally, and opportunities for environmental work which are provided indirectly and mainly through teaching.

A comparison of these three surveys shows that the teaching model of management is widely used. However, with the shift to an environmental focus, most SLTs are predominantly providing an indirect individual approach with a reduction in the direct approach (group and individual). There is a great amount of variety between SLTs and trusts and this reflects the flexible and needs-led approaches taken by SLTs to deliver a combination of the most appropriate models in the most appropriate locations.

Jones (2000) described the progress of the Somerset 'total communication' approach. She concluded the following learning points from their experience:

- Recognition of the fundamental importance of communication is vital and involves 'everyone'. This needs a very high level of co-operation across agencies, professionals and services.
- SLTs train, monitor and support staff and carers, alongside providing accurate specialist assessments.
- No matter how many National Collections of signs and symbols are available, there will always be a need for local and individual person-specific vocabulary.
- Training and resources need to be free or inexpensive, accessible, locally and personally relevant.
- Clients with LD benefit from developing their comprehension, choice, relationships, participation, self-advocacy, independence, literacy and opportunities for inclusion; 'total communication' can facilitate these.

Van der Gaag (1998) reviewed models of 'total communication' and felt that four main aspects were important for its success:

- It is driven by the individual's communication needs.
- It depends on the involvement of everyone in the service user's environment.
- Speech and language therapy concentrates equally on the partner's and user's skills.
- SLTs focus on detailed assessments and planning, empowering others and letting go of their control of communication development.
- It has the full support of management.

From the available research evidence it was clear that within Nottinghamshire (Trent Region), improvement of the communication environment was needed, and that this required a planned strategy together with management, staff and service users (van der Gaag, 1998; Jones, 2000). From our SLTs' subjective and objective experiences, and reports in the literature, a 'total communication' approach involving all augmentative means of communication from objects of reference, through to signs, symbols, photos and gestures seemed to be appropriate (Jones et al., 1992; Jones, 2000).

Currently, an evaluation strategy of the pilot year of the Nottingham Signs and Symbols Linkworker Network is under way. It has been time-intensive for participating SLTs but a positive experience of working together across NHS trusts. The issue of developing service user involvement in the network from an individual unit level to the planning level and membership of the steering group will need to be addressed. It is early days for seeing any changes in service user communication as a consequence of our service initiative. However, this combination model of service delivery is planned, evidence-based, and could be subjected to an action-research approach, combining longitudinal, single case study and qualitative methods (Purcell et al., 2000).

Research supporting management models

Unfortunately, there is limited published research or information available supporting different models of management. This is despite the fact that there is undoubtedly a wealth of knowledge and experience that exists within the profession, which is evident from the development of special interest groups (SIGs) and other networks. Historically, SLTs have made service delivery recommendations and decisions on the basis of their local expertise and their own subjective evaluations. Some of these have evolved to cope with the high caseloads and resource constraints, including models based on screening the population jointly with key staff (Law and Lester, 1991; Law et al., 1994). Others reflect local policies, procedures and practice. This has led to a variety of models of care, use of staffing, different work practices and patterns of intervention, which are both striking and imaginative (Dobson, 1990).

Many of these models can be considered valid and successful. However, regardless of the model used, it is essential to have a clear underlying philosophical and theoretical framework. The emphasis, in both assessment and management, must be directed towards the functional communication needs of the person and their communication partners within the context of the communication environment. Evaluation must indicate whether both the staff and the service users are benefiting. If staff are to become communication facilitators, the quality of the interaction between each staff member and service user needs to be assessed and there must be changes in staff communication aimed at facilitating changes in service user communication.

Research evidence to support models of management will always be difficult within the LD field. It has to be conducted within the 'real world' in order to make valid recommendations. However, although this may increase the external validity of research projects it will always reduce the internal validity. It would be very difficult to match staff in terms of age, sex, experiences, skills, length of service, let alone service users. Most research is carried out in specific settings at one moment in time, often with an observer or a video present. Often staff are volunteer subjects. These factors combine to make researching management models very daunting. None the less, we need to find effective models of management. McConkey et al. (1999b) warned us that failure to attend to this issue runs the risk that service users are given little opportunity by staff to enhance their communications, with the inevitable consequences for their capacity to advocate for themselves and enjoy a better quality of life.

Evidence for training models

Current research varies regarding how often staff training is effective. An in-depth review of the literature on staff training would have to result in an answer of 'sometimes' (Ziarnik and Bernstein, 1982). Staff training 'on its own' rarely has any long-term effects on staff behaviour (Cullen, 1987). The ultimate benefit of staff training procedures must be evidenced in positive changes in the lives of people with LD. Many staff trainers are content with evaluating changes in staff practice and views, during and after training exercises, without seeing how these relate to changes in the person with a LD (Cullen, 1988). Staff trainers assess variables such as numbers of training sessions attended or held, and how much the sessions were liked or valued by those attending (Woods and Cullen, 1983). Cullen (1987) pointed out that there will almost certainly be short-term effects on staff behaviour, such as immediate improvements in staff morale, and positive evaluations of the training programme by participants, but there is virtually no reliable evidence that such changes are related to benefits to people with LD. Applying these principles to the field of speech and language therapy, van der Gaag and Dormandy (1993) recommended that teaching is most effective when:

- The techniques used include the ongoing use of feedback: video, verbal and written.
- Management support is secured.
- Training is moulded as closely as possible to the individual staff members.
- Training is practical and straightforward.

Purcell et al. (2000) concluded that effective communication training has four main features:

- It should take place in the work place and be based around situations and contexts within staff's daily work.
- It should focus on clients who staff frequently interact with.
- It should be guided by a more experienced colleague who knows the client and has the opportunity to work alongside staff.
- Communication styles that facilitate clients' communication should be assessed, documented and evaluated and then shared with a wider staff group.

Evidence for combination models

Money (1997) compared three different intervention approaches to service delivery:

- working directly on a one-to-one basis with the person and partner
- working indirectly by providing teaching for partners
- a combination of these two approaches.

Within the direct group there was no statistically significant difference in the number of staff initiations or service user responses after intervention. However, there was a trend for staff to decrease their use of closed questions, and subsequently, a decrease in service user yes/no responses and an increase of single-element responses. There was statistically significant increased use of modalities for both staff and service users.

Within the teaching group, as with the direct group, there was no statistical significance post-intervention, in the amount of staff initiations, or service user responses. However, there were different trends which reflected the different emphasis of the style of intervention. For example, staff use of statements decreased, but they used more multi-uttered initiations and open questions. The number of yes/no and single-element responses by service users increased, and there was a corresponding decrease in the number of action responses. The teaching group was the only group with no increase in the overall use of modalities by staff. However, there was a statistically significant increase in staff use of formal modalities and an increased use of modalities by service users with a high and significant positive correlation.

Interestingly, the combination group was the only group with statistically significant differences after intervention, in terms of staff initiations, service user responses, and their use of modalities. In the combination group, statistical significance was found for the (a) increased use of open questions by staff; (b) overall increase in the number of responses by service users; (c) increased use of yes/no and action responses; and (d) decreased number of nil responses. Staff significantly increased both their overall use of modalities, and their use of formal modalities. The increased use by service users was also significant, with a significant positive correlation between staff and service user use.

Money (1997) concluded that in order to maximise the communication skills of both person and partner, the two approaches of direct and indirect teaching need to be combined. Jones (2000) described an evaluation of the Somerset Total Communication Approach which found that, despite considerable emphasis on training, staff had not recognised the importance of verbal comprehension. This was supported by Hodgkinson (1998:4) who summarised that although training achieves much in raising awareness of communication, it is necessary to 'combine the best from the consultative model and the less fashionable but nevertheless still valid therapist role.' These findings are supported by recent case studies and research whereby training is a major component of communication intervention, but is individualised and targeted (McLeod et al., 1995; Thurman, 1997; Bradshaw, 1998; Purcell et al., 2000). For successful management models such as the Somerset Total Communication Approach, the role of the SLT has to be a combination of jointly assessing, training, monitoring and supporting.

Recommendations

The main aim of all speech and language therapy models of management is to maximise the communicative competence of a person with LD. This can be achieved by working together with communication partners to develop means, reasons and opportunities for communication for both the staff and carers and for service users. To achieve this, communication must interface with the service users' specific, vocational and residential needs and every attempt must be made towards increasingly integrated models of speech and language therapy management (Calculator, 1988). Van der Gaag (1998) described this as a paradigm shift for both SLTs and staff, away from traditional therapy approaches based on medical models, to an integrated environmental approach based on a social model of disability.

The limited research evidence suggests that speech and language therapy service delivery should be based on an environmental, or ecological, approach, which combines teaching both general and specific skills together with individual work. Comparing the results of the surveys, there has been a shift in speech and language therapy models of management in terms of both areas of intervention and approaches. In order to reflect the social model of communication and the available research, SLTs are predominantly delivering indirect speech and language therapy services, either targeted at individuals or groups, or through teaching. SLTs are working indirectly as a choice, not because of service constraints. In Trent Region, indirect models account for more than 70% of intervention. Almost half of speech and language therapy intervention involves supporting and teaching staff, targeted at individuals or groups. With children the indirect approaches also accounted for the most frequently used management models (57% in special schools; 61% in mainstream schools). Indirect-individual was the most frequently used model across all the children and adult services. It is probably the same pattern across other regions in the UK.

The training model is another indirect management model consistently used across NHS trusts in the UK. This is in spite of varied research findings on the effectiveness of staff training and the huge commitment in terms of cost and time for both SLTs and staff to plan, organise, facilitate, attend and/or provide cover. For training to be effective, the research suggests it has to be practical with the aim of developing specific communication strategies. Specific communication strategies include developing staff's means, reasons and opportunities of communication, in terms of their own language, question styles, using and sharing additional modalities, attending, reducing, pre-empting and providing time. Staff need to understand that communication is a two-way process with both partners having an equal role in making the communication exchange successful. This is a crucial part of breaking the cycle of negativity that colours many communication experiences for service users (van der Gaag, 1998).

Within the current political climate, all speech and language therapy services need to be able to justify their service provision to the purchaser. The need for further evaluation of service delivery, in order to make recommendations for effective management models, is evident. Different models of management have implications for both speech and language therapy practice and training, as well as for the service providers with whom we work. Although the research suggests environmental approaches to developing communication, there is little research evidence to suggest that changing the focus of intervention from the service user to the staff, or carer, will facilitate service user communication. Future research needs to address this deficit and provide objective data which can drive the planning of future speech and language therapy services. There is some evidence that changes in staff communication positively affect service user communication, especially in terms of use of additional modalities. Staff need to demonstrate that they can develop the quality and/or quantity of their interactions, thus providing more opportunities for successful communication by service users. In turn, service users need to demonstrate that they respond to these improvements in staffs' interaction skills, by developing their own communicative competence.

The surveys of management models demonstrate that there is great variation in terms of the areas and styles of intervention delivered by both individual SLTs and NHS trusts. Research into these different models needs to operationally describe the models in detail, evaluate them and publish the outcomes. It needs to be replicable, large scale and generalisable. The communication exchange structure between staff and service users needs further investigation and communication strategies that help or hinder communication need to be identified. Only then will there be a clearer definition of what dimensions contribute to a positive communication environment and/or acceptable skills for a communication partner. It remains to be explored whether staff, managers, speech and language therapy students and graduates are prepared for this paradigm shift to an integrated environmental approach based on a social model of disability.

Such research is however, increasingly difficult within the context of a real world with a gradually increasing staff and service user movement, reflecting positive policies for promoting community presence and choice, with greater opportunities for training and employment. One solution is to encourage more action-research to investigate the effects of small-scale interventions in real-life situations. Action-research is a problem-solving approach that involves the team in a process of identifying problems and possible solutions, implementing the change and evaluating the effects. It combines qualitative and quantitative data, using a combination of research methods, such as case studies, surveys, and longitudinal studies.

Conclusion

In conclusion, there is a variety of models of management that can be considered valid and successful that have evolved from SLTs' local experiences and knowledge. However, until this evidence is available, SLTs working with people with LD will find it difficult to deliver evidence-based practice, and models of management will continue to be based on a consensus of practice.

CHAPTER 4

Early Intervention

SAMUEL ABUDARHAM

Abstract

The concept of early intervention (EI) is not new. However, a fresh and urgent interest in EI is currently palpable in the UK. Though the benefits of EI have always been suspected, they have also been debated. Empirical arguments such as poor methodology, small samples, or inappropriate evaluation techniques have often been the main reasons for the criticism expressed.

In this chapter, a number of issues are discussed. These are the definition of EI, its general and cost-effectiveness and the prerequisites, content and structures of EI programmes. Most studies evaluate progress made by children with learning disability (LD) and the benefits accrued by their parents. However, there is much less focus on children with LD whose parents also have LD and who themselves need specialist help to enable them to help their children. This chapter contains some discussion of this issue.

A case study reflecting many of the issues discussed is presented.

Introduction

In Chapter 2, 'Assessment and Appraisal of Communication Needs', we noted that a number of studies have concluded that the qualitative development of communication in most individuals with LD is developmentally rational. That is to say, such individuals progress through stages of communication development in the same way as individuals without any LD, until they reach their potential for language learning. However, their communication development is likely to be delayed. The amount of delay depends on a number of factors or combination of factors, such as cognitive skills or deficits, environmental factors, the existence or non-existence of sensory deficits and so on. The logical implication of the existence of a developmentally rational progression in communication would, therefore, appear to be that intervention should be based on a developmentally rational approach. The other implication is that if all relevant factors are considered, it is often possible to make predictions about what the next stage in the development of communication might be for any one individual. We return to this issue later in the chapter.

Though the existence of a 'critical period hypothesis' for children without a LD learning language is often fiercely debated (see later in this chapter), its existence for children with LD may be much more doubtful. However, it nevertheless seems logical to hypothesise that if intervention should be developmentally rational, then the earlier the intervention and subsequent learning starts, the more one can capitalise on early developmental experiences and stages. By so doing, those skills which are established earlier in life can be promoted and in turn used as a basis for future 'scaffolding' (Reason, 1993) of further experiences and learning. EI is thus indicated.

As we shall see later in this chapter, the prognosis for children who receive EI has been reported to be better than for those who received 'late' intervention. This should not be surprising, given that it is generally accepted that experiences and opportunities in the early years are crucial for subsequent development and learning. There are many possible reasons for this, not least the positive effects an EI programme may have on the child's family. EI can also pre-empt the development of difficulties in other areas such as non-verbal and verbal (i.e. speech and language) communication, reading or writing, given that knowledge is accumulated incrementally.

EI is now an accepted and well-established strategy in best practice, though research regarding its efficacy is still being conducted. It aims at providing LD clients and their parents or carers with opportunities for maximising learning contingencies such as optimum language learning environments, the early facilitation of language learning related skills and motivation.

Review of the literature

Definition

The term EI can relate to different contexts or client groups. For example, it may apply to starting intervention soon after a client has *acquired* a communication impairment. One can thus refer to EI after a stroke or road traffic accident, for a client who was able to speak well before the accident but then lost the ability to so do. In this chapter, however, EI relates to the process of deciding to commence intervention soon after a LD has been predicted, or identified, and the programme implementation. This diagnosis may even be made at the prenatal stage, for instance when amniocentesis tests have shown that the foetus has Down's syndrome (DS), or any other disorder which will result in a LD. However, a LD may not manifest itself until some years after birth either because early assessment and identification procedures are poor or lacking, or because the LD does not present until later on in the child's development, sometimes because of a progressive disorder. The success of EI therefore depends on many factors, not least on accurate and reliable early assessment and identification (see later in this chapter).

EI itself comprises the provision of services to pre-schoolers and children aged 0–6 years, already attending school, who have or are at risk of having or developing a special need that may affect their development. An EI programme may thus begin at any time between birth and school age, though there are many reasons for it to begin as early as possible. EI services include assessment and identification in hospitals, or school screening and referral services to diagnostic and direct intervention programmes. Such services are not just offered to, or focused on, the children themselves, but also on their families, in an attempt to lessen the adverse effects of the condition. The nature of an EI programme can be remedial or prophylactic (preventative). EI programmes may operate in different settings such as at home, in a centre, hospital, school (e.g. kindergarten or playschool) or combination of these.

Rationale for early intervention

The concept of EI is by no means new. Among pioneers of EI in the UK were Rex Brinkworth, Cliff Cunningham (see for example, Cunningham, 1987), Roy McConkey, Dorothy Jeffree (see for example, McConkey et al., 1979) and their colleagues who worked and researched primarily with children with DS, from the 1970s onwards. But claims about the efficacy of EI programmes were being published even earlier, in the 1960s. The American programmes HeadStart and Portage (Bluma et al., 1976 – the original Portage Early Education package was started 7 years earlier in Wisconsin) were well on their way in the 1970s.

There are four primary reasons for EI:

- to provide support and assistance to the family
- to empower parents
- to enhance the child's development
- to maximise the child's and family's benefit to society.

All these objectives are mutually inclusive. Research has established that human learning and development is most rapid in the pre-school years. If a child is to avoid running the risk of missing an opportunity to learn during a state of maximum readiness, the timing of the intervention becomes particularly crucial. A child may have difficulty learning a particular skill at a time later than the optimum for the learning of that skill. Other factors such as motivation, reasons and opportunities for learning some skills may be missed in later years. Karnes and Lee (1978:1) have noted that 'only through early identification and appropriate programming can children develop their potential'.

EI services have been reported to have a significant impact on the parents and siblings of children with special needs (see later). The feelings of disappointment, social isolation, added stress, frustration and helplessness that a family of a child with special needs (SN) often suffers may, directly and indirectly, have an adverse and sometimes irreparable effect on family relationships, dynamics, and well-being. The incidence of family dysfunction, divorce, suicide (see OERI, 2000) and affective disorders in clients and in members of families with a child with SN has been well documented (see Parker et al., 1987; Bryan, 1998; Burke and Cigno, 2000). Furthermore, a child with SN is more likely to be abused than is a child without SN (see OERI, 2000). A well-planned and well-resourced EI programme can enable parents to develop improved attitudes about themselves and their child. The programme should also better inform parents and family about the nature of the LD, the child's strengths, potential and needs. Parents and family can acquire skills for teaching their child, thereby avoiding frustration and feelings of inadequacy, helplessness and sometimes despair. Managing the child more effectively and successfully, and knowing how best to nourish the environment for the child, may have other benefits such as releasing more time for leisure and employment for the parents and family. If EI is successful, society will also gain maximum benefit. Economic as well as social benefits are more likely to result with the child's enhancement of developmental and educational gains, and decreased dependence upon social institutions. Similarly, the family's increased ability to cope with the presence of a child with SN, and perhaps the child's increased eligibility for employment, may also provide benefits for society.

Despite all this optimistic argument, the question often asked is whether a client with LD is likely to have an inherent ability to benefit from EI. Clearly, one would expect that, all other factors being equal, those with a milder LD should benefit more than those with a more severe LD. It was Lenneberg in the mid-1960s who posited that there was a critical period during normal development when language learning is optimised. His rationale for this was that language learning was significantly determined by biological (or maturational) factors. The critical period for language learning, he suggested, was between 2 years of age and puberty (Lenneberg, 1967). Earlier, Lenneberg et al. (1964) had studied 61 children with DS. They concluded that various aspects of language (e.g. vocabulary, comprehension, expression, early sentences) progressed in a developmentally rational continuum and this progression was thus unaffected by the syndrome. Another finding by Lenneberg was that progression through stages of language was more related to general maturation (e.g. motor and physical development) than to intellectual development. The implication of this was that unless such maturation occurred, there was little point in trying to teach language. When such teaching was initiated, it should follow a developmentally rational format.

Rondal and Edwards (1997:116–17) provided an in-depth review of work published in the last four decades related to the critical period hypothesis. They hypothesise that 'the critical period for language development exhibits *modular characteristics*'. They define modularity as

> the characteristics of an organic system in which constitutive parts, although interacting with each other in several ways, are special purpose devices dedicated to particular tasks.

So, for example, phonology and grammar are both constituent parts of 'language', and they can develop autonomously although there are relationships between them. For example, an individual who is not able to 'produce' an 's' cannot signal the plural form of most English nouns, or a possessive morpheme. Rondal and Edwards refer to a personal communication with Lenneberg (1975) and report on his own conclusions that there are several critical periods (in the 'normally' developing individual) which relate to different aspects of the development of verbal communication. Examples given are the termination (Rondal and Edwards, 1997:129; use the term 'plasticity') of a critical period for phonological development of 6–7 years of age, a critical period for voice setting and control by 2 years of age, and age 10–12 years marking the approximate age for the end of the critical period for acquiring morpho-syntactic skills. Rondal and Edwards (1997) suggested, however, that some learning can continue after the end of the 'critical period' and that rather than a 'sudden drop-off' in learning, a 'marked decline' takes place. They further concluded that it is 'only hard core aspects of the linguistic system, i.e. phonology and morpho-syntax [which] exhibit critical periods' (p. 129). Aspects such as lexical development, pragmatic skills and discursive abilities may continue to develop after age 10–12 years.

The discussion so far relates predominantly to 'normal' development. However, if we are to adhere to the earlier argument that language learning correlates with maturational development, that unless an appropriate maturational level is reached learning a corresponding aspect of language is not possible, and that language learning in most individuals with LD is developmentally rational from the sequential perspective, does all this mean that EI may in some cases yield little or no benefit? Despite Rondal and Edwards' (1997) view about plasticity – a small amount of learning after the critical period for hard-core aspects of language – is there room for pessimism and a feeling of impotence about continuing attempts to teach such skills beyond a certain age? And then, what 'age' are we referring to with regard to the client with LD – 'mental' or 'chronological' age? How do other factors come into play, such as the severity of the LD or the quality of the environment for the stimulation of language development, and how such factors may counteract others or interact with each other, and possibly justify or contra-indicate some elements of EI?

Efficacy of early intervention

There seems to be a general consensus in the recent literature that EI has many advantages. The evidence is not solely related to the client group with LD (see Rosetti and Kile, 1997). Among others, de Graaf (1995) found that EI was effective with children with DS. Spiker and Hopmann (1997:275) also conclude that

> It is generally assumed that EI is beneficial for infants with DS and their families – both in the ways it serves to improve the child's rate of early development and in the opportunities it provides for parents.

The Office of Educational Research and Improvement, US Department of Education (OERI, 2000) claims that

> after nearly 50 years of research, there is evidence, both quantitative (data-based) and qualitative (reports of parents and teachers) that EI increases the developmental and educational gains for the child, improves the functioning of the family, and reaps long-term benefits for society.

It goes on to claim that as a result of EI, it has been shown that a child:

- needs fewer special education and other (re)habilitation services later in life
- does not need to be retained in a grade more frequently
- in some cases, children who have had this intervention are indistinguishable from classmates without LD, years after intervention.

EI has also shown benefits with other client groups. For example, Berrueta-Clement et al. (1984) reported that longitudinal data showed that disadvantaged children who had participated in the Ypsilanti Perry Preschool Project had maintained significant gains at 19 years of age. More commitment to schooling was demonstrated by these children. Furthermore, more of them completed high school and continued to post-secondary programmes and employment than those who did not attend pre-school. Their performance on reading, arithmetic and language achievement tests at all grade levels was higher and the children showed a 50% reduction in the need for special education services throughout their school years. Furthermore, they manifested fewer anti-social or delinquent behaviours outside of school.

The literature reports on the effect of EI on specific targets which may or may not form part of the whole programme. For example, Girolametto (1999) studied the effects of training parents to administer focused stimulation intervention to teach specific target words to their toddlers (age 22–33 months) with expressive vocabulary delays. Slower, less complex and more focused language input from mothers in the experimental group was reported after training. The children in the experimental group were found to use more target words in naturalistic probes and more words in free-play interaction. According to reports from the parents, the children also had larger vocabularies overall. Furthermore, they used more multi-word combinations and early morphemes than children in the control group. On a different targeted skill, Girolametto (2000) confirmed that 'instructional context is an important mediator of teachers' directiveness' and suggests that 'subtypes of directiveness have differential effects on child language output'.

A vast amount of literature is available regarding the efficacy of programmes such as HeadStart (HS) in the USA. Law (1992:156) comments that

> the results from major experiments in the provision of stimulating environments such as the Headstart programmes . . . have been equivocal in some respects.

Advantages of this programme have, however, been reported in several areas. For example, Schweinhart et al. (1993) reported that at-risk children spent 1.3 years less in some form of special education placement. The cost implications of such a result cannot be lost on the reader (see next section). They also found that such children were 25% less likely to be retained a grade. Much of the literature related to the efficacy of HS is not on children with LD. For example, benefits in economically deprived children's cognitive development at the end of the first HS year were reported in over 70 studies (see Devaney et al., 1997). This does not mean, however, that similar benefits do not apply to children with LD, especially since the EI programme includes the development of parental skills and collaboration which are so crucial to the success of their child's development.

Social benefits have also been reported as a result of EI programmes. For example, Schweinhart et al. (1993) found that young women who had experienced a quality EI programme during childhood were one-third less likely to have out-of-wedlock births and 25% less likely to be teen mothers. Similar benefits are reported regarding criminal behaviour, medical conditions, school problems, etc.

The beneficial effects of EI on children are compounded by its positive effects on parents. Abramson and Jarvis (1993) found that parents involved in HS participated in more activities, including transition and comparison kindergartens, than non-HS parents. Plutro (1990) found that HS parents made positive changes in their personal lives, behaviours and attitudes.

In the UK, a programme entitled Sure Start is equivalent to HS. Efficacy research for Sure Start is not as advanced as for HS, which is not surprising as the former was only launched as recently as 1998 in the UK, having been first introduced by the US Department of Defense Education Activity (DoDEA) in 1991 for families living and working at military installations overseas. However, a web search indicates that there is an ever-increasing number of current research activities in the UK aimed at studying the effectiveness of Sure Start. For a large number of SLTs in the UK, their role in Sure Start may seem somewhat nebulous. More SLTs are becoming involved in Sure Start research projects and are identifying a clear role in the approach (see for example Lees et al., 2001; Pickstone, 2001). Pickstone (2001:10–11) was quite clear about the SLT's role. She stated that SLTs are used to working with young children and with parents:

The challenge for therapists recruited to work on Sure Start. . . is to develop models for new service provision.

and

to be clear about the strategic direction of local Sure Start work and the implications for SLT services to children across the age range, as well as to explore.

Pickstone stated that Sure Start managers and SLT planners need to 'review the impact of changes in Sure Start areas and the effect on the current provision'. She believed that SLTs do not have 'a monopoly on knowledge about language in the under threes', and other professionals such as pre-school teachers and health visitors have their own perspectives.

This results in a blurring of roles and a need to define the key areas of knowledge and skill which will bring added value through therapist involvement.

A recent study conducted in Belfast and involving the delivery of an EI programme via video-conferencing was reported by McCullough (2001). As part of the European ATTRACT project, she conducted her Teletherapy intervention programme with four pre-school children with special needs, two with Down's syndrome and one with Cornelia de Lange syndrome who were attending a MENCAP nursery, and one DS child attending mainstream nursery school. The children in the MENCAP nursery received one home-based and one nursery-based 'televisit' per week. The child attending the mainstream nursery school received a weekly home-based 'televisit'. The SLT worked from her clinic and communicated with the children's parent or carers via video-conferencing. The results of the study indicated that

the children in the pilot made significant progress in their communication skills, parents reported increased knowledge and ability in developing their child's communication and the system was reliable and easy to use. (McCullough, 2001:48)

She concluded that 'Teletherapy has been demonstrated to be an effective, reliable and exciting addition to a new era of therapy provision'.

Cost-effectiveness of EI

Recent and current developments in the UK indicate that the awareness of the concept of cost-effectiveness in professions allied to medicine has never been keener, nor more paramount for the survival of their services. No doubt, the devolution of funds to NHS trusts and GPs has forced upon the professions a clear view of the need to ensure that all services must be cost-effective. As the rosy, albeit naive, view that the NHS is a financial bottomless pit becomes a distant memory, the professions are having to learn ways of evidencing that cost-effectiveness which is being constantly audited. The results of such audits are crucial in determining which services receive what levels of the limited NHS funding available, and which may not be funded at all, and possibly closed down. The competition between all the different services within education, social and health services in the UK is palpably heating up. In the USA, however, the issue has been uppermost in the minds of the medical professionals and educators for at least two decades (see Schweinhart and Weikart, 1980; Wood, 1983; McNulty et al., 1983).

Despite the many claims that EI is essential and effective, especially to ensure that the potential of individuals with LDs is maximised, and that if it is not implemented, opportunities to secure this will have been missed, the value of some of the published programmes does not escape debate and criticism. Claims about the success of particular EI programmes, for example, are often tested over too short a period of time and sometimes discarded as a result of inadequacies experienced either in their effectiveness, as indicated by outcome studies, or cost-effectiveness. The effectiveness of EI cannot be measured in the short term, and most studies will show that there are in fact long-term cost savings in EI programmes. Some evaluations are likely to indicate that short-term gains are more costly than traditional service delivery models. This is bound to be the case, when often it takes years to witness substantial progress in some clients with LD. Despite all these considerations, some EI programmes are still being evaluated after a short term.

Claims and counter-claims about the (general and) cost-effectiveness of intervention programmes may be futile if judged by short-term rather than long-term gains. Paradoxically, perhaps, the opposite is sometimes true: short-term gains may sometimes become apparent but not long-term ones. In the UK, Ward (1992, 1994, 1999) studied 122 children, aged 8–21 months, with language delay. These children had been diagnosed in their first year as having language delay, through a screen previously developed by Ward, and had received intervention in the first year of life. Ward (1999) claimed that after intervention, 85% of the 61 matched paired controls showed language delay whereas only 5% of the peers who had received SLT showed a delay. Furthermore, whereas 30%

of the controls had been referred to SLT, none of the experimental group had been referred. Oakenfull et al. (2001) documented their decision to withdraw Ward's EI programme, Ward Infant Language Screening Test Assessment, Acceleration and Remediation (WILSTAAR – Ward, 1992, 1994) from their Early Years Service. Their two-year study (1996–98) revealed early gains with nearly 90% of the 177 children receiving intervention in their first year of life achieving scores on the Receptive and Expressive Emergent Language Scales (REEL – Bzoch and League, 1971) of 85 or above. Oakenfull et al. (2001) claimed, however, that

> an audit demonstrated that we could be effective in producing early gains in infants completing intervention programmes, but in the longer term, the efficiency of the programme was questionable. (p. 138)

More recent research, albeit sometimes with equivocal findings, has been reported by Evans (2001) and Coulter and Gallagher (2001a). However, none of this research has been conducted specifically with children with LD.

Studies in cost-effectiveness can themselves be very costly. The NHS Executive, through its Research and Development Programme Health Technology Assessment, made £5 million available for research in the year 2000. Many of the projects funded are about evaluating cost-effectiveness. One of several criteria necessary for a project to be funded relates to the methodology proposed for costing effectiveness. One needs to ensure that a cost evaluation process is not methodologically flawed, or lacking in validity or reliability. Such projects often require a team comprising researchers in the subject matter, research assistants, experts in other fields (particularly economists), computer software to conduct cost analysis and, not least, a large number of subjects to be studied over a period of time. Other expenses such as accommodation and transport for the subjects also need to be allowed for. The funding required for many cost-effectiveness studies can be in six and even seven figures.

The debate will certainly continue, and an increasing number of both cost-effectiveness and general effectiveness studies will be conducted. Recently (RCSLT, 2001) a report appeared in the Bulletin of the Royal College of Speech and Language Therapists announcing that the UK Department for Education and Employment had 'commissioned a two year development and evaluation project' under the Sure Start programme which would look into improving speech and language development; due to report in the autumn of 2002, the study will be led by an SLT, James Law, of City University, London.

Criteria for the effectiveness of EI programmes

There seem to be few attempts to determine the critical features of effective EI programmes. However, a number of factors can be identified in many of the efficacy studies that report the greatest effectiveness. Among critical features identified in EI approaches are:

- the child's age at the time of intervention
- active parental involvement
- the intensity of the intervention and/or
- the amount of structure of the programme model.

There seems to be a consensus that the earlier the intervention, the more effective it is likely to be. Services in the UK are not always well enough resourced to ensure a speedy and proactive EI response as soon as a child is predicted to be, or identified as, at risk of needing special needs help. And yet, this speedy response may be crucial and could well set the foundation for successful outcomes for both the child and family. The need for intervention at birth, or soon after the diagnosis of a disability or high risk factors, has long been recognised (Cooper, 1981; Garland et al., 1981). The developmental gains are also reported to be greater, as is the reduction of a likelihood of developing problems.

Clearly, the decision to start EI is not just determined by biological, maturational factors. EI should not need to focus solely on a client's communication skills or deficits, but also on their communication and related needs. The needs of parents, family and carers may well be the first and most important focus of attention. Gompertz (1997) joined other authors in advocating that the EI programme may well start before the child is born. Modern medical technology allows antenatal identification of conditions such as DS which will more than likely result in LD, and it is now common for parents to be aware that their child is likely to be born with a disability.

In an ideal situation, relevant members of the team (SLTs included), would have a role to play even at this stage. This role does not seem to be recognised or well understood by the predominantly medical team involved at this stage. However, health visitors can be alerted to the SLT's role. With the increasing openness and education about LD that western society is exposed to, it should be less difficult to confront certain issues and needs and how these can be addressed. It is hard to corroborate the assertion by Gompertz (1997:65) that mothers who have been pre-warned that they will be giving birth to a child with LD, and have subsequently decided to continue the pregnancy, do not 'usually start off with a positive attitude and are ideal candidates for early intervention from birth, or even before birth'. She implies that the situation is less optimistic. The fact is that one can never assume how a mother may react after the birth, whether she knows of the LD before or not. The same applies to the rest of the family. Shock, feelings of social isolation, denial and other affective factors can be experienced at any point.

The SLT needs to be aware of all the potential psychodynamics involved and how these can change over time, and not always in a positive direction. This is illustrated in a case study later in this chapter. Issues such as general development, 'intelligence' and possibly future schooling may initially attract parents' attention. However, partly because a newborn infant is not yet expected to communicate verbally, speech and language development may often not feature highly in the hierarchy of parents' concern, except perhaps in a tokenistic way. Sooner or later, the child's communication development assumes priority. Advising parents as early as possible on what to expect in relation to their child's potential communicative proficiency, the sequence and stages through which the child may progress and what they and others can do to enhance the development of verbal and non-verbal communication, is often the first step in an EI programme. Anxiety is often due to a fear of the unknown. By discussing what may be achieved, the parents' fears and anxieties may be substantially reduced. Persuading parents, family and carers that they are empowered to effect change allows them to take on responsibilities and reduce any sense of inadequacy or impotence. They need to know they are equal members of 'the team', and key figures in their child's development and achievement of his or her true potential. Encouraging them to be 'therapeutic allies' should thus be one of the first aims of the SLT.

Gompertz (1997:67) stated that 'Early speech and language therapy intervention must . . . be viewed as a priority'. From a biological, neurolinguistic viewpoint, it has been established that the brain's plasticity for learning is greatest in the early years. Skills established early on become a base for the development of further skills. However, identifying when the brain is at its optimum state of readiness to acquire a new skill is not always easy. Often, the optimum point is revealed through trial and error. Furthermore, biological readiness is not everything, as has been demonstrated by studies of children deprived of language, social and intellectual stimulation.

Parental involvement in their child's treatment is also paramount. We agree with Gompertz (1997:67) that 'Communication, by definition, cannot only be confined to the child'. Working with parents and family and making appropriate changes in the child's communicative environment is essential, and requires for its success a careful appraisal of many factors such as the child's physical environment, and the parents' and family's attitude to the child and his/her disability. Parents also need to recognise the child's abilities and potential; relationships between family members, and between the child and family members; communication styles between mother and child, family and child, and so on. The results of such assessments and appraisals should indicate how the environment might best be modified. If EI succeeds in helping the child to communicate more effectively, by verbal or non-verbal means, many pressures on the family and on the child can be significantly reduced. Very often challenging behaviours have a genesis in poor communication skills (see Bradshaw, Chapter 9 in this book). The degree of success with which this may be achieved often depends on how realistic any plan for change is, how well it is presented to the child's family, and how receptive the family is to changes which may on occasions require major modifications to their lifestyle, environment or attitudes. If parents and family are encouraged to involve themselves in the planning, such changes often have a great chance of success.

Parents of pre-school children with LD thus need the support and skills necessary to cope with their child's special needs. In an EI programme, objectives of family intervention must include the following.

- The encouragement of parents and members of the immediate family to participate in an EI programme. In order to achieve this, they need to be made aware that the child is educable and probably has more potential than they fear, that this potential cannot be achieved without them, that everyone will benefit if they take an active and interested part in the EI programme, that joint planning will take place and that realistic and achievable objectives and tasks will be set.
- The parents' ability to implement the child's programme at home – to achieve this, parents have to be consulted on their expert knowledge of the child, and together with the members of the team they will learn more about the child, develop appropriate programmes and train to implement them.
- The reduction of stress in order to facilitate the health of the family – this can be achieved through counselling, team effort, confidence and trust building, and demonstrating to the parents and family that not only are they part of the EI team but that everyone works together to maximise the child's potential and the child's and family's well-being. Unrealistic and frequently broken promises to families militate against the achievement of these objectives.

All these factors appear to play an important role in the success of the programme with the child (see for example, Karnes, 1983; Shonkoff and Hauser-Cram, 1987). Abudarham (see Brinkworth and Abudarham, 1984) studied the development of communication in 15 children with DS, aged 3 months to 6 years, over a period of 5 years. An essential feature of the research programme was to train parents as 'research assistants' in collecting relevant data on their children. Very early on in the research, it was noticed that all parents were reporting observations of their children's development which did not appear in their brief, as defined by the research project. It was concluded that having to report their observations between six-weekly sessions made the parents better observers and encouraged interaction between them and their child. Parents also became more curious about their child's development, demanded more information about development and how to enhance it, and offered insights and suggestions regarding ways to deal with their children's communication needs.

An EI programme can only be as good as its appropriateness, its structure and the will and efficacy with which it is co-ordinated and delivered. Successful programmes are reported to be those which are more highly structured (Strain and Odom, 1986; Shonkoff and Hauser-Cram, 1987). Maximum benefits are reported when programmes:

- Clearly specify child and family behaviour objectives – this can only be achieved after discussing a particular approach and its rationale with parents, therapists, carers, or teachers, and opportunities are provided for parents to demonstrate their ability to implement the tasks involved; so often, parents are just 'told' to do a piece of set work at home, sometimes with no *aide memoire* other than brief, unclear (and often rushed) instructions, or at best a written list of bullet points to help them – such strategies are not likely to inspire confidence on the parents nor motivate them to do the task(s).
- Frequently monitor child and family behaviour objectives – if parents know that the next session will start with such monitoring, they will be more inclined to feel they have a responsibility to carry out the tasks at home; the monitoring can also be a feedback session for the parent and an opportunity to evaluate what they have done at home and the outcomes and consider the next step.
- Precisely identify teacher behaviours and activities that are to be used in each lesson – this should be done during and after the planning stage; everyone must know how they can identify that the objective has

been achieved and share the same operational definitions regarding outcomes.

- Utilise task analysis procedures – this can be demonstrated and taught throughout the EI programme, during monitoring and feedback sessions, etc.
- Regularly use child assessment and progress data to modify instruction – this can be achieved by joint collaboration between parents, carers, or teachers, at appropriate intervals, continuous reflection and a preparedness to change a particular task or direction in response to the child's emerging needs or following a decision that something has not worked as expected, is crucial to the success of the programme.

Particularly for children with severe LD, the intensity of the services seems to determine outcomes. Individualising instruction and services to meet a child's needs is also reported to increase effectiveness. This does not necessarily mean one-to-one instruction; rather, group activities are structured to reflect the instructional needs of each child.

We referred earlier to the view that intervention programmes should be based on a developmental framework. Some researchers, however, query whether this is appropriate for all clients with LD. With reference to EI for children with DS, Guralnick (1999:51) acknowledged that a 'general developmental framework can accommodate most empirical findings' and that there is a correspondence between such a framework and EI programmes. He decried the fact, however, that there has not been adequate appreciation for 'specific and to some extent unique developmental patterns exhibited by children with Down's Syndrome'. Such discrepancies are often noted during the implementation of EI programmes. As a consequence, a developmental framework for EI may not work and other (i.e. non-developmentally based) intervention strategies need to be employed. One example of this might be adopting a more functional approach to intervention such as work on relatively advanced pragmatic skills when the client may not have attained communication skills which, on the developmental framework, should have been achieved earlier, e.g. one-word utterances.

In Chapter 2 of this book, we refer to possible feeding difficulties in the LD population. These can occur in adults, particularly those with severe LD, but they are more likely to occur in babies whose articulatory organs may be weak. Though it is not widely documented, babies with LD may be born with structural abnormalities such as a cleft lip or palate. This condition may exacerbate their feeding difficulties. The parents may need help and advice sometimes given by a health visitor from a SLT, (see case study below). The development of feeding patterns is a precursor to the development of speech. EI when feeding is not developing 'normally' is essential, as there are a number of other skills such as chewing which take place at critical periods in the child's development and which may be difficult to remediate later on if they are missed.

An area of work in the management of clients with LD which does not seem to appear often in the literature is the effectiveness of EI for children whose parents themselves have a LD. Feldman (1997:183–84) reviewed 20 papers published on this subject between 1983 and 1994. He concluded that 'a socially valid and effective training technology for parents with mental retardation is evolving'. Primarily behavioural approaches were used in training strategies. He suggested that 'out-of-home training may need to be conducted in a home-like environment to maximise generalisation'. He observed that the performance of parenting skills probably did not improve with increasing knowledge, e.g. of correct verbal responses. Feldman also reported on the outcomes of child-focused intervention projects designed to help parents with LD. He briefly critically discussed the outcomes of the Milwaukee Project initiated in the 1960s (see Garber, 1988). Although the results indicated that a decline in the children's IQ was prevented, 'school achievement scores were not as impressive' (Feldman, 1997:185). Garber et al. (1991) reported, however, that only half of the children in the control group needed to repeat a grade or required extra assistance. The numbers involved were small: 10 and 5 children in the experimental and control group, respectively. Feldman concluded that the studies he reviewed indicated that mothers' (with IQ of less than 75) positive interactions with their children increased as a result of the direct training of the mothers, and the children's language and cognitive abilities also improved. He did not mention, however, whether the children's progress may have been partly or entirely due to any EI they may have been receiving though he stated that 'it appears that improvements in mother child interactions can occur via parent- *or* child-focused interventions and can be precipitated by either the parents or the child' (p. 185).

Current EI programmes

It is not within the scope of this chapter to discuss EI programmes in detail. However, there are two in particular whose popularity is accelerating in the UK and these will be discussed in some depth. Neither of them is a recent newcomer, as they have both been implemented in the USA for well over a decade. The Hanen Parent Programme (Manolson, 1992) was developed by Ayala Manolson in 1974–77 and the Picture Exchange Communication System (PECS; Bondy and Frost, 1986) was developed in the mid 1980s. Both have attracted an inordinate amount of interest, with courses being popularly attended by SLTs in the UK. Essentially, each programme utilises material and approaches traditionally employed by SLTs for some decades, the only difference being that they are packaged, structured and marketed mainly via training courses. Two other programmes are also discussed briefly.

The Hanen Parent Programme

In the introduction to her book about the programme, Manolson suggested that Hanen focuses on the parent of a child who has 'a limited ability to communicate' (Manolson, 1992:iv). Hanen is an example of a 'naturalistic' or 'transactional' communication approach. The approach aims to teach the parent how to

> overcome . . . barriers to good communication . . . his negative emotions, his perceived lack of power, his scepticism about the benefits of communicating.

Manolson explored some of the reasons why a child may not communicate or wish to communicate. She urged parents to consider these reasons and to reflect on their own reaction to their child's lack of communication, which is often one of taking over, or withdrawing, exerting direct pressure on the child and rejecting the position taken by the child. She believed that 'In trying to break our child's resistance, we usually increase it'. Another reaction as a result of parents' disappointment and frustration with the 'child's limited desire or ability to communicate' is to give up. She warned, however, that if this happens 'not only will we lose, but our child will not have an opportunity to improve his ability to communicate and learn'.

Manolson expressed the view that the Hanen approach is 'counter-intuitive' because it urges parents to do the opposite of what may come naturally when communication breaks down.

> The essence of this approach is to encourage communication by direct action. We go around the child's resistance. Rather than telling him what to do, we let him figure it out . . . make it easier for our child to enjoy the pleasures and benefits of communicating.

From this position, Manolson developed her '3a Way' which incorporates the principles to:

- allow our child to lead
- adapt to 'share the moment'
- add language and experience.

An essential philosophy of Hanen is to make use of naturalistic settings to enable the child to learn language meaningfully. The programme may be used for a number of young client groups. Awcock and Habgood (1998) briefly reported on their work with children with autism or autistic traits. They reported on the positive results regarding the benefits for their children as witnessed by parents, and the benefits experienced by the parents themselves. Wicks (1998) also reported on the use of Hanen (and WILSTAAR – see Ward, 1992) with SN children. More recently in the UK the results of several other studies have been published, though the authors have sometimes acknowledged equivocal outcomes (see Baxendale et al., 2001; Papagna et al., 2001; Coulter and Gallagher, 2001b). Again, most of the studies are about the effect of the EI programme on children who do not have a LD.

There is a relatively large body of published research into the effectiveness of Hanen and other approaches involving parents. Hanen's principal researcher is Dr Luigi Girolametto. He and his colleagues have published extensively (see Girolametto, 1988; Tannock et al., 1992; Girolametto et al., 1996). Results from these studies indicated that compared to mothers in a control group, mothers attending a modified version of the Hanen programme:

- decreased their directiveness and increased their responsiveness as well as their commenting and contingent labelling (related to the child's topic of conversation); these changes were maintained over a period of time
- used target words spontaneously and repetitively during interactions with their child
- used more target words when interacting with their child and used them repetitively
- used fewer words per minute and shorter sentences.

Children in the experimental group demonstrated:

- an increase in their social assertiveness and joint attention when compared with children in the control groups
- a more diverse vocabulary and greater verbal turns, thus reflecting quantitative and qualitative changes in turn-taking as compared to the control groups

- use of significantly more utterances and a higher rate of words per minute
- larger vocabularies and a greater variety of words
- use of more target words in structured and play situations
- that they had learned more words which had not been targeted
- use of more sentences, containing two or more words
- accelerated vocabulary and language development
- use of significantly more utterances
- use of a higher rate of words per minute.

Regarding the interaction between mother and child:

- The interactive episodes between mothers and children in the experimental group lasted longer and occurred more frequently than they had prior to intervention; this change was linked to changes in the mothers' interactive behaviour.
- Changes in the mothers' interactive behaviour and language use were related to significant improvements in their children's language skills.
- There was no change reportedly in the control group's length or duration of interactive episodes (Girolametto et al., 1994).

Changes in length and duration of interactive episodes have implications for the child's future learning of vocabulary. Children's expansion of both receptive and expressive vocabulary can benefit from mothers' labelling during these episodes.

The authors of these studies claim that these results demonstrate unequivocally that the change in both mothers and children was a result of their participation in the Hanen Programme. Several other conclusions may be drawn:

- the importance of early language intervention
- that parents can provide this intervention effectively, when taught how to do so
- the development of later difficulties such as educational/academic problems, social, behavioural, emotional and language disorders.

Given the frequently reported difficulties in persuading some parents to take an active part in their children's speech and language therapy programme, and current demands for service users' and their family's satisfaction, it is important to establish whether parent involvement and user/family satisfaction have been achieved. Girolametto et al. (1993), following a study of 32 Hanen families on their satisfaction, found that parents were highly satisfied with the programme's content and format. They also acknowledged the effectiveness in improving their communication with their children and in maintaining their continued use of programme techniques and strategies.

The Picture Exchange Communication System

PECS originated in the USA over a decade ago and PECS training was introduced in the UK in 1998. It is a behaviourist approach which teaches children with little or no speech and language how to utilise pictures in order to acquire what they want. The publicity material states that

> PECS offers a clearly structured approach to teaching functional communication skills to young children, older pupils and adults with autism and other communication difficulties.

The programme developers, Andrew Bondy and Lori Frost, initially used the programme with autistic children (Bondy and Frost, 1994) and provided a rationale for their approach. They referred to traditional approaches in teaching language, when after capturing a child's attention he/she is rewarded for making sounds, imitating and eventually, blending sounds to make words. Success takes time, and until it is achieved, Bondy and Frost claimed, the child continues to be unable to communicate wishes and needs. They argued that other approaches require prerequisite skills similar to those required with direct speech and language training. Furthermore, the choice of tasks is often dictated by the adult. PECS requires that the wants and needs of the child are determined from the start. Once this is done, one of the two 'trainers' holds an item the child is interested in or wants. The child is not prompted by the adults to select the item. When the child reaches out for the desired item, one trainer physically helps the child to pick up the relevant picture and to place it in the hand of the trainer who has the item. This is immediately followed by a short verbal reference to the item. The process progresses to stages when the child has to use more initiative, and more pictures of the desired items are presented. The pictures are first placed one at a time on a Velcro board, eventually progressing to more than one picture. One of the aims is that when the child wants something, they can choose it from the board, put the picture on an adult's hand and be given the requested item. The child thus needs to initiate the process of communication and does not need to depend on the adult to provide verbal prompts. The programme moves on in similar ways to teach sentences, though the child is still required to hand the pictorially represented 'sentence' to an adult. Making requests and simple comments are also taught using the same approach and the 'sentences' are expanded as the child progresses through each of the programme's 'phases', as are the number of communication functions.

The main claim for the efficacy of the approach came from Bondy and Frost. They claimed that many pre-schoolers using PECS also begin developing speech. The system has been successful with adolescents and adults who have a wide array of communicative, cognitive and physical difficulties. The children's motivation for learning lies in the fact that they can quickly obtain what they want. Despite their criticism that other approaches take a long time, they celebrated the 'large' number of children who have developed speech a *year or two* after starting the programme. They reported that children who use 30–100 pictures often start to speak when handing the picture over to an adult. They acknowledged that the overall communicative and education prognosis is 'strongly' related to a child's overall level of intellectual functioning.

Bondy and Frost stated that learning to implement PECS is relatively easy, and it does not involve expensive material, equipment, staff or parent training, nor comprehensive testing. However, they warned that 'training is effective only within an educational environment that incorporates the full range of strategies associated with applied behaviour analysis and a behaviour management system'.

Portage Early Education Programme

The Portage Early Education Programme, referred to earlier in this chapter, deserves a mention as it is still being used in the USA and the UK (Cameron and White, 1987; see also White and Cameron, 1988). This training programme is aimed at teaching parents to teach their pre-school children. The parent training is supported by Portage teachers who visit homes. They both jointly assess the child in a number of developmental areas, i.e. 'language', 'self help', 'motor skills', 'socialisation' and 'cognitive development'. The programme comprises many specific tasks to aid the parent to help the child through the different stages. One of the criticisms about Portage is that it is almost entirely behaviourist. Gompertz (1997:70) reported that

> Proponents of the 'naturalistic' approach argue that while a behaviourist structure can
> be highly effective in dealing with . . . social behaviours, it does not lend itself to the

development of cognition and communication, which require a more interactive framework.

Swedish Early Language Intervention Programme

The Swedish Early Language Intervention Programme (Johansson, 1994), which can be introduced at birth, uses an augmentative sign system and

> employs a highly controversial auditory bombardment technique, whereby the baby is frequently exposed to the phonological units of sound which make up his or her native language (Gompertz, 1997:71).

Johansson (1994:4) stated that her

> intervention method is based on a theoretical model of speech, language and communication development in which the child's participation during the learning process is seen as fundamental.

The basic training is towards achieving 'performative communication' which she defined as 'the speaker's deliberate, conscious and goal oriented use of communication' (p. 9). Essentially, the programme focuses on very early 'interaction' between adult and child, the development of 'vision' (e.g. eye contact, mutual gaze between adult and child, shared gaze, mutual attention), 'listening' (including auditory stimulation and discrimination), 'motor skills' (including hand function as a communication tool), 'play' (including enabling cognitive skills e.g. cause and effect, object-constancy, relationship of objects) and 'imitation' (e.g. of movements made by the adult). Johansson (1990, 1994) claimed that children with DS perform better after this intervention than with conventional speech and language therapy. However, Gompertz (1997) commented that Johansson did not statistically analyse her results and wonders whether the same results might have been achieved if only one aspect of the programme had been implemented.

Practical issues

A typical EI programme can draw from the discussion presented above. There is, however, no rational reason why one cannot adopt an eclectic approach as there is no guarantee that *all* clients with LD will benefit from solely one approach. In a sense, though not denying that the process is important, Hanen and PECS seem to focus more on the strategies one can use. Such strategies can be employed within other delivery models. For example, Awcock and Habgood (1998) evaluated the effectiveness of the WILSTAAR approach (and the Hanen) but also provided their children with language-rich environments in play groups

> focusing on Hanen principles of language stimulation plus the provision of direct speech and language [therapy] individually and in small groups (p. 504).

In summary, several issues need to be considered when deciding on, and planning an EI programme. In Chapter 2 of this book we discuss a holistic model for assessment. The same applies for intervention. The child's and family's needs have to be assessed. The assessment and appraisal must be conducted jointly so that parents feel free and confident to express their own views and share their 'expert' knowledge about their child with carers, teachers, special educational needs co-ordinators (SENCOs), SLTs and anyone else involved. It is very likely that in the early stages parents will need a lot of moral support and encouragement so that they can cope not only with handling their infant and his or her disabilities but also deal with any social, cultural and religious stigma, isolation, marital and other family conflicts, and so on (see Lambe, 1998). Parents whose first language is not English may experience added difficulties. A bilingual co-worker may be needed to aid the work of the SLT (see Abudarham, 1987, 1998; Mahdani, 1996). Complex management decisions will need to be made, such as whether to use both the parent's first language and English, or whether one should focus on one language only and if so, which language should be adopted as the medium of intervention and which language to encourage. The decision is rarely an easy one and will depend on many factors, not least the severity of the child's LD (see Abudarham, 1987, 1996; Ara and Thompson, 1989).

The ultimate objective of the exercise is to enhance the child's communication skills via verbal or alternative and augmentative strategies. In order to learn, the child needs means, reasons and opportunities (see Money, Chapter 3 in this book). Perhaps reasons and opportunities need to be considered first, and here the child's parents and siblings are likely to be among the main facilitators. They need to feel and see that they have very significant and key roles to play and that they are part of the team. They need to be empowered to achieve through joint discussion and planning and by receiving training to enable them to implement programmes. Strategies such as 'micro-teaching' and 'teach–reteach' used by Abudarham (Brinkworth and Abudarham, 1984), as briefly described in the case study below, may be of benefit not only to parents but also to teachers and SLTs. The environment of the child and family has to be enabling, meaningful and motivating for both. One prerequisite for this is to ensure that work is done in naturalistic settings. Communication must be pleasant, as devoid of stress and frustration to all parties as possible, and rewarding for all, not least the child.

It would not be wise to think that the only objective is to get the child to signal their wishes. Other skills, such as social, pragmatic and cognitive ones, need to be developed. Objectives in an EI programme must relate to the child's subsequent or actual educational needs (e.g. as prescribed by the National Curriculum and the school's own programmes), developments and achievements. In this book, Hurd (Chapter 5) discusses an approach to enhance a client's pre-symbolic and pre-linguistic skills. She and Dobson discuss working with parents in Chapter 8. Grove (Chapter 6) presents a comprehensive review regarding a child's progress from one word to phrase to sentence and how this can be assessed and facilitated. All these issues need to be considered in an EI programme, especially since programmes such as PECS seem to be geared to children with severe or less severe difficulties who may or may not acquire much language. Some children with LD may only have a mild impairment, and the prognosis for their acquisition of verbal, functional adult language may be more promising.

Case study 4.1

In this case study we illustrate the importance of EI, how important it is to contact parents as early as possible and the role the SLT plays in working with the parents to facilitate the development of a number of abilities and skills in the child.

Becky was born with DS and a cleft lip. Her parents were in their twenties and unemployed. Becky was their first child and at first they had found it difficult to accept a 'handicapped' child: 'this was not the child we were expecting so we did not feel we were rejecting her'. Within a fortnight of Becky's birth, the parents were visited by Rex Brinkworth. They were shown a photograph album of many young children born with DS and also photographs of them at different stages of development (infancy to adulthood, in many cases). The parents were given brief life histories of these individuals and their achievements, both educational, and where appropriate, at work. One in particular had learned to type, albeit not at the speed required by an office typist or secretary, but fast enough to allow her to take on some small, part-time paid jobs.

The parents were told that there was no guarantee that their child would achieve all this but that she might have more potential than they had been told by hospital staff. The important thing was that whatever potential Becky had could only be achieved if they and the professionals worked together to help her progress throughout her life, but especially in her early years. A couple of months later the parents agreed to attend a group, once every 6 weeks, for a whole-day session for advice and help by a psychologist who himself had a teenage daughter with DS, and a SLT researching into the development of communication skills in infants with DS (see Brinkworth and Abudarham, 1984).

At the first session, twelve other children aged 3–18 months and their parents were present. After an appropriate amount of time of informal 'getting to know you' activities when they all had an opportunity to relate their experiences, concerns, fears and aspirations, they realised that they had much more in common than having a child with DS. The aims, objectives and nature of the programme were discussed with them. It was mainly a research project which was to last up to 5 years. However, they would be given advice on as many aspects of their child's needs as we were competent to give and they would also be helped with EI. They were advised that team work was crucial and that they were very important members of that team. They would be partners throughout the whole process of assessment and planning of intervention.

Other than advice on developmental norms and how Becky was likely to follow these although she would be delayed, advice on the (reported) development of communication skills in children with DS, and how they could stimulate such development, Becky's parents were also given advice on the difficulties she was experiencing feeding, because of her very hypotonic tongue and cleft lip. This was a major and the most immediate concern for her parents.

At the beginning of every half-day session, Becky's progress since the previous visit was reviewed. The parents were required to inform the SLT in quite a lot of detail how they had implemented the plan, the outcomes, what worked and what did not, and any other issues that the parents wished to raise – some of these were sometimes concerns about matters outside the brief of the project. The SLT recognised the need to allow parents to express their concerns, some of which were personal and marital, others medical. At no time, however, did the SLT overstep his professional brief. At the end of a session, the parents and SLT agreed on a written plan for the next 6 weeks. The psychologist who saw them for the rest of the session did the same and both SLT and psychologist had input into each other's plan.

Both parents attended until a year later when Becky's father started a job. They were both very keen. Following discussion of the last week's progress, objectives for the following week were discussed and set. The SLT demonstrated where necessary, how to achieve the objectives. This was video-taped. The parents were then given the opportunity to repeat the activity, using the strategies they had observed the SLT use or those they felt would work best for Becky. This was also video-recorded, with their consent. Using the techniques of 'teach–reteach' and 'micro-teaching', the recording of the parents' work was then watched by the parents on their own, to avoid any feelings of threat, inadequacy or self-consciousness. Their task was to evaluate their performance and outcome of the session and to suggest how they might have achieved the objectives more rewardingly. The SLT would then join the parents and watch the video of his interaction first. He provided evaluative comments, such as suggesting when an activity could have been achieved more effectively and how. The parents were also invited to make comments, especially as they knew their child better than the SLT did. They were then invited to take part in a similar exercise for their session, but this time sharing their comments with the SLT.

This was a little difficult at first because they were not always aware of how to evaluate the session. However, having witnessed the SLT making comments on how his own session could have been improved, they felt less threatened at commenting on their own session. Immediately after each evaluation, and as a result of discussion on how the session could be improved, the parents incorporated the recommendations in another attempt. This was videoed again for subsequent feedback and evaluation. This is the 'teach–reteach' process. The advantage of such an approach is that not only does feedback to the parents take place within the same session, and is thus fresher in their mind, but they also have an opportunity of trying out new ideas almost immediately and evaluating any gains. There were times when it was necessary to focus on one very small part of the intervention session, either because it represented a complex activity, for example, or because it was essential to refine it as the success of the rest of the activities in the session depended on getting this one right. The particular part would be identified by either the SLT or the parents, watched on the video, discussed, re-planned and re-enacted (i.e. 'micro-teaching'). Again, the activity would be videoed for later review and discussion.

Over the period of the project Becky's parents co-operated all the way, and by the end of the project Becky was able to produce phrases. The parents reported that they had experienced a process of 'demystification' about the needs and potentials of their child. Attending once every 6 weeks allowed them more time to see any progress and raise any issues. The interval between visits and the length of the visit enable us to explore many factors and allow time to help the parents develop observation and intervention skills early on. Travelling time was less than it would have been had they needed to attend once a week. There were also opportunities to meet with other parents of children with DS and share experiences. They reported that by being encouraged to take responsibility for their child's learning, and by being helped to develop appropriate skills, they did not feel impotent and felt empowered to help their child progress. Being able to discuss issues freely helped them understand, place matters in perspective and not fear unduly for Becky's future.

The success of this approach depended very much on an EI policy. EI helped the parents to come to grips with the initial problems, prevented the undue development of negative attitudes towards their child, and provided a network of professional support.

Conclusion

A number of issues regarding EI have been presented and discussed. More empirical work needs to be conducted to establish the existence or true extent of the effectiveness of EI, its intensity, frequency, programme structure and contents, theoretical underpinnings, and so on. EI needs to be implemented as early as possible. If there is only one benefit that EI achieves, it is the partnership which is formed with the parents and family. If the intervention is started as early as possible, much of the frustration, negative attitudes, missed opportunities for the child and family and subsequently society, can be minimised, if not prevented totally. The child's learning potential and the family's well-being and other health benefits can therefore be maximised.

CHAPTER 5

Development of Pre-symbolic and Pre-linguistic Skills

ANGELA HURD

Abstract

Historically, the emphasis for speech and language therapists (SLTs) has been on the precision of the system. However, in recent years there has been a radical shift in work with clients with learning disability (LD), to place more emphasis on the consideration of pragmatic aspects and the need for clients to acquire a means of communication that they can use. This implies that the skills of the interactive partner are crucial in developing and maintaining communicative exchanges. The SLT's more traditional approach in developing communicative competence, that is, the 'means' of communication, is also critical to success. A management plan should therefore include work on comprehension, syntax and semantics.

An effective programme requires the integration of 'form', 'content' and 'use' to ensure that all aspects of the client's communication development are addressed and that areas of mismatch in terms of the client's developmental language and communication profile are identified within this model. Other models such as the 'means, reasons and opportunities' (see Chapter 3 in this book) may be appropriate for looking at functional communication but do not always provide the specificity about language and communication skills also needed when working with this client group. It is also important to ensure that the client is given the best possible chance of developing functional and meaningful communication.

In this chapter we explore how successful communication can be developed with children and adults with LD before there is 'any true verbal understanding' (Cooper et al., 1978:32). We discuss the importance of having small, graded objectives for learning as well as a facilitatory environment. How communication develops before first words has been extensively researched. Some of this body of knowledge is discussed in order to help SLTs starting work with pre-verbal clients with LD to identify the starting point and to maximise learning opportunities for the client.

Early communication development using the 'form', 'content' and 'use' model is also discussed. Pre-verbal communication is broken down into five stages to allow adequate focus to be placed on the objectives within each, and also to look at stage-appropriate activities. Interactions are considered within each stage to facilitate integration of all areas of communication.

Introduction

Work with children and adults with LD is in its infancy. Within this client group, it is only relatively recently that people with profound and multiple learning disabilities (PMLD) have been given equal access to appropriate services. There still remains a large amount of discrimination and a belief that there is little the SLT can offer. This has been particularly prevalent in adult services such as day centres and institutional settings. However, as carers are becoming more aware of the needs of this client group, and an increasing number of people take an active part in using local community facilities, so the role of the SLT in enhancing and developing communication skills in this client group becomes more recognised and essential.

In contrast to some other client groups, there is relatively little written and little research has been done on how communication skills actually develop in people with PMLD (but see recent works such as Rondal and Edwards, 1997; also Chapter 6, by Grove in this book), and even less on what the SLT should actually do with the client and their environment. Evidence about efficacy of intervention with this client group is in short supply, and studies centred on children have rarely considered the impact of LD and sensory impairments on both the development of communication skills and the outcome of intervention. However, SLTs *are* equipped to deal with this client group. They have skills in observation and behavioural analysis, and perhaps most importantly, in working and communicating with a range of carers, parents and other professionals who are crucial to facilitating communication throughout the child's or adult's life. There is thus cause for optimism. This is an exciting and constantly evolving area, and as the world opens up to the client with LD, so the SLT can become part of a much wider set of aims and aspirations than was the case even 10 years ago.

There can be a large number of potential interactors in the daily life of a person at a pre-symbolic level. This can make consistency difficult to obtain and maintain, but it also means that the challenge to the SLT is both stimulating and rewarding. Opening up the world for clients with LD, and being part of the team showing them how they can make an impact on the world around them, perhaps for the first time, is a rewarding experience. As many more people move from long-stay hospitals to smaller, more receptive communication environments, perhaps in group homes, so opportunities arise for the SLT to be instrumental in changing the lives of people who may have become very passive communicators, by facilitating more active communication, where individuals are keen to seek out new experiences and relationships. The needs of both children and adults who are at a pre-linguistic/pre-symbolic stage of communication development need to be considered. These stages relate to the time before clients have a linguistic system for acquiring language at their disposal. The stages pertinent to achieving this are described later in this chapter. Much of what is outlined is relevant to all age groups, because the emphasis is on the developmental stage that the individual has reached in terms of their communication development, rather than their biological or chronological age. 'The key to success is engaging in person appropriate rather than age appropriate behaviour' (Evans, 2000:7).

Very relevant to this client group is a range of issues that face SLTs working in the area, such as the role of carers. Some practical suggestions for direct work with clients, including the use of objects of reference and sensory stimulation, are discussed later.

Review of the literature

'Communication as a process, an experience and a strategy is pivotal to the inclusion of people with severe disabilities' (Butterfield et al., 1995:7). This statement marks a shift both in society's view of communication and about people with LD that has predominated over the last twenty years or so. The emphasis, as demonstrated in this chapter, shows the move to functional communication, enhancement of pragmatic skills, generalisation of learned skills and considering partners' skills as vital to the interaction. However, as mentioned earlier, writing an effective programme also involves focusing on the 'form', 'content' and 'use' paradigm of communication. This is because we also need to be specific and have detailed, quantified and measurable objectives rather than general statements about enhancing communication skills. The 'form', 'content' and 'use' model can be used to achieve this by ensuring that the SLT is much more analytical and focused on identifying the precise level of breakdown within each area or stage, and then addressing each skill objectively. Despite the fact that this model is predominantly a linguistic one, Hurd (1991) has been able to employ it to assess and plan intervention at a pre-linguistic stage (see below). In addition, in this model, it is also possible to identify clients who are progressing well in the areas of 'content' and 'form' but need much more focused work on promoting their skills of language 'use'. In the absence of specific and quantified objectives, which this model can help the SLT to identify, it can be difficult to demonstrate progress with this client group. Unless SLTs are much more precise in the way they operationally define intervention variables and learning outcomes or objectives, then their claims about the efficacy of their intervention can be called into question, particularly by other professionals and carers.

In early development, it is vital that equal emphasis is placed on each area of communication development, e.g. use of the senses, imitation skills, etc. In the 1970s for example, speech and language programmes were criticised for placing 'over emphasis on the precision with which a system is used, at the expense of the function or purpose of the communicative attempt' (Butterfield et al., 1995:7). However, it is also possible that the consequent shift from direct work with the client to indirect therapy with the carers (van der Gaag and Dormandy, 1993; see also Chapter 3 in this book) has placed unequal emphasis on other aspects, e.g. work on modifying the environment only. Perhaps the pendulum has swung too far the other way, or else a combined approach would be preferable.

Two approaches have traditionally been used with clients with LD. The first is generally directed at children and involves teaching pre-symbolic skills before moving on to a more symbolic communication approach. The second begins with symbolic communication and is essentially more behaviourist (i.e. stimulus–response) than cognitive in focus. There is wide disagreement about whether a behaviourist or a cognitive approach is more effective. Owens and Rogerson (1988) found that there is agreement in the literature regarding the need for functionality, in relation to a client's needs, in any programme. They state that:

- language training should be functional
- trainers are crucial
- the developmental approach needs to be considered.

Owings (1985) went as far as to say that, despite obvious differences, there is reason to believe that pre-symbolic and pre-verbal behaviours of adults with severe to profound retardation follow a sequence of development similar to that of infants without LD. In recent years, there has been considerable interest in how communication develops before single words in children without LD. However, there is a paucity of literature on what SLTs and teachers can do to enhance communication skills in people with LD, and who often have additional sensory disabilities. For the SLT new to the area, findings such as those reported by Leeming et al. (1979:32), who identified 26.5% of pupils with severe LD and who were not at the stage of imitating single words, can often be a daunting situation. However, as suggested earlier, SLTs do have knowledge and skills to bring to this client group and do not need to feel any sense of inadequacy in formulating intervention programmes for clients with LD. As in other areas of work with young children generally, for example, a developmental perspective may be considered appropriate. In the past some SLTs were equally fazed when faced with adults with LD, especially those at a pre-symbolic level, and many shied away from working with these adults. Broadly speaking, a developmental approach can be considered appropriate, thus enabling adults to benefit from SLT services. Fortunately, there has been considerable progress from the time when SLTs placed children on review until they reached prescribed levels of attention/listening and symbolic play. There has been a thrust to capitalise on this crucial early time through early intervention (see Chapter 4 in this book), and enhance the development of communication as much as possible.

Owens and Rogerson (1988:190) pointed out that

> The population with severe to profound retardation is a heterogeneous group of individuals, as varied as the general population that it mirrors.

This makes functional communication even more of a challenge, particularly because a large proportion of the population with LD live in institutional settings. Some studies have shown that the nature of the environment (e.g. how supportive, stimulating and facilitatory it is) is crucial for the development of communication. When daily routines are predictable 'there is little need to make decisions, to ask questions, to comment' (Owens and Rogerson, 1988:191). In order to develop their communication skills further, and also to see that they have an influence over the environment, clients need a supportive context. For example, Owens and Rogerson (1988:191) summarised the needs of pre-symbolic adults as being:

- a responsive communication environment
- an initial communication system for reliably expressing individuals' intentions

- a generalisable communication system suitable for the communication environment of each individual
- a more conventional sign or symbol system.

When planning intervention, the difficulty is knowing which specific area to select, especially at the start of an intervention programme. It is not clear from the literature which skills are essential for an adult with severe learning disability (SLD), for example. Kahn (1982) found that cognitive work was essential for a good outcome and he particularly identified 'cause and effect' (the outcome of a particular behaviour) and 'object permanence' (the cognitive awareness that objects and people exist even when out of sight) as learning objectives for adults with profound learning difficulties (PLD). One essential criterion for successful intervention is an analytical approach to the communication skills of the individual.

Three main stages have been described in the literature, and these are referred to in different ways by different authors.

- The first can be described as *pre-intentional*, where it is up to the client's partner to assign communicative intent. This, in the view of Bates et al. (1979), is described as the 'pre-locutionary' stage.
- The second main stage is *intentional communication*, where the client's partner reads the intent that the client is trying to express and responds accordingly. In Bates et al.'s (1979) frame of reference this is called the 'illocutionary' stage.
- The third is *symbolic*, where conventional symbolic communication systems are used. Bates et al. (1979) refer to this as the 'per-locutionary' stage; it is the point at which single words or signs are used by the client.

Coupe O'Kane and Goldbart (2000) divided language learning into six stages, but otherwise their work has many similarities to that of Bates et al. (1979). Their framework describes the transition from communication development to the interrelated development of speech and language (for further detail, see Coupe O'Kane and Goldbart, 2000). The stages briefly span the 'pre-intentional reflexive' to the 'development of intentional/referential communication' where single words are being used for a variety of purposes. At the pre-intentional reflexive stage, for example, reflexes such as crying communicate the behavioural and affective status to an observer. At this stage, the child who manifests this reflex is not able to communicate intentionally and it is up to the caregiver to interpret (or misinterpret) the child's response. The onus for interpretation thus rests with the caregivers and depends on their observation skills and sensitivity to the child's behaviour.

It is therefore important that appraisal identifies the linguistic stage at which the child is functioning. This enables intervention to be targeted at the appropriate level. However, it is also important to note that these stages refer to the normally developing child and it is important to take into account, for example, the sensory abilities that clients with LD have and their potential implications for learning language and communication skills.

In order to devise a programme containing specific objectives, it is important to consider all available models of language and communication development and profile language skills appropriately (see Chapter 2 in this book). There are a number of assessments currently available, such as Assessing Communication Together (Bradley, 1991b), which look at the earlier steps in the development of language and communication skills. The Affective Communication Assessment (Coupe O'Kane and Goldbart, 2000) is also a useful tool, as is the Caller Azuza H form designed for the assessment of deaf, blind and multi-sensory impaired children (Stillman and Battle, 1985). However, detailed observation is also critical. Most of the available published assessments take a developmental approach and some SLTs may feel at times that this approach is artificial and not appropriate for the assessment of functional communication, particularly with adults. However, it must be stressed that a developmental approach can still be used and applied in a 'total communication' environment. Total Communication was described by Jones (2000) as involving all modalities of communication from objects of reference through to signs, symbols, photos and gestures. Only when a detailed profile of the client is obtained (see also Chapter 2 in this book) can we determine exactly what the level of functioning is and what the client's needs are, and these can then become transparent to others such as parents and teachers. This detailed profile is particularly important when answering parents' questions, such as 'when will my child talk?' For some parents, detailing steps and stages allows them to see the range of essential elements that are necessary for 'talking' and helps them to focus on goals that are both realistic and achievable, while remaining motivated. It also enables them to understand the broader picture of communication and its development. For the carers of an adult with LD who is first beginning to respond with predictable patterns of behaviour, it can be difficult to see that they have a crucial role in developing consistency, perhaps through response to gesture or facial expression. It is even more difficult for some carers to recognise that their responses are important for the development of more advanced communication skills across all modalities, particularly when the focus may be on 'when can John tell us when he needs the toilet?'

There is some debate about what intervention should actually focus on. Beukelman and Mirenda (1998) noted 'attention seeking', 'acceptance' and 'rejection' as the initial focus for the SLT's intervention programme. For example, the client first needs to know how to gain the attention of people in the environment. This is very important in initiating interaction with others, and provides the foundation stone for building further communication skills. These areas outlined by Beukelman and Mirenda (1998) are more functional in focus than those outlined by Haring and Bricker (1976) who felt that intervention should focus on development of communication skills from a more developmental perspective. They recommended a methodology for working through the early stages of language and communication development. They pointed out that the developmental model has three important principal tenets:

- development or change follows a developmental hierarchy
- behaviour change goes from simple to complex
- complex behaviour results from co-ordination or modification of simpler responses.

It is then down to the analytical skills of the SLT, based on a sound knowledge of normal development, to determine the specifics of the intervention programme. These will be addressed in more detail later in this chapter.

Research has found that 'linguistic input in joint attentional focus facilitates noun acquisition' (Yoder et al., 1998:47), so the 'social responsiveness' of the communicative partner is influential in the development of language and communication. The debate about which methodology is most effective for clients at the pre-verbal level is reviewed by Kaiser (1993) and Kaiser et al. (1992, 1997a,b). They considered the role of incidental and milieu teaching in developing functional communication.

During the development of communication, adults or competent communicators often respond to behaviours that they consider communicative, but which technically are still considered unintentional. However, these behaviours (i.e. actions involving toys, or gazing towards people or objects) are very important. The response from the competent communicator is generally immediate.

Two different types of adult responsiveness have been identified:

- *Non-linguistic contingent responses* – here the behaviour is acknowledged predominantly through imitation or commenting; this behaviour, which essentially consists of 'allow your child to lead' (Manolson, 1992:9), builds 'joint attention'.
- *Linguistic contingent responses* – this generally involves talking about the focus of interest using key word labels. The principles of 'motherese' apply here; for example, the use of pitch, exaggeration, employing a slower rate of delivery but with enhanced rhythmic features, keeping sentences short and simple, exaggerating the use of volume, highlighting key words.

In addition, gestures can be used or objects of reference added to the caregiver's verbal communication.

The role of the senses in learning

Before 'normally' developing children achieve their 'first words' (see Chapter 6 in this book), they are already skilled communicators. The acquisition of many skills is dependent on the development and use of the senses. Input modalities at the pre-linguistic/pre-symbolic stage include hearing/auditory, visual, smell/olfactory, taste, touch (tactile, kinaesthetic/proprioceptive/vestibular), and it is vital that these are considered in programmes for clients at the earliest stages of communication development. These fundamental skills are then built on, or 'scaffolded', and extended in subsequent stages (Rosen, 1997) and continue to be important input channels for learning throughout the client's life.

The proprioceptive sense

This sense allows us to understand our body and its movement and position in space. For clients with limited movement, these experiences need to be provided by people around them and to be further developed through work aiming at sensory integration, which will in turn enable clients to build a complete picture of information about their sense of position, movement and orientation. Activities can include swinging (e.g. in a hammock), swimming, horse riding, 'crawling' with help, or use of equipment such as a resonance board, ball pool, softly inflated airbed, or toys to move on, e.g. rockers, physiotherapy ball.

The tactile sense

Feeling and touching is vital for learning language content. It helps in the development of an understanding of the world around us. For children with sensory impairments, these experiences are particularly crucial and are often part of the normal child's 'incidental' learning experience. The opportunity for incidental learning, i.e. 'passive' learning in everyday situations, is very restricted for the child with multi-sensory impairment. For children with sensory impairment, who may also have additional motor difficulties, tactile and other sensory experiences need to be deliberately provided by adults around them. This requires caregivers to adjust their interaction styles and provide appropriate opportunities for the client. For example, the adults need to take toys to the child that encourage the development of exploratory play – the opportunity to touch and feel a range of textures. It may also be necessary to help the child reach out and touch the items by giving physical support and assistance. For normal children, this happens almost by accident, as they learn to reach out and move around their environment.

Tactile experiences can be divided into five areas:

- Use of touch by adults introducing themselves to clients with LD (e.g. bracelet, watch), establishing a personal symbol that allows the client a consistent cue for that particular adult.
- Providing a tactile detection of sound for the client, e.g. allowing the client to feel the beat or rhythm by, say, drumming while they are lying on a resonance board, or feeling the vibrations from a loudspeaker, vacuum cleaner, etc.
- Enabling tactile detection of speech by encouraging clients to feel their own larynx and also the adult's.
- Employing tactile signs as communication. In this case, consistency between interactors is vital; often a number of different people are involved with clients but it is essential to ensure that everyone uses the same sign for the same referent: for example, clapping the client's hands together means time for a play activity.
- Using tactile objects as clues to events. Objects of reference (i.e. objects used for communication – see Ockelford, 1994) can be introduced to the pre-verbal communicator initially to help them anticipate events; these objects may be crucial for enabling the client to communicate with the environment. This issue is discussed later in the chapter.

Smell and taste

The role of smell is important. It is often the least emphasised sense, but it can be a crucial input for the person with multi-sensory impairments. Certain smells will elicit aversive reactions and this can help carers and others recognise a client's 'like'/'don't like' response. Such responses may be in the form of a particular vocalisation, facial expression, or movement. Smell can also be used to signal different environments around the house, e.g. by the use of different (but consistent) cleaning fluids and air fresheners. Much of what we learn about smell and taste comes from our experience with food. For most people, eating and drinking are highly rewarding and motivating experiences. Communication at mealtimes, or around food-tasting sessions, is vitally important, and choice is particularly necessary because if mealtime communication is not sensitively handled it is very easy to develop feeding problems that can last a lifetime. Being fed can feel quite threatening and invasive. Mealtimes should be seen as central to the communication curriculum because food can be particularly motivating and there are multiple opportunities for practice throughout the day. For some multi-sensory impaired children and adults, on the other hand, mealtime experiences may often be very frightening and demotivating. It is vital that clients are never forced to eat or drink, and are never rushed. Smell and taste can be used in the general intervention programme, but it is very important that associations are positive.

Vision

Very few clients with LD have no vision at all. It is vital that vision is stimulated, however, and that the SLT's intervention programme emphasises learning to use vision, especially for functional purposes. This is very much the role of the SLT, and developing use of vision can be achieved in a variety of ways. As a starting point, we need to know how the client uses vision functionally and in a variety of settings, rather than conducting a scientific analysis in a vacuum regardless of functional use. It is important to determine the type of visual impairment, e.g. whether it is central, peripheral, or a combination of both. Clients with peripheral visual lesions particularly can be encouraged to use their vision more if a few simple strategies are employed:

- providing materials with regular markings or consistent patterns
- placing items against a contrasting coloured background, e.g. red doors against white walls in the general environment; orange toys in front of a black background.

With central lesions, perception is more important than visual acuity, and clients with what appears to be severe damage can in fact often demonstrate a good ability to take in visual information (Hyvärinen, 1995). Equally, people with a hemiplegia may well present visual inattention on one side, and the SLT may need to work to help the client learn to scan visually and to develop awareness on the blind side. Intensive work may be necessary to encourage midline looking.

Occulomotor function is essential for tracking, and it is possible to stimulate occulomotor function and facilitate development through smell and taste. Training in visual tracking skills should begin with the visual tracking direction the client already has. In the absence of this, work on horizontal tracking first is essential, followed by vertical tracking, as this follows the normal developmental pattern. In addition, when presenting items, the visual field is important. Visual attention work needs to come first, however, because the client needs initially to look at an object that is introduced into their visual field and be aware that it is there before developing distance-related visual skills, for example watching people as they move around the room.

Any form of visual stimulation needs to be well structured, otherwise it may present just as visual 'noise' to a client. Too much information bombarding the client can be chaotic, and can be so disturbing and distressing that the client may avoid using vision at all. One of the major developments of early visual use is the focus on developing early scanning skills. Alternating glance, between two visually presented objects, slowly at first, provides the starting point for 'choice making'. Unless clients can scan, it is difficult for them to communicate preferences.

Hearing and listening

It is also important to work on developing listening skills and functional use of hearing. Learning to listen is something that all of us develop through experience and practice. The same is true for children with hearing impairments. Again, functional use, i.e. making sense of what we hear and doing something with that knowledge, can be quite different from what a formal audiogram might suggest. When we learn to use hearing, it is reinforced by the visual sense. Thus, when someone comes into a room, we turn to the sound of the door opening. For a child with additional visual impairments, responses may be quite different, as this visual reinforcement does not exist. Skilled observers will be looking for a stilling to hearing sound, for example, as a sign that the child is aware of the sound and is displaying early listening skills. Some children may respond by a whole body movement, or change in behaviour, rather than an active turn by the client to look at the sound source. When developing programmes to work on hearing, it is important to remember that the client may not turn towards a sound for signal localisation, but this does not necessarily mean that localisation is not happening.

In general, a key route for learning is through all of these sensory modalities. They are thus vital for early development and for laying the foundations for future development.

It is important to acknowledge that few clients with LD are either completely deaf or completely blind. Children and adults with PMLD may appear to be deaf or blind, but they may in fact be severely delayed in learning how to process, interpret and respond to the sensory information they are receiving.

The influence of cognition

There are basic steps in cognitive growth that need to be developed. This includes development of the object concept, i.e. knowing what objects are all about (see Gratch 1979 for more details concerning development and levels of analysis), particularly object constancy (Bee, 1981), object permanence (Piaget, 1973), spatial relationships, information about how things are organised in the world, vocal and gestural imitation, means–end causality, purposeful problem solving and play (Dunst, 1978, 1981). All this early cognitive learning about the environment is not discrete but is primarily learned through play and links with other developmental areas.

Play

Play skills are vital for language learning. Learning about the world and learning about self in space is essential. Thus, through play behaviours, clients are working on a range of cognitive skills. Early exploratory play actions – for example, touching, feeling and mouthing – also aid the development of object knowledge. For visually impaired children, the tactile sense may be the primary means of exploring and learning about the world around them. It may also be important to bring exploratory experiences to the child. Mouthing may also continue throughout life as the first exploratory behaviour for a visually impaired client presented with a new object. To the trained observer, watching play can provide an insight into what children actually know about objects and events around them. Play can be used as an excellent medium for intervention. Theoretical knowledge about play has been largely influenced by Piaget. In his view, play was essentially 'a happy display of known actions' (Piaget, 1963:93). Piaget's original notion has been modified by later researchers who see play as a means for acquiring new knowledge. Thus, Lifter and Bloom (1998) proposed a new definition of play:

> the expression of intentional states . . . the representations in consciousness constructed from what young children know about, and are learning about, from ongoing events . . . and consists of spontaneous naturally occurring activities with objects that engage attention and interest.

Caregivers may be involved in facilitating this process and, as the child develops, their role as teachers demonstrating new possibilities and experiences becomes increasingly important in expanding the child's world.

From Lifter and Bloom's definition, the link is made that

> both play and language are expressions of the contents of the mind, interventions that contribute to developments in play also may contribute to developments in language. (Lifter and Bloom, 1998:164)

These intentional play behaviours include elements of communication using gesture. Gesture in play can include activities such as showing and giving in order to involve someone else in the play process. In the pre-speech phase, play activities involving 'separating' (e.g. taking things apart) dominate. The next step is when basic relationships between objects in real life are reinvented, e.g. children act out things that they have experienced directly, and constructing dominates, again involving putting objects together in ways that they have learned either through direct experience or observation and imitation. As they are learning about the world, learners also have more opportunities for practice. For most children, play is effortless, or appears to be so. However, for children with developmental disabilities, this learning about the world through play is not easy (Fewell and Kaminski, 1988). In teaching, however, it is important to note that new actions can be taught. Vygotsky (1978) extensively addressed the 'zone of proximal development', i.e. how more able interactors could lead and support the client to the next stage of development and learning. With this in mind, it is vital that individuals are taught at a developmentally-appropriate level rather than at an age-appropriate level. This is particularly important to note when working with adults because these clients have sometimes been denied play activities when they are not seen as age appropriate, and yet all of us play and continue to learn new skills through the medium of play.

It can be noted that relating objects to self, e.g. pretending to drink from a cup, which is the first symbolic stage, is particularly important because it demonstrates to the observer that the client is able to reinvent activities that take place in the world, showing the beginnings of symbolic understanding. The learner has, through symbolic play, the opportunity to practise observed actions with objects, i.e. everyday objects that form part of their daily life, for example, pretending to drink from a cup or feed themself with a spoon. These symbolic actions with the objects become elaborated further (i.e. into pretending with other people and other objects giving an adult a pretend drink and then giving a toy, e.g. a teddy, a pretend drink), as language develops involving the verbal understanding and use of single words. Getting to this stage of single-word understanding is complex and difficult because for the client with LD it can represent a very long, challenging and time-consuming learning journey, and requires that the SLT or carer is clear about what they are aiming to achieve. Careful and accurate gradations of stages for the development of play and communication are the starting point for breaking down tasks and teaching specific objectives where there is evidence of attention to the context.

The role of parents and carers

When working with pre-linguistic young clients, parents and carers need to know the reasons for what needs to be taught because only by understanding why something is important do people feel a sense of ownership for the outcome. This is essential for motivating the carers and sustaining their commitment to maximising communication development in the client. They need to be told what to teach, ideally work in partnership with the SLT (see Chapter 8 in this book), and be shown which skills need to be taught and how to develop these in their children. It then becomes rewarding for them to follow a developmental curriculum and be continuously making progress, no matter how small the steps. Burford (1989:190) pointed out that 'the basic emotional communication is similar to that observed between non-handicapped infants and their primary care givers'. Although the needs of adults with LD are often different, the role of the caregiver is just as vital. A caregiver can be anyone who spends time with the individual client and thus has the opportunity for developing specific skills and interacting in natural environments.

Involving the parents and carers in the SLT intervention programme starts with the initial assessment process when the SLT has the first contact with the family, and is crucial for the development of 'ownership' (Beukelman and Mirenda, 1998). This ownership is important for later decision-making and intervention choices and also for finding out more about the individual client. Using caregivers to help with the assessment process also increases efficiency. A number of studies (Bricker and Squires, 1989; Dale, 1991) have shown that caregivers often know a great deal about the individual's level of development and they also know about likes and dislikes and so on, which means that more information can be gathered about the client. This information is essential in putting together a 'personal passport' for the client, as discussed further, later in this chapter.

Rosenberg and Robinson (1988) pointed out that in this client group, activity levels, of both children and adults, are often low. There is decreased responsiveness, limited use of initiation and, overall, fewer affective cues and communicative signals. Being involved in the process also helps caregivers understand what their child's strengths and needs are, and also come to terms with the individual's disabilities. Often caregivers of clients with pre-intentional or pre-symbolic communication are under a lot of stress, and having something positive to do can be helpful. Butterfield et al. (1995) detailed the skills of the competent communicator:

- empathy, perception and insight
- constant analysis of his or her own behaviours and those of the client
- taking particular account of behaviour which leads to particularly intense periods of interaction where the client is completely 'engaged' in the interaction
- recording and interpreting behaviours which involve consistent responses from the client
- attempting to interpret consistent responses in a meaningful way
- recording of unsuccessful behaviours.

Carers thus have a varied and extensive role in both assessment and intervention, and this requires the SLT also to adopt a range of roles, for example, counsellor, facilitator, educator and supporter.

The importance of attitude, knowledge and opportunities

The onus for a successful communicative exchange therefore sits firmly with the competent communicator, and requires them to develop an appropriate 'attitude' and 'knowledge' and to generate appropriate 'opportunities' for the client to facilitate pre-linguistic development. Butterfield et al. (1995:8) felt that a successful intervention programme 'is based on the belief that these features are linked'. Attitude has to be the initial focus because if carers do not 'accept that all 'clients' are capable of communicating' then there is no motivation to facilitate communicative behaviours. All too often, the public perception of people with LD, particularly adolescents and adults whose communication is at a pre-linguistic level, is negative. We need to start with the basic premise that all human beings are capable of communicating at some level, however unsophisticated, and by whatever means. The communication observed may be very personal and idiosyncratic to a particular client, but with a positive attitude from the caregiver, the communicative power of the client has been shown to increase (see Butterfield et al., 1995). Butterfield et al. (1995:74) noted that 'partners who have high but realistic expectations will bring out the most in students'. Caregivers also need knowledge of what to look out for, and what is important (Wilcox, 1992). When communication is idiosyncratic, it is possible to miss the communicative attempts that the person with LD is making. For example, a fleeting look at a wanted item may signal a request, yet in the course of a busy day when carers may have a number of other demands on their time, this could be overlooked. Thus, the SLT has a primary role in providing the carers with the information and knowledge that they need to enable carers to become better communication partners. Closely linked to knowledge is the ability to provide appropriate opportunities throughout the day for the client to develop and enhance their communication skills and also to improve the 'quality and quantity of interaction' (Butterfield et al., 1995:8).

What seems to be crucial is the issue of 'critical communicative match'. But how can carers match their interaction unless they know what to look out for? This 'knowing what communication is all about' makes eminent sense, but again means that we must be more specific and consider an appropriate balance. The development of observation skills is vital for parents and caregivers. Understanding another's behaviour requires a high level of analysis and evaluation of the interaction to provide the context for communication on the part of the caregiver. A number of studies have found that teachers, for example, have failed to recognise pre-verbal children's behaviour as communicative. For example, Houghton et al. (1987) found that students initiated communication at the rate of one initiation per minute but these were only responded to 7–15% of the time, whereas students responded to the staff's initiations 99% of the time. Also students used a range of behaviours, primarily body movements, but more attention was paid to verbal behaviour. Successful intervention programmes are often based on approaches where observation skills are critical. For example, the carer is required to identify and interpret potentially communicative behaviours.

SLTs are fond of extolling the values of naturalistic strategies. But for these to work, it is not enough to tell people to 'do it' – they need knowledge of what to do and most importantly, why. Kaiser (1993:190) rightly pointed out that 'natural events occasion and reinforce the behaviour' but people need to know what to do, and when and how to so do. Otherwise, without explicit tasks and feedback indicating that the caregivers' efforts are not being wasted, it becomes a token exercise. Sigafoos et al. (1994:263) found that the 'observational studies repeatedly report missed opportunities for communication where teachers fail to recognise student behaviours as communicative', and this obviously has damaging effects on the client who becomes more and more 'passive' (Calculator and Jorgensen, 1991:208). One approach which focuses on the natural communication context is Intensive Interaction (Nind and Hewett, 1994), but specificity is also important because when considering efficacy there is more to a successful intervention programme than a positive interaction between the client and the caregiver. Schwartz et al. (1989) reported success in training teachers to apply incidental teaching techniques as part of the daily classroom routine, but Mirenda et al. (1990) found that more structured approaches are also necessary and can be complementary to one another. A comprehensive review of a range of instructional strategies can be found in Butterfield et al. (1995). Caregivers often need clear goals to work on, so it is possible to identify and work towards specific objectives. Objectives need to specify the target behaviour carefully, have a criterion for success and ensure that the role of the communication partner is highlighted. For example, when given the cue 'show me what you want', the client will independently look at the wanted item from a choice of two and maintain gaze for five seconds. The carer will then give the client the item.

The two-way nature of communication is essential from the earliest pre-operational level, otherwise it is impossible for the client to see that they can have an impact on the world around them. Through seeing the results of their behaviour, clients are facilitated to develop intentional communication. Clients typically need to learn a range of communicative functions at an intentional level – for example, requesting, rejecting, greeting – before a more formal symbolic system can be used.

Thus, several principles seem to apply to the pre-verbal population. These are:

- develop consistent responses
- watch and listen to any behaviour that could be potentially communicative
- limit the number of care givers so that supportive relationships can be developed
- promote security of attachment.

For children at school, adults attending day centres or any other client with LD living in a care situation, these principles are particularly important because there is potentially a huge number of interactors.

Personal passports

One very valuable tool in deciding what the individual is actually doing may be the creation of a 'personal passport' for the needs of the particular client. For example, if a person moves between a number of settings, or carers, and perhaps goes to respite care where it may be more difficult to build long-term relationships, then it is important to have a comprehensive passport so that no communicative attempts are ruined. A 'personal dictionary' is a similar concept and comprises the client's lexicon and other communication skills. The passport might detail the client's feelings and wants, as well as their individual signals for interest, involvement and response. For example, the following observations about (several) clients' non-verbal behaviour have been noted by their parents:

- 'She flares her nostrils when she's really interested in what's going on.'
- 'He opens and closes his mouth when he wants a drink.'
- 'She lifts her head and clasps her arms together when she wants a cuddle.'

Anything the client does spontaneously to initiate communication is particularly important because these non-verbal behaviours can be used to reinforce the value of communicating, but it is important to ensure everyone acknowledges these communication initiations.

Objects of reference

Using objects for communication (Ockelford, 1994) is becoming increasingly prevalent with the pre-symbolic client group as a tool for supporting spoken language. In the beginning, key events need to be signalled. One should not choose too many items at once. It is also important to think about the words used to pair them with the particular object(s) of reference. For example, holding a 'cup' could signal 'time to go for a drink'. Often, the selection of objects of reference is idiosyncratic to the needs of the client. At this stage, the object needs to be taken by, or with, the client to the activity to make the representation level as concrete as possible. Objects of reference need to be introduced before the client is expected to use them as a means of communication themselves, and there is no reason why signing and objects of reference cannot be introduced at the same time. When considering the different input and output modes to communication from a psycholinguistic perspective, it is not surprising that for some clients the best modality is tactile as a result of their multi-sensory impairment. For clients with visual and hearing impairment, the dominant sense and their main input mode for learning tends to be tactile because it allows them to get the best-quality information from their surroundings.

The tactile sense tends to be particularly favoured as the primary input modality by individuals with a significant visual impairment who have limited responses to light except in conditions where introducing a light source makes it appear more intense, i.e. in a dark room. A number of reasons have been proposed for the success of objects of reference with this client group, one being that objects involve a reduced memory load and are therefore more concrete. However, for some clients, objects of reference are not the answer. For other clients, symbols might be introduced early on (e.g. symbols or pictures of reference as two-dimensional representations). The use of symbols or pictures is more successful with some clients even though it might be argued that cognitively pictures are more symbolically difficult, because they are two-dimensional representations and remain perceptually more constant (see Cooper et al., 1978:54–5).

Similarly, as for spoken language, the client needs to see the objects being used functionally many times to develop meaning for themselves. The objects need to be carefully selected according to the routine and personal needs of the individual. Frequent exposure to the objects or pictures of reference selected is also important. The object chosen must also be meaningful for the client and it must also be sufficiently motivating otherwise, at best, random choice operates (see Cross and Park, 2000) which does not have a communicative function. Despite the number of times parents or carers request that the child knows how to ask for 'toilet', for example, going to the toilet is rarely a motivating experience for the clients. A small cup may be what carers or SLTs might consider appropriate, but the client may not share this choice. It is vital to consider the selection of objects carefully, on the basis of a full analysis of the client's strengths and needs and involving observations from all members of the multi-disciplinary team.

Using objects or pictures of reference can also be problematic for a number of reasons. They get lost, misplaced, damaged or forgotten and are left behind at home, for example, rather than being taken with the client at all times. It is important to keep objects of reference safe and accessible without them getting mixed up with other objects in the environment: for example, a paintbrush which is someone's symbol for painting might get used by another client.

Consistent vocabulary must also be used with objects or pictures of reference. Otherwise, there are multiple possibilities for 'drink', for example, and this can be potentially confusing for the client when the aim is to promote consistency. This can be particularly difficult when there are several carers involved and people refer to things in different ways (e.g. mug or cup).

Overall, it is important to ensure that objects of reference are used continuously, and it is therefore necessary to have multiple sets of objects, or pictures, in all the locations used by the client so that they are never without a communication system. This means that even when the client's bag is left behind at the day centre, carers at home still have a back-up set of identical equipment to use over the weekend.

Case study 5.1

This case study highlights the use of objects of reference and demonstrates the positive impact that their introduction can have for an adult who has not had the opportunity to express his choices or had an impact on his environment in such a structured way before.

John is 28 years old, with severe visual impairment and profound hearing loss. He has recently transferred from a hospital environment to a small group home. Members of staff have been very positive in introducing objects of reference, with a twofold purpose:

- to communicate to John what his day is going to consist of
- to encourage John to make some choices.

Initially, John was extremely passive. He had no real use for communication. He spent many hours rocking in the corner and had little to communicate about. Initially, objects of reference were selected for key events during the day, so rather than things just happening to him and having no idea what or where, John was given an object to represent five different daily living activities. For example, at mealtimes, he was given a spoon to hold, touch and take with him to the dining room. He was also taken along the same route. Even though this was a short distance, he was helped to feel and negotiate his own way around the furniture. Similarly, John had objects of reference for bed, bath, music and shopping (trip out in car). The objects of reference were kept in one box which was labelled for John, and were accessible to him at all times. John is just at the stage of pairing meaning with his objects, and he is beginning to hand over the music object of reference (an empty cassette tape box) to request this activity. He has become more animated, less passive and is beginning to explore objects in the environment. The staff involved, some of whom had moved with him to the new environment, were astounded that he was actually capable of requesting an activity as they felt he was 'not cognitively able enough' to do this before the introduction of objects of reference.

Progress

Progress in terms of the development of language and communication skills with this client group can be slow but change can, however, be demonstrated if the SLT or carer makes skilled and detailed initial observations in a range of settings with a range of people. It may be that the frequency of responses changes, such as when touching is allowed more frequently by a particular person in a particular situation. This ultimately means that informal assessment procedures are very important. In order to monitor progress, observations need to be very specific and objective. The person who is with the client all the time does not always notice change taking place and this can be potentially demotivating. Over the first few stages of the communication development, it is important to take video evidence or photographs to support and monitor change.

The 'form, content and use' model applied to pre-linguistic and pre-symbolic development

As stated earlier, it is essential to identify specific objectives to focus on and develop. For the purposes of clarity, Bloom and Lahey's (1978) 'form', 'content' and 'use' model will be used to illustrate the need to work on all these three aspects in parallel. For 'normal' language skills to develop, all three areas need to be inter-related and balanced.

- *Form* is defined as the shape/sound of messages – including the earliest stages of sound production and imitation; what mode/s of communication is/are used.
- *Content* is 'what individuals talk about or understand in messages' (Bloom and Lahey, 1978:11) – which could be said to include the development of concepts, play at all stages and the steps towards symbolic understanding.
- *Use* focuses on the reasons why individuals speak – this is communication from a pragmatic perspective – how the individual uses communication and how 'content' is used to initiate.

Bloom and Lahey (1978) did not delineate the early steps of communication development of the stages in such detail as Hurd (1991). Such detail has developed from the current author's practical application in the field working with a range of children and adults all described as being pre-verbal or pre-symbolic. Obviously, developmental skills are discrete entities and language and communication do not solely develop in this manner in a straightforward step-by-step manner. This means that there is no one right answer, and a cookbook approach just will not work. However, it is perhaps helpful to divide early communication behaviours into stages within the areas of content, form and use. This may assist the SLT in profiling and understanding the client's range of skills. The Hurd (1991) model, which is based on the principles of form, content and use (Bloom and Lahey, 1978) proposed that before words, at both the receptive and expressive levels, there are five stages through which the child needs to progress (see Hurd, 1991 for full details). The boundaries between the stages are somewhat artificial, as communication development is a continuous process. However, there is a pattern, or trend, within each stage. By considering the stage in which the client is functioning, objectives can be identified and principles for working with clients generally at this stage can be described. This type of approach is most appropriate for the SLT new to the area, but for the more experienced SLT, it provides a format that is easy to understand and can help SLT and carers develop a shared frame of reference for joint working.

Stage 1

The earliest stage of development corresponds to children learning to use their senses. Any degree of sensory impairment can affect the development of language and communication. Furthermore, as stated earlier, a client may have multi-sensory impairments. At this point, we focus primarily on the child responding to external stimuli. Cognitive development, as discussed earlier under the section entitled 'The Influence of Cognition', plays a crucial part throughout the development of communication. For the learner, cognitive development of any type should be a pleasurable activity, so learning should be fun and highly interactive. This remains the case throughout the development of communication and language skills, but for the beginning learner it is perhaps even more crucial to build that initial motivation. For example, being close to a client when engaging in an interaction is very important; this applies to adults as well as children. At this stage, the slightest movement, look or sound from the client, is very important because all the client's behaviours must be viewed as potentially communicative. Long pauses by the client may be expected, giving them time to respond to the communicative partner's communication behaviour. However, it is important at all times that there is close face-to-face gaze because at this stage eye contact and interest in faces in close contact predominates (McGurk, 1979). This also allows the carer to respond more immediately to the client. Progress at this stage may be slow and the behaviours observed idiosyncratic to the client. One particular movement, or facial expression, is not necessarily a better form of communication than another and it is important to take into account the physical status of the individual. For example, a blind child may communicate primarily through body movement. Body movement for this child may be just as valuable as when a child with low muscle tone communicates through eye gaze.

In Stage 1, the aim is for clients to use their senses more fully. Objectives which can be specified further for each client may include:

- fixate on object held 20–25 cm above eyes
- increase or decrease activity level on seeing a visually presented object
- attend to a grand gesture performed by an adult, e.g. arms up
- respond to sound at ear level
- grasp finger when offered
- vocalise in response to speech.

During this stage, the client should be developing first responses to interaction (e.g. looking at the carer) which can be built up to monitoring of imitation skills. During this stage also, strategies used primarily focus on the differentiation of sensory responses, for example presenting objects for the child to look at is the best way of achieving visual fixation.

There is evidence (Fantz, 1963) that about 17.5–20 cm is the best focal distance, but here obviously watching the child's response to the stimuli is critical. Similarly, brightly coloured objects and black and white are better for this purpose than pastel shades. Response to sound, and in general the child's responsiveness, can be shown by an increase or decrease in their behaviour level (Eisenberg, 1976). Building relationships and social consequences of communication are also essential for language use, and response to voice can be established through a range of reinforcing social, tactile and additional verbal behaviours on the part of the interactor.

All of the areas within Stage 1 need to be actively facilitated through appropriate communication contexts. The interactions at this stage need to focus on general essential areas, for example, 'making the response to the behaviour clear and consistent to allow the child to predict in all situations', and 'sensitive phasing of time and rhythm with the adult rewarding responsiveness with social, tactile and auditory behaviour' (see Hurd, 1991:11, for full details).

Stage 2

Within Stage 2, the overall aim is for the client to produce differentiated, potentially communicative behaviours (e.g. making a specific sound to signal pleasure) which can be reinforced by the sensitive caregiver and the competent communicator in the interaction. The use of specific sounds or vocalisations to signal particular emotional states is seen by many researchers as almost vegetative at this stage. However, without these vital behaviours it is difficult to develop communication, in its broadest sense, any further because as with a number of areas of learning, development follows a sequence whereby one set of skills supports and underpins the development of the next step.

Recognising the communicative behaviour that leads to social interaction and joint attention is crucial; joint attention, for example, is fundamental to later language learning because it allows the client and the carer to engage in referential communication, whereby the carer can interpret and enhance the client's interaction with the environment (Adamson and McArthur, 1995). It takes many months for the normally developing child to master the skill, but it seems to be crucial in making the later transition to symbolic understanding. It is also important to recognise the function that any particular behaviour serves for a client. Several areas need to be considered, and at this stage the expression of feelings is vital. This is defined as the expression of happiness, sorrow and/or pleasure and could be represented by a whole body movement and/or a vocalisation. For example, one knows if someone is in pain because they have real tears in their eyes. At other times, there may be a moan but there may not be any tears.

Nind and Hewett (1994) stressed that interaction at this stage should involve the competent communicator responding to sounds as if they are meaningful. The adult also needs to be 'attentive' and 'focused', and should scan 'constantly for signals and feedback' (Nind and Hewett, 1994:64). It is important to focus on the development of turn taking and laying the foundation for the development of imitation skills. Imitation is an essential part of learning throughout our lives and this is, therefore, a very important skill for life-long learning.

Stage 2 objectives may include:

- turning and looking at an object silently introduced into visual field
- mouthing object placed and held in hand
- watching others within visual field
- squealing, screaming or shouting if frustrated.

During this stage, strategies used need to focus on helping the client to integrate the senses. This continues further and to a greater extent into Stage 3. However, these strategies and activities are appropriate and relevant to all of the early stages. Using sensory experiences provides the client with as much information about the environment and their place within it as possible. Interactions may include 'imitation of the sounds produced' as this is a particularly effective way of increasing vocalisation, developing interactions in a 'my turn, your turn' manner to foster vocal production within the context of mutual, reciprocal interactions, rather than under demand conditions.

Stage 3

This stage is characterised by greater exploratory play behaviours, particularly of the immediate environment (Lifter and Bloom, 1989). Here, communication is quite idiosyncratic to the client and the competent adults in the environment need to respond to any and all potentially communicative behaviours. Ware (1996) pointed out that the response needs to be immediate, every time and appropriate. The best teaching environment is the natural communication environment so that the individual can learn the complexities of language and communication and realise that they have an impact on the environment.

Within this stage, the foundations of imitation are further laid down. The focus is on encouraging selective looking and use of vision that has been adequately stimulated previously. It is important that the client has many opportunities to experience this very specialised behaviour because visual input channels are highly important for learning and monitoring the response to one's own communicative behaviour. The focus needs to be on all later forms of imitation, as imitation is a primary means through which we acquire new skills throughout life. Motor imitation is thus vitally important as a starting point because it is important that the client learns the skill of intermodal mapping. Meltzoff and Moore (1991:124) stated that 'imitation reflects a process of active intermodal mapping' in which the client 'uses the equivalences between visually and proprioceptively perceived body transformations as a basis for organising their responses.' It was considered by Meltzoff and Moore (1991) to be a prerequisite for speech, language and communication development and also for the future development of cognitive and social skills. There is a developmental pattern from the newborn's ability to imitate faces to physical/whole body imitation and then vocal imitation. Motor imitation is the first main stage in the skill acquisition process and this is then refined into finer behaviours (e.g. fine motor imitation, vocal imitation, etc.). Imitation is also a social behaviour and although it is more difficult to achieve this skill in the visually impaired child, for example, it is still important to teach imitation skills as a route for subsequent learning. This could be done through using the proprioceptive sense, for example, but it will take longer than in a child who has additional sensory impairments without LD.

Interaction behaviours are also very important because communication is essentially an interactive skill and remains so throughout all of our lives. The focus is on enjoying interaction with other people and signalling likes and dislikes, as these functions enable the client to exert some choice and control over the immediate context. There is also a focus on looking at a wanted object as opposed to looking at a person to get something, marking the shift from a fixed interest in people to bringing objects into their world of experience. Until this point, the person will normally display an intense and predominant interest in the interpersonal realm, such as focusing on people (Wetherby et al., 1998). Moving to objects signals a developmental leap forward.

Objectives in this stage may include:

- rotating objects, examining the various sides
- emptying/tipping out box/container

- imitating cooing sounds
- looking at liked object in midline for 2 seconds to be given it.

At this point, the development of interactional skills needs to highlight the 'adult imitating the child's actions and vice versa to encourage prolonged interactions because feedback and further perceptual matching is thought to be essential to the further development of imitation' and 'the adult providing opportunities for increased initiation and control by the child' again because initiation is seen as critical in the development of functional communication (see Hurd 1991:13, for further details).

During this stage, the shift from self-oriented behaviours more to objects and events near at hand begins (Kaye and Fogel, 1980). Adamson and Bakeman (1997) identified the stage of supported joint engagement. The client's working partner thus needs to take a lot of control of the situation and ensure that a shared attention focus is monitored. Being able to take over control of the communication exchange, and be instrumental in the focus of their language learning, can take the client a considerable time; in the normal child it can take at least 7 months. This major 'take over of control' that is ongoing through Stages 4, 5, and 6, signals the ability to 'penetrate the symbolic realm' (Wetherby et al., 1998:4), where symbols can stand for and represent things and events around the child. This is crucial for the development of language as a symbolic and social behaviour because language development is essentially a symbolic experience and movement into the symbolic stage marks the start of much quicker learning from then on. This also tends to be mirrored by the stage of linguistic as opposed to pre-linguistic development.

Stage 4

This is an appropriate stage during which to attempt to use sign consistently. Natural gesture is important to all of us, but for children with LD signs can be particularly important in building understanding. It is important that the client will tolerate 'hand-over-hand' work for co-active signing. If necessary, desensitisation work should be carried out beforehand. This type of work is often necessary with this client group because there is a high incidence of tactile defensiveness, particularly with clients with additional visual impairments. As with all children without LD, understanding precedes expression, so it is vital that as well as co-active sign work, spoken language used for commenting or narrating is accompanied by sign. Lee and MacWilliam (1995) have adapted signs for multi-sensory impaired children. Their advice includes:

- making a specific contact point for the sign on the body
- using hand-over-hand signs so that the person can feel where the sign is being made and how movement is involved
- ensuring the signer is very close and, if appropriate, within the visual field.

This may initially involve the carer sitting behind the client to provide whole body security. However, hand-over-hand signing is not always appropriate. For some clients, being physically manipulated in this way may be a damaging experience and it is better to build signs through visual or proprioceptive imitation skills, i.e. direct copying of the adult's gesture of 'arms up', to be picked up, rather than working on helping or teaching the client through the necessary movements. It is important to sign key words, and carefully consider and choose the level of vocabulary chosen and the need for consistency. The use of objects of reference, as mentioned earlier, has also been found to be beneficial for individuals at this stage of development, and now is an appropriate time to introduce them.

The driving force within Stage 4 is development of further play skills, problem-solving skills, and helping the client to work out what objects can do in terms of relational play. This enables the development of the essential 'content' which gives clients something to communicate about. It also ensures that their observations about the world are internalised and, thus, the beginnings of inner language start to develop, which is important for the later development of single-word understanding and use. Visual skills and physical exploration are developed further by work in this stage, and there is much more emphasis on the role of objects and pictures in the learning process. Imitation skills are particularly important at this stage as they are becoming more refined and can thus be used to facilitate greater use of sign and vocalisation. Within Stage 4, enabling the client to acquire the concept of 'cause and effect' is important and this does not have to be just between people and objects. Cause and effect toys have long been used by SLTs, but communication aids such as the Echo 4 or Bigmack (see also Chapter 7 in this book) are also very valuable for individuals in developing more intentional communication, i.e. seeing the impact of their communicative attempts and then deliberately repeating the action.

It may be more exciting for an individual to see that when they press the Echo 4 switch their carer jumps up and down, rather than the carer (or client) getting a toy dog to bark. Use of a communication aid of this type also reinforces the link with the communicative behaviour of requesting rather than just focusing on cause and effect as an end in itself. There may, however, be some drawbacks. Electronic equipment can break down and often needs to be transported from one situation to another. Furthermore, everyone involved with the person must be willing to take part.

In fostering language use, natural gesture and facial expression are highlighted as intentional communication is developing. Although the emphasis of the SLT intervention programme at this stage is primarily on basic meanings, these can be expanded to ensure that semantic functions are addressed as part of any intervention programme. There is no problem in having a range of different means of communication. For example, we all use gesture, vocalisation and facial expression: the client, at this stage, is no different. It is important that if, for example, signs and objects of reference have been introduced, the use of natural gesture which is spontaneous on the part of the individual is still encouraged. What is vital is celebrating and capitalising on the fact that the individual can express some aspect of their feelings or wishes and that this is getting more and more consistent.

Objectives within Stage 4 may include:

- pulling a string to obtain an object attached to it
- securing a hidden object by pulling off a cloth
- imitating large facial movements, e.g. opening mouth wide
- lifting arms up to be picked up
- vocalising to draw attention to an object – equivalent to 'look, there it is'.

For example, interactions should focus on:

- pairing vocal and gestural imitation
- encouraging imitation of simple words and social meanings, e.g. 'bye-bye'
- pairing the word with the gesture and engaging in using eye contact to achieve a desired goal, e.g. takes adult to toy or eye points.

Case study 5.2

This case study illustrates the importance of working on a number of areas within an intervention programme in order to facilitate the integration of form, content and use.

Andrew is 18 months old and has been diagnosed as having a cortical visual impairment, moderate hearing loss and severe LD. He is, however, learning how to use his vision and has worked through a programme to encourage sensory use at Stages 1–3. He is using his residual vision to monitor familiar people in the environment and is beginning to look from one object to another. He explores new objects primarily by mouthing and holding and uses some babble sounds and crying to signal emotional states. Andrew is ready to work on a number of activities within Stage 4. He needs to extend his play skills from an exploratory to a relational level, e.g. bang drum, develop cause and effect relationships further and engage in the beginnings of a more formal communication system. Andrew has recently been introduced to co-active signing. The first sign, to be used across all events in a range of situations, is 'MORE'. This was chosen because of its value as a 'request' and also because it has a range of movement within Andrew's physical capabilities. Initially, Andrew was introduced to the sign 'MORE' in play situations. He loves rough and tumble, and 'MORE' was established when bouncing on the bed. After only a few examples of the adult moulding his hands from behind and saying 'MORE' when there was a long pause, Andrew began to bring his hands into the midline. The sign is still being used co-actively in all situations but Andrew is beginning to show active participation and imitation.

Stage 5

At this level, 'use' emphasises the crucial role of the caregiver as the client's development in this stage primarily involves another person. The further fostering of joint attention is essential. A solid foundation is vital for the development of intentional communication as later development of communication is highly dependent on this. Essential for the achievement of intentional communication is the caregiver. What is important in order to avoid a 'cumulative deficit' is introducing early intervention (Hart and Risley, 1995). Hart and Risley (1995) explored the 'cumulative deficit' hypothesis and looked at the number of interactions during the first 3 years of life. They pointed out that at a time when most basic communication and language skills are acquired, it is possible to create an experiential lag that may be virtually impossible to overcome by later intervention efforts. Yoder et al. (1998) further pointed out that, given lower rates of initiation and responsiveness in children with developmental delays, this, added to the difference in quantity and quality of input from caregivers, could add even more significantly to the 'cumulative deficit.' Over a three-year period, there can be an immense difference in the client's opportunities for communication. If progress is to be made, there needs to be a two-pronged strategy:

- teaching carers to be more responsive
- directly teaching the client communicative functions by prompting modelling, providing appropriate consequences, requiring an ongoing analysis of content, form and use and an evaluation of the specific functions displayed within specific contexts.

Objectives within this stage may include:

- waving hand for 'bye bye' in imitation
- wriggling fingers for example on top of an ocean drum, in imitation
- relating cup to self spontaneously and appropriately
- looking at an object a person is pointing at when the object is within 1 metre
- anticipating action in very familiar action rhyme/song.

The need for specificity has been stated, but it is also important to think about the principles behind all language learning: 'The optimal environment for acquiring communication skills is interactive' (Ostrosky et al., 1998:438).

Thus, at this stage, interactions, for example, should focus on:

- consistently using a new word in all contexts
- encouraging symbolic play
- encouraging the client to imitate gestures by gradual approximation.

The success of any intervention programme rests on the expectations and the opportunities for the client that are provided by their communicative partners. The Hurd (1991) approach has been shown to work with all age groups, and with clients with a range of sensory impairments in addition to profound learning disabilities. However, as Warren (1988:295) pointed out, 'context is more important than who is present, when, with what objects and in what environmental setting'. There is also the relationship between the communicative partners, the climate established and the influence of prior learning experiences. Unless we address all these variables, then efficacy of SLT intervention and progress for the client is seriously challenged. The intervention approach rests within a particular model of service delivery and SLTs may need to re-think the types of services offered and their frequency etc. to better fit the needs of the client rather than trying to fit the client into a particular model of service delivery or method of working. The communication needs of the individual are paramount.

Conclusions

Working with clients at a pre-symbolic or pre-linguistic level can be immensely rewarding. The crux of the issue is developing specific behavioural objectives within the context of supportive communication relationships. It is not always easy for carers and other professionals to see the value of speech and language therapy intervention with this client group. There are often a number of preconceptions that need to be overcome to foster positive working relationships for the benefit of the client. It is not uncommon, for example, for this client group to have a low priority in the context of wider service delivery. However, by using their skills of observation, analysis and evaluation, SLTs and carers have an enormous amount to offer. There is also increasing awareness that offering speech and language therapy services needs to be sooner rather than later in an individual's life – we have a considerable amount to offer this client group. Wetherby et al. (1998:6) concluded that 'the provision of early intervention to increasingly younger children has created the impetus to view communication as a multi-modal process' and so SLTs are urged to 'utilise the most efficient communicative means in the context of a wide range of environments.' This is no less the case for adults.

Research in the area is increasing and as theory influences practice so it becomes a more satisfying field in which to work.

CHAPTER 6

From First Words to Phrase and from Phrase to Sentence

NICOLA GROVE

Abstract

This chapter provides an overview of research on the acquisition of sentence structure by typically developing children and by children with learning disabilities (LD) in the modalities of speech, manual sign and graphic representations. In order to move from a purely lexical to a grammatically organised system, the child needs to develop a range of skills, some cognitive (such as working memory and sequencing) and some linguistic. Evidence suggests that the existence of an intellectual impairment *per se* is not necessarily a barrier to the acquisition of language structure, but that specific difficulties may be associated with particular syndromes. Some children have difficulties developing language through speech, and make use of Augmentative and Alternative Communication (AAC). Research suggests that although they may be able to link signs or graphic symbols together, they appear to have problems in mastering syntax. However, they can sometimes make use of their existing resources to create complex meanings through novel combinations or inflections. Issues of assessment and intervention from a multi-modal developmental perspective are considered and a range of approaches to the teaching of sentence structure are discussed. It is concluded that the search for meaning should be the guiding principle in speech and language therapy with children with LD.

Introduction

By the age of 1 year, children have gained the insight that things, people and events in the world can be referred to by name. A small vocabulary of first words rapidly appears. A few months later, children acquire a new insight: that words can be combined to form phrases and then sentences. The best illustration I have ever found to show how word combinations are more than the sum of their parts comes from Tamsin, a young girl with severe LD. I went one day to fetch her from her classroom, and as we left, I said and signed 'Say goodbye to Rick' (her teacher). Tamsin looked at me, waved briefly, and then turned and moved towards Rick. She had understood the meaning of the two individual words in sequence – 'bye-bye' and 'Rick' – but not the meaning created when they were combined within a single utterance.

Review of the literature

In order to understand the problems of acquisition of language structure for children with LD, we need to analyse the differences between single words and word combinations, and to identify the skills involved at each level. This area has been well documented by authors such as McNeill (1970), Fonagy (1972), Nelson (1973), Branigan (1979), Scollon (1979), Anisfield (1984), Greenfield et al. (1985), Bates et al. (1988), Veneziano et al. (1990), Bloom and Capatides (1991), Lieven et al. (1992), Morford and Goldin-Meadow (1992) and Locke (1997).

The main skills appear to involve:

- working memory sufficient to retain a sequence of items
- a productive lexicon of sufficient size to allow for the combination of different items
- a range of meanings expressed through relations between items
- mastery of the linguistic rules involved
- the ability to link two items within one prosodic contour, rather than producing several single words with several contours.

For children with LD, it can be concluded that language development is characterised by late onset, a slower rate of development and lower final levels of achievement, than for their peers matched for chronological age (Rondal and Edwards, 1997). However, this picture is complicated by aetiology. The compounding effects of neurological impairments and/or particular syndromes appear to constrain development in quite specific ways (Bowler and Lister Brook, 1997).

It is equally important to recognise the effects of the environment. Much of the early work on language development in children with LD was carried out with populations for whom expectations were very low, many being institutionalised. More recent work suggests that environmental factors play a significant role in facilitating or inhibiting development in this population (Greenbaum and Auerbach, 1998).

The following review of the literature focuses on specific aspects relevant to the acquisition of language structure by different groups of children with LD.

Sequences

It might be anticipated that cognitive limitations would have some effect on the ability to link words in sequence. Individuals with LD are impaired in their ability to pay attention to, memorise and recall relevant stimuli (Brewer, 1987; Torgesen et al., 1988). General deficits in categorisation, integration and organisation of information seem bound to have an impact on language as well as on other skills (Johansson, 1994). Sequential cognitive processing has been found to be lower than simultaneous processing for individuals with Down's syndrome (DS), Fragile-X and 'non-specific' LD (Hodapp et al., 1992). In addition, neuromotor impairments may make it relatively more difficult for individuals with LD to produce the complex co-ordinated movements which underlie mature sentence construction. There is a growing body of evidence indicating that deficits in working memory may be associated with difficulties in the development of morpho-syntax (Fowler, 1998). However, because word order tends to be preserved by children with a range of LD, there can be no simple equation of sequential processing difficulties and language disorders.

Lexical development

Children with LD seem to develop vocabulary in very similar ways to controls matched for mental age (MA). Researchers have found overwhelming similarities in the processes of acquisition and generalisation of object names (Cardoso-Martin et al., 1985; Fowler et al., 1994; Mervis and Bertrand, 1999). However, receptive and expressive vocabularies are often smaller than would be predicted from MA, and more dominated by concrete, basic category terms (Bellugi et al., 1990a; Tager-Flusberg, 1986).

Children with LD do not seem to experience the same naming insight and consequent lexical expansion as do typically developing children (Barrett and Diniz, 1989; Singer et al., 1994), although this may occur at a later stage (Oliver and Buckley, 1994). Early word combinations appear to express the same underlying semantic relations and ideational complexity as in typically developing children, although again there may be a lag in development (Dooley, 1976; Duchan and Erickson, 1976; Coggins, 1979; Rosenberg and Abbeduto, 1993; Fowler, 1998). Rondal (1985:332) suggested that this is because 'the sensori-motor cognitive knowledge on which the basic semantic structure of language appears to rest is a pre-requisite for the onset of combinatorial speech'. However, lexical delays may have long-term consequences for the activation of the analytical linguistic system (Locke, 1997), given that this seems to be triggered in part by lexical size. Locke (1997) hypothesised that, for some children, by the time the lexicon has increased to the point where storage of individual items becomes impossible, the critical period for grammar has already passed.

Morpho-syntax

Up to a MA of about 20 months, and a mean length of utterance (MLU) level of 3.0, the similarities between individuals with LD and their typically developing peers are more striking than their differences (Tager-Flusberg et al., 1990). After this point, however, divergences occur. As MA increases, language delay becomes more pronounced, particularly in the area of morpho-syntax which develops slowly and remains incomplete for most people with moderate and severe impairments. Studies of children with DS indicate that the characteristic pattern is for grammatical development to plateau at the level of simple sentences, with little evidence of knowledge of complex constructions and the more advanced functional categories of language (Comblain, 1994; Fowler et al., 1994). For example, Comblain found that at MA 3.7, MLU was 2.08.

Tager-Flusberg et al. (1990) and Fowler et al. (1994) reported on the acquisition of two-word combinations by children with DS. For some children, these appeared at around 4 years of age and were followed by a relatively rapid increase in MLU, whereas others, with IQs below 50, progressed at a much slower rate.

Rondal and Edwards (1997) reported in detail on the problems experienced by individuals with LD in both receptive and productive acquisition of grammar. Receptively, understanding of morpho-syntax is more delayed than would be predicted from MA (Bartel et al., 1973; Barblan and Chipman, 1978), and this is particularly marked at MA levels above 5 years (Abbeduto et al., 1989). It is difficult for them to process sentences if the order of clauses is in conflict with the temporal order of events, e.g. 'Mary started dinner after she answered the phone' (Kernan, 1990). Children with DS have particular difficulties with the comprehension of articles, personal pronouns, negative and passive sentences (Rondal and

Edwards, 1997). However, their comprehension strategies appear to be no different from those of young typically developing children. For example, they tend to interpret passive sentences as though they were active and rely on word order as the cue to meaning (Bridges and Smith, 1984; Natsopoulos and Xeromeritou, 1990). Children with DS also appear to be sensitive to the same types of constraints on argument structure as typically developing children, taking longer to act out ungrammatical sentences than grammatical ones (Naigles et al., 1995). Processing difficulties increase when the task involves stretches of discourse, such as narrative (Chapman et al., 1991).

Productively, individuals with moderate and severe LD tend to speak in short simple sentences, with reduced morpho-syntax (Lackner, 1968; Miller et al., 1981). Word order is conventionally expressed, both in early word combinations and in longer sentences (Dooley, 1976; Rosenberg and Abbeduto, 1993). Rondal and Lambert (1983), who analysed the language output of 22 adults with LD, found that only half of their utterances were grammatical clauses.

Morpho-syntax appears to be a particular area of difficulty for individuals with DS. The proportion of function words in their speech (articles, prepositions, pronouns, modals, auxiliaries, copula and conjunctions) is reduced compared to typically developing peers, although performance is variable, and some youngsters may approach the norm in their patterns of use (Rutter and Buckley, 1994). They are more likely to omit morphemes than peers matched on MLU (Bol and Kuiken, 1990; Fowler et al., 1994; Chapman, 1995). It has been hypothesised that the underlying reason for these difficulties is a specific impairment in phonological working memory, which may affect the ability to perceive, take in, store and retrieve morpho-syntactic information (Fowler, 1998). However, morpho-syntax may be spared in individuals with LD. Rondal (1985) provided a detailed report on the case of Françoise, a woman with DS and a global IQ of 65, who developed normal production and understanding of grammatical speech, although she appeared to have some problems at the level of discourse cohesion. Morpho-syntax is also a relative strength for people with Williams' syndrome, whose difficulties lie more in the realm of semantics and pragmatics (Bellugi et al., 1990b). Other exceptional cases have been documented by Curtiss (1988), Yamada (1990) and Smith and Tsimpli (1995), and are suggestive of a dissociation between the computational aspects of language (phonology and morpho-syntax) and the conceptual and social aspects (semantics, lexicon and pragmatics).

In conclusion, research into the development of spoken language suggests that LD *per se* is not a sufficient explanation for delays and difficulties. The early, pre-grammatical stages of language appear very similar to the norm, with MA predicting the emergence of lexical categories and the semantic relations underpinning word combinations. A certain level of sensori-motor cognition seems to be critical in order for the activation of analytic, computational language mechanisms. Rondal and Edwards (1997) suggested that this is about the level of 24 months, which concurs with Locke's (1997) schedule for the shift from a semantic to a structurally based system. As MA and chronological age (CA) increase, delays in both semantic and morpho-syntactic aspects increase compared to typically developing children. Conversely, morpho-syntactic skills may be far higher than MA would predict. However, the evidence suggests that the general pattern is one of delay rather than deviance. Fowler (1998:311) concluded that individuals with LD are systematic in their grammatical knowledge, follow the normal course of development, show a similar order of difficulty, but can usually only cope with limited levels of syntactic complexity.

The pervasive nature of these difficulties in the acquisition of spoken language has led to increasing use of alternative and augmentative (AAC) systems to facilitate the development of language. There is plenty of evidence that individuals with LD can acquire a functional lexicon, used communicatively, through alternative modalities (see for example, Kiernan et al., 1982; Launonen, 1996; Møller and von Tetzchner, 1996). However, the evidence for acquisition of grammatical structure is more equivocal and suggests that the relationship between modality and linguistic competence is highly complex, for both manual sign and graphic symbols.

Language acquisition through manual sign

There are several reports relating to the acquisition of multi-sign combinations in children with LD. They yield a consistent picture suggesting that this stage of language development is problematic. Firstly, relatively few individuals seem to reach this stage. In the survey by Kiernan et al. (1982), only 16% of children using sign were said to use two or more signs per utterance. In a follow-up survey by Grove (1995), only 61 children in 100 schools for pupils with severe learning difficulty (SLD) were reported to regularly combine signs. Bryen et al. (1988) reported on the outcome of sign programmes with 118 individuals and found an average of only 2% of utterances were more than one sign in length. These results do not, however, make it clear whether the individuals concerned are using single signs in conjunction with spoken sentences. More detailed information is available from three studies which examined sign production in children who used sign as a primary means of communication.

Grove and McDougall (1991) studied 49 children, the majority of whom were sign reliant. Thirty of these children produced sign combinations, but MLU ranged from only 1.1–1.5. Many were combinations of signs and points. Udwin and Yule (1990, 1991) studied 14 manual sign users with cerebral palsy over a period of 18 months. At the end of this period, MLU was only 1.6, and only 12% of utterances on average involved more than one term. Grove and Dockrell (2000) analysed structural aspects of language development in 10 multi-signing children with moderate LD. Six children had an MLU in sign of 1.54 (SD = 0.24) and four of the children an MLU of 2.30 (SD = 0.22).

These levels of development correspond to MLU stage I–II (Brown, 1973), reached by typically developing children at approximately 18–24 months. This is well below what would have been predicted from the MAs of the children concerned, which ranged from 2;9 to 5;3. Since children with LD who are developing spoken language appear to attain the stage of word combinations at the equivalent MA to typically developing children, this appears to be a significant delay. Sign combinations are, therefore, produced relatively rarely and seem slow to develop.

Semantic relations in sign combinations have been studied by Fenn and Rowe (1975) and Grove and Dockrell (2000) and have found to be those characteristic of children functioning at the stage I period: actions, locations, attributes predominating, with occasional evidence of later patterns such as negatives and causal relations. The children in both studies also produced numerous examples of the repetition patterns which are typical of stage I – ABA type within turns (e.g. 'WATER ME WATER') and vertical sequences across turns (Veneziano et al., 1990). So far, although development is severely delayed, it is similar to the norm for both typical speakers and speakers with LD.

When we come to syntax, however, the picture changes. Several studies have revealed high levels of word order errors in sign combinations (Fenn and Rowe, 1975; Light et al., 1989; Grove et al., 1996a). Both Fenn and Rowe, and Light and his colleagues, reported that word order is erratic and did not respond (in the case of the study by Light et al., 1989) to specific and intensive training. Fenn and Rowe (1975), however, point out that noun phrase integrity was retained by their subjects. Error analyses by these authors, and by Grove and Dockrell (2000), showed that the most common errors involve the placement of objects (semantic patients) after the verb, and attributes after the noun, errors which are also found in typically developing children. Locatives may also occur before verbs or nouns.

However, Grove and Dockrell's (2000) participants showed some sensitivity to the category of agency. First, they preferentially retained the subjects of intransitive verbs and dropped the subject of transitive verbs in their two-sign utterances, as do typically developing children (Goldin-Meadow and Mylander, 1990). Second, they rarely made the error of placing the subject after the verb. It has been suggested that sensitivity to agency, which develops into the syntactic category of subject, is the first to develop and is present at the point when children start to combine words (Bates et al., 1988). However, grammatical development beyond this early stage appears to be extremely limited. Udwin and Yule (1990, 1991) found no examples of clause expansion, and very few of questions, commands, negatives, adjectives and auxiliary verbs.

The somewhat bleak picture of language acquisition in manual sign is mitigated by evidence of creativity by the children in the study by Grove and Dockrell (2000). We must never forget that language is a means to an end, namely the expression of meaning. These children spontaneously introduced contrastive changes to the forms of their signs to convey different meanings: for example, using two hands rather than one to pluralise ('LIGHT-S' vs. 'LIGHT') or to intensify ('REALLY-BAD' vs. 'BAD'), changes in handshape to convey different sizes and shapes of objects ('LITTLE-HOUSE' vs. 'BIG-HOUSE'; 'GIVE-SWEET' vs. 'GIVE'), and changes in movement ('VERY-FAST' vs. 'FAST'). This gestural or sign morphology suggests that the children were in fact capable of some level of segmental analysis which they employed effectively in relevant contexts.

If children are having problems in developing grammatical structure in sign, are they any more successful in their accompanying speech? Kouri (1989) studied the development of language in speech and sign in a young child with DS between the ages of 2;8 and 3;6. The child's first words were mostly in sign, but by the end of the programme she was beginning to combine spoken words, suggesting a shift in modality preference. Grove and Dockrell (2000) analysed the spoken language output of the six children in their study who had some functional speech. In most cases, the structure of the accompanying speech exactly paralleled their signing, including word order errors. However, one child showed evidence of separation of the two systems, with some use of morpho-syntax in spoken phrases such as 'give it', 'boy eating' (Smith and Grove, 1999). This suggested that we need to pay close attention to what is happening in both modalities.

The above findings relate to children with LD who are taught a form of signs supporting speech (e.g. the Makaton Vocabulary; Walker, 1980) rather than a true sign language. Woll and Grove (1997) reported on the case of hearing twins with DS whose parents were deaf and who acquired sign as their first language. The children had acquired a wide vocabulary of signs which they used appropriately to fulfil different pragmatic functions, and they combined signs in short sentences. However, sign-based assessments of language suggested that they had some difficulties in expressing spatial syntax – a tentative indication that verbal short-term memory deficits may not account for all the difficulties children with DS may experience in the development of the computational aspects of language.

Language through graphic representation

Less information is available on the acquisition of language structure through graphic rather than manual systems. Kiernan et al. (1982) provided data on 46 symbol users in 33 ESN(S) (educationally subnormal – severe) schools where 17.4% of pupils could use more than two symbols per message, and 34.9% more than two. This is considerably higher than the comparable figures for manual sign (see above). It is worth noting that over half of the 46 youngsters were using Blissymbolics charts of 100 or 200 symbols. Nine children were said to make use of the 'opposite' symbol, 3 the 'combine' symbol, 3 the 'make descriptive' symbol, and 10 the 'make action' symbol. Soto and Toro-Zambrana (1995) have also found evidence of the use of the linguistic conventions of Blissymbolics by individuals with LD.

The more pictorial Rebus and Picture Communication Symbols (PCS) systems do not employ specific linguistic conventions, making it difficult to tell whether or not children are developing morpho-syntax through these media (Sutton and Morford, 1998). However, children may be creative with symbols and picture use, as with signs. Detheridge (personal communication, 1998) cited the example of a child who did not have the symbol for 'very', but who wrote '*WINDY WINDY*', using doubling to intensify in a similar way to one of Grove's signing subjects (who used two hands for the one-handed sign 'BAD').

Wilkinson et al. (1994) and Romski and Sevcik (1996) have analysed the multi-symbol combinations produced by adolescents with LD. The majority were two symbols in length, were creative in the sense that novel combinations were formed from lexical items to convey different meanings, and seemed to reflect distributional regularities similar to those identified by Braine (1976). For example, one item ('*WANT*') functioned as a 'pivot' to which others could be added ('*BISCUIT*', '*ICE-CREAM*').

Soto (1999) analysed the structural characteristics of graphic symbol messages reported in the existing literature for individuals with and without LD, finding a predominance of single-symbol messages, failure to utilise available morpho-syntactic structures, word order differences and predominance of simple clauses. Combinations often employ different modalities simultaneously, such as the use of eye gaze and symbol, symbol and gesture, gesture and vocalisation. These characteristics are similar to those reported for manual signers and suggest that qualitative differences exist between the organisation of messages in speech and in AAC systems. However, far more information is needed about the language output of users before any firm conclusions can be made about the course of development through alternative modalities.

The problems that children have in developing language structure in the alternative modality of manual sign may be due to a number of interacting factors.

- First, children with LD are provided with pretty impoverished sign input; typically the adults around them use only one key sign per clause (Grove et al., 1996a), which means they are exposed to limited contrastivity in ordering patterns.
- Secondly, they have access to limited lexicons. For example, Grove and Norwich (1997) found that most pupils in SLD schools using manual sign or graphic symbols were reported to use vocabularies of less than 50 items. Given that lexical size seems to play a role in the activation of analytic and combinatorial language skills, it may be that children simply do not have control over sufficient items to afford contrastivity at either syntactic or morphological levels.
- Thirdly, lexicons are dominated by nouns. This is problematic because mastery of a range of verbs and their argument structures seems to be central to linguistic development (Tomasello, 1992). Udwin and Yule's finding (1990, 1991) of a limited range of sentence types may also reflect a paucity of lexical items needed to ask questions,

hypothesise, predict or reflect causal relationships. Signs and graphic symbols to express these functions are available in most existing vocabularies but may not be prioritised in teaching.

Assessment

It is apparent that the transition from single words to sentences presents a major challenge for many children with LD, who may have specific difficulties in the acquisition of morpho-syntax. One of the implications for assessment and intervention by speech and language therapists (SLTs) is that it is important to adopt a multi-modal developmental perspective.

Multi-modal perspective

The adoption of a multi-modal perspective on language acquisition for children with LD requires close analysis of the ways in which different modalities are used in communication, both independently and combined. One problem currently facing SLTs is that there is no common approach to transcription, although von Tetzchner and Jensen (1996) have proposed a notation system that has been adopted by the International Society for Augmentative and Alternative Communication (their suggested conventions are employed in this chapter). The CHILDES system (MacWhinney, 2000) has been successfully adapted by Slobin and his colleagues for the transcription of sign (the Berkeley Transcription System), and it would certainly be helpful if this were extended to cover the use of graphic representations (see Hughes, 2000; Hunt-Berg, 2000)

When we look at modalities in combination, we often find that children are producing more complex utterances in this way than in one modality alone (Heim and Baker-Mills, 1996). MacDonald (1984) and Grove (1995) found that children sometimes produce combinations of signs and spoken words, or symbols and signs, where agents (nouns) are likely to be spoken or symbolised, and actions (verbs) are more likely to be signed, perhaps because signing is inherently dynamic. Early combinations are likely to involve words and gestures, such as points, for all children, and this suggests a starting point for teaching them to link ideas. Points continue to provide very effective ways of signalling deictic pronouns for children with limited speech skills. We therefore need to be aware of all the possible ways in which children are expressing meaning.

In parallel, we need to look in detail at the specific ways in which children are making use of particular modalities. For children with functional speech, the recognition of the link between phonology and grammar underlies the importance of continuing to work on speech perception and production, even when augmentative systems are introduced. In the manual modality, we need to be aware of the ways in which meaning can be varied by changes to the formational properties of sign and gesture. With symbol systems, we may need to make sure that we are introducing some linguistic conventions to enable children to change or elaborate meaning, such as negatives, question words, tense markers and modal verbs.

Two case studies illustrate how a multi-modal perspective may inform assessment.

Case study 6.1

Andy was 15 years old, and had athetoid cerebral palsy and moderate LD. His understanding was at about a 4-year-old's level. He communicated predominantly through responses to 'yes–no' questions, vocalisations and whole body movement. He had recently acquired a communication aid which he used for topical single messages, and a chart on his wheelchair tray with pictures and symbols for his favoured communication topics.

Assessment of his expressive skills showed that he frequently combined several modalities in a sequence to communicate complex meanings. Thus, a gaze upwards (towards the room where the hamster lived) indicated 'hamster'; gaze at the window indicated 'outside', 'da' vocalisation meant 'Dad'; touching his hair might indicate 'I've had a hairwash', or 'get my hair out of my eyes', lipsmack meant 'food'. A look out of the door, for example, combined with the sound 'da' + lipsmack, meant 'Dad is coming home to supper'.

Case study 6.2

Pardeep was a 15 year old girl of Punjabi origin, with a MA of 4;6. Although English was not her first language, she spoke it consistently at school, paired with sign, and there was no evidence of interference from Punjabi. On the Derbyshire Language Scheme (DLS) (Knowles and Masidlover, 1982), her understanding of receptive language was assessed by her SLT as five or more Information Carrying Words. She reportedly knew and used around 250 signs, and about 50 intelligible words. Analysis of her expressive language, elicited in conversation, picture description and story recall, illustrates the importance of integrating information about sign and speech, and how modality dependence can vary with context (Smith and Grove, 1999).

In conversation, Pardeep used predominantly speech, with a MLU of 2.03. She produced 22 single-word utterances, 10 two-word utterances, and six utterances of 3–4 words. By contrast, MLU in sign was only 1.32, and signs were used mainly to back up her speech. In the story recall task, however, she made far more use of sign. Here, MLU in speech remained at the two-word level (2.2) but in sign it rose to 4.6. The modality dependence was reversed, with speech appearing to back up sign. Pardeep's speech showed some evidence of phrase structure (e.g. ' my little baby', 'bite it', 'at home') and word level morphology (e.g. 'pulling/pulled'). In conversation, she was using mostly single uninflected signs, but in the story recall context, she frequently changed the form of signs to indicate complex meanings. For example, she modified the handshape of the sign 'GIVE' from a flat hand (the citation form) to a bunched hand, indicating that something small (a sweet) was given. She also produced the sign 'RUN' with intensity, indicating a meaning of 'RUN-FAST'.

Developmental perspective

We need to make full use of the techniques available to us from the study of spoken language to enrich our approaches to working with children with LD. In particular, we need to look at different aspects of language use, across modalities.

Semantics

We need to consider:

- The range of *lexical categories* available to the child, and used by the child; for example, the proportion of lexical (nouns, verbs, adjectives) and functional (prepositions, pronouns, modal verbs, negatives, intensifiers, interrogatives, conjunctions) categories.
- *Generative semantics* – the ways in which children create novel meanings, for example through compounds or the creation of verbs from nouns or adjectives; for example, Jayesh used 'RED-APPLE' for tomato and 'DOCTOR-SHOP' for hospital. Penny, a teenager with moderate LD, coined the phrase 'cry-eye!' for any sad experience (this has been adopted for its expressive power by everyone who has ever worked with her).
- *Semantic relations* underpinning combinatorial utterances: the earliest combinations typically involve agents, actions and patients ('boy eat'), ('eat cake'); locatives ('Marianne school'); attributes ('orange bus'); later, children use more complex relations such as interrogative

('where Mum'?), temporal ('party after dinner'), causal ('because I big'), quantitative ('lots tree') and epistemic ('think man box', i.e. I think it's a man in a box) (Grove, 1995). The range of semantic relations is obviously influenced by the diversity of categories available in the lexicon, suggesting that we should avoid too much focus on nouns in teaching.

In some cases, it is difficult to discern any specific relations in the child's output, which looks more like a string of signs, words, or symbols, as though the child were just listing discrete aspects of an event. This is the category referred to by Lahey (1988) as additive, and was extremely prominent in the 10 children studied by Grove (Grove et al., 1996a; Grove and Dockrell, 2000). Typically, the child would produce a string of signs, one after the other, with no discernible structure as might be indicated by a pause, or stress. For example, in response to the question 'What does Daddy do?' Adam signs 'CAR TRAIN TRAIN MUMMY'. Jayesh, describing a picture of a mother reaching out to a little boy who is running towards her, signs 'WALK REACH CUDDLE'. Jonathan is relating what happens in a video story where a girl makes a spider sandwich for her brother, and signs 'SPIDER HUNGRY SQUASH EAT (point to television)' (Grove, 1995). The story makes it clear that it is the brother who is hungry and who eats, and the girl who squashes the spider. In these examples, however, it is impossible to infer what the relationships are between the constituents. This suggests that although children have mastered the productive ability to sequence lexical items, they are not always able to organise them into coherent representations of events. The same children were often able to generate semantic relations in shorter utterances, in response to less complex stimuli. This suggests that we need to find ways of helping children to select and organise information in more complex scenarios, such as narratives.

Syntax and morphology

Contrastive word order

In a language such as English, children need to be able to signal contrasts in meaning through word order, as represented in the two sentences: 'John hit Mary' and 'Mary hit John'. Some children develop this sensitivity very early, but others do not seem to perceive its significance, suggesting that they need more explicit exposure to word order contrasts. Note that word order is of less importance in languages which rely more on morphological inflections to signal meaning, such as sign languages.

Complex clauses

Use of co-ordinate and compound sentences is often signalled by conjunctions, such as 'who', 'when', 'if', 'then', 'because'. Again, they seem to be rarely produced by children with LD who use AAC, and are likely to need specific teaching.

Changes to meaning (morphology)

These may occur within words and signs or gestures, or through adding elements to symbols or pictures, and inflections. The children in Grove's study (1995) were most likely to innovate when they were describing personal events important to them, or in narrating a funny story they had seen on video. Relatively few examples were seen in a picture description task. Again, this argues for assessment and intervention contexts which challenge children to explore the potential of their existing language. We should be alert to creative innovations, and the extent to which these are productive for individual children. Using the criteria proposed by Pine and Lieven (1993) we can look for contrastivity and consistency. At the level of the word and the level of the sentence, new forms stand in contrast to old, established forms. Thus, the child may start with 'sit down' and subsequently produce 'sit up', 'sit there', and the words 'down', 'up' and 'there' will appear in other combinations. At word level, she starts with 'sit', then produces 'sitting' and 'sits'. With sign morphology, the child should be seen to produce the citation form of the sign correctly, before being credited with the introduction of a formal change. Changes must also have some clear relationship with meaning. For example, if the child only produces the sign 'GIVE' with a bunched hand, this could be a production error. However, if she usually produces 'GIVE' with a flat hand, and the bunched hand is used for a class of objects for which this would be the appropriate handshape (e.g. a bunch of flowers or a stick), then she has probably introduced a morphological change.

The second point to look for is the consistency with which structures are employed to express similar meanings. In spoken grammar, we look to see if verb particles ('up', 'down') are employed with verbs other than the original one ('sit') – such as 'stand', or 'look'. With sign or gestural morphology therefore, we would look to see if the child can produce the same changes with other signs – increasing the dimensions to indicate 'BIG' or 'LITTLE' not only within the sign 'HOUSE', but signs such as 'TABLE' or 'PICTURE'; increasing or decreasing the speed on signs such as 'RUN, WALK, SWIM' to indicate 'FAST' or 'SLOW'.

Pragmatics

This refers to the range of uses to which children put their available 'language', in different communicative contexts. There is an understandable tendency to focus on the development of requests in initial communication training, because these are intrinsically motivating and relatively easy to facilitate. However, if children are to engage actively in interactions with other people and their environments, they need to develop the ability to name and describe, to ask questions, to negotiate, deny and confirm, to play and to narrate.

The developmental perspective can be used to provide a framework for the planning of therapy. This is appropriate, given that all available research suggests that children with LD follow a typical path, although the trajectory may be slower, and there may be plateaux in development. However, we also need to bear in mind what is functional for the child at particular points in time, by keeping the focus on meaning, rather than on linguistic targets for their own sake. As children grow up, the focus of assessment and intervention may need to change from the acquisition of language structures to the functional use of language in contexts which promote participation and inclusion.

Intervention

Early intervention is of prime importance (see Chapter 3), but because of the protracted nature of language development in children with LD, intervention may need to continue into adolescence and even adulthood. Rondal and Edwards (1997) point out that although dramatic developments in phonology and morpho-syntax are unlikely to occur after the age of 12–14 years, there is considerable scope for development in lexical and pragmatic aspects well into adulthood. It is also worth noting that some level of intervention is critical to encourage individuals to use the language skills that they have developed across all relevant contexts. This has implications for prioritisation in the management of SLT services.

A range of strategies is available for teaching language structures, only some of which have been formally evaluated.

Derbyshire Language Scheme (DLS) (Knowles and Masidlover, 1982)

This remains the most comprehensive programme available for the teaching of semantic relations underpinning early combinations, and for basic morpho-syntax. Although the materials have mainly been developed to suit younger children, it is possible to make the programme more

age-appropriate for older pupils and adults, by substituting real objects
and cartoon dolls with timeless appeal (e.g. Wallace and Gromit, or South
Park figures). Perhaps surprisingly, there have been few direct evaluations
of the DLS. However, a similar approach appears to have been taken in a
successful study by Leonard (1975 – reviewed by Rosenberg and
Abbeduto, 1993) to teach children with mild LD to move from single-
word to two-word utterances.

Matrix training

This procedure has proved effective in teaching children the principle of
productive combination of words or signs (Karlan et al., 1982; Romski and
Ruder, 1984; Goldstein et al., 1987; Light et al., 1989). A matrix is
constructed to provide exemplars of two-term sentences, with one term
(e.g. nouns) represented on the x-axis, and another (e.g. verbs, adjectives or
locatives) on the y-axis. The children progress through the matrix in a
stepwise fashion, so that one set of combinations is directly trained, and
the remainder are used to test for generalisation. For example, the x-axis
might consist of 'car', 'plane', 'bus', 'bike', and the y-axis of 'red', 'blue',
'green', 'yellow'. The child learns to produce 'red' + 'car'; 'blue' + 'plane',
'green' + 'bus', 'yellow' + 'bike', in a game format. Although children may
quickly learn the principle of combination, they may not necessarily pick
up on the linguistic significance of word order (Light et al., 1989).

Script training

'Script' was the term used by Nelson (1986) to describe formulaic
language forms which are consistently associated with particular events:
for example 'Can I help you?', 'How are you?', 'Happy birthday', 'Good
to see you'. Holistic production of formulaic phrases is mastered quite
early on in typical language development, and should therefore be within
the capacity of children who have a range of single words. Scripts have
been successfully taught to individuals with LD in a variety of social
contexts (Tae-Kim and Lombardino, 1991) and can be programmed into
voice output devices. Scripts extend language output from single words to
sentences, but the generalised use of a script does not imply understanding or productive control of the language structures which generate the
particular phrase or sentence used. However, scripts can be combined
with creative language. Having routines within the home or classroom
where there is a common framework, e.g. a sentence starter such as
'Today I'm doing . . .' or 'I went to . . .', may help children to make the
bridge from single words to short phrases.

Didactic teaching

Didactic interventions based on operant principles have been used quite extensively to teach language structures to children with LD. They rely on learning by imitation through massed trials. For example: 'Look at this picture. The girl is sitting. You say the girl is sitting'. Rosenberg and Abbeduto (1993), in a review of language teaching strategies, concluded that the main problem with didactic approaches is that although the target structures may be learned to criterion in the instructional context, research shows that they have little impact on the individual's language performance in everyday life. However, it has been suggested that didactic approaches are the best suited to the teaching of specific syntactic and morphological forms, which appear resistant to more subtle forms of intervention (Connell, 1987).

Incidental teaching

Incidental, or *milieu*, teaching (Hart and Risley, 1980) is built on the principle of using child-directed language, based on what is known about facilitative early parent–child interaction, such as following the child's lead, providing models of target structures just in advance of the child's current level of functioning, including increasingly more specific prompts to elicit target structures, and using natural reinforcers. When this approach is employed with children with more severe LD and language delay, it is usual for more didactic elements to be included, to allow for the fact that incidental teaching relies heavily on child initiations, which are often infrequent in this population. Kaiser et al. (1997b) concluded from a review of interventions employing incidental teaching that it may have a dramatic effect, but only for the particular structures which are targeted. Furthermore, these are limited, because some linguistic forms (e.g. morphology) are difficult to teach through this approach.

A general caveat regarding all forms of incidental teaching is that the style of social interaction appears to have little impact on the development of linguistic structure, as opposed to the development of language use, where it is a key factor (Rosenberg and Abbeduto, 1993). Variants of incidental teaching approaches (not always identified as such) can be seen in programmes such as FOCAL (Kiernan et al., 1987).

Reading and writing

Buckley (1992) has demonstrated that teaching children with DS to read can have a beneficial impact on their grammatical development. This is probably because written language offers visual feedback and a permanent representation of the functors which can easily be misperceived or mispronounced by children with hearing and articulatory impairments and phonological memory deficits. The recent emphasis on literacy development, and advances in technology in both mainstream and special schools, means that more children with special needs than ever before are being provided with the opportunity to develop reading and writing skills. SLTs need to be making active use of these opportunities for language development. Children who find conventional orthography too difficult as a first step may start to read through graphic symbols and pictures (Detheridge and Detheridge, 1997) and these too offer opportunities for the construction of simple sentences. Carpenter (1987) demonstrated that young people with LD could use the visual feedback afforded by symbol sequences to build up sentences and self-correct when terms were omitted or wrongly ordered.

Creative writing offers children a genuinely motivating context for extending beyond single-word utterances. Activities such as writing frames, or sentence completion, can also be used to develop sentence structure. Children select symbols or words, and say or sign the complete unit. For example, 'I went (to the shops/in the sea)'; 'I saw (a new dress/a big shark)'.

Focus on verbs

Because verbs are so critical to the development of language structure, they should be a central focus of intervention designed to develop morpho-syntax. Early vocabulary teaching, for obvious practical reasons, tends to be dominated by nouns. The context of verb teaching is highly important. To start with, children' s own actions may provide the best stimuli, e.g. 'tickling', 'rocking', 'jumping', 'falling'. To develop verb tenses, dynamic images may be more useful than pictures or photographs. Videos of children in action can be used to develop verb tenses in spoken language, or to illustrate different types of movement that can be mimed or signed (manner of action is marked on signed verbs, whereas tense is not).

Focus on phonology

Work by Buckley (1993), Cholmain (1994) and Comblain (1994) with children with DS has shown that working on phonology can have a direct impact on the development of grammatical morphology. Given the known difficulties of phonological short-term memory, it is important to focus on perception and recall as well as on production. Comblain (1994) used amplification techniques, whereas Buckley (1993) used printed language. Such therapy can proceed in parallel with the introduction of augmentative approaches to increase functional communication and assist the child in processing auditory information.

Focus on working memory

Since working memory deficits seem to be reliably associated with difficulties in perceiving, recalling and producing phonological and morpho-syntactic structures, several authors have recently proposed that this could prove a fruitful area of intervention for children with LD. Rondal and Edwards (1997) suggested that the priorities should be to increase memory span, accelerate speech rates, and develop good overt rehearsal strategies (see Hulme and Mackenzie, 1992 and Broadley et al., 1993 for reports on the successful use of some of these techniques).

Focus on meaning

When language is developing along typical lines, children seem to utilise complex structures to express meaning as naturally as breathing. When language is severely delayed, however, children seem to take the route of least effort. Observations indicate that they are unlikely to employ two words where one will do. This means that we need to create complex, motivating opportunities for meanings to be extended in the contexts of everyday life. The principle of informativeness is helpful here (Greenfield et al., 1985). Children in the early stages of development are likely to encode comments and to leave topics unstated. Things that change, are unexpected, funny, frightening or out of the ordinary may be more successful in eliciting descriptive language (attributes and adverbs) than things that are routine and predictable.

Case study 6.3

Rebekah, a 10 year old girl who used a small vocabulary of routine words ('mum', 'hallo') and signs ('goodbye', 'drink') was taking the role of the guard in *Macbeth*. As I went around the group checking who had 'blood' on their hands, and whose hands were clean, she vocalised urgently to gain my attention, raised her hands in the air for me to see and simultaneously shook her head to tell me 'No, not me! My hands are clean!'

We need to encourage children to formulate and interrogate their experiences, creating stories about things that happen to them, predicting and explaining events and reactions. By working closely with teachers,

SLTs can identify the range of language opportunities presented within the curriculum; for example, prediction, description and explanation in Science; feelings and motivation in Drama; locations and their descriptions in Geography; verbs and prepositions in Physical Education. One of the most important things to establish is an expectation of creative language use within the peer group, so that children become accustomed to meeting a variety of linguistic challenges.

Enriching language

The multi-modal perspective offers an alternative route to increasing the effectiveness of communication, particularly for children whose development reaches a plateau before the emergence of morpho-syntax, at expressive language levels of 1–3 words. They can be encouraged to amplify meaning through creative use of facial expression, body language, vocalisations, mime and gestures. This may involve the kind of gestural morphology described earlier, or simpler approaches. For example, in Grove's study (1995) negatives were almost always expressed by headshakes, rather than the lexical sign 'NO'. Points to people, places and things in the immediate environment can be combined with signs, symbols or words – either functioning as deictic pronouns, or to indicate complete events. These enrichment strategies may allow individuals to work from their strengths as communicators, rather than their deficits.

Conclusion

The study of the acquisition of language structure by different groups of children with LD remains an underdeveloped area of knowledge. We need to learn more about the particular problems associated with particular syndromes, and the effects of new interventions, particularly those concerned with literacy and computer enhanced language intervention. The context of intervention is changing, as more children with LD are educated in mainstream schools, and we have yet to discover what impact these new opportunities will have on the developing language skills of this population. Review of the research literature suggests, however, that morpho-syntax is one of the areas most at risk of severe delay, and that if intervention is to be effective, it probably needs to be:

- early
- intensive and specific – hence needing specialist input
- associated with rapid lexical development

- associated with the development of verb systems
- associated with visual feedback through the teaching of early reading
- associated with work on phonological short-term memory.

When augmentative and alternative forms of communication are introduced (see Chapter 7 in this book) it is important not to assume that because the child now has a functional means of communication, the development of language structure will automatically follow. Children probably need extensive models of how to combine and sequence signs and symbols. We need to be alert to the significance of their innovations in whatever modalities they are using. Finally, we need to keep in mind that the acquisition of structure without meaning is a hollow achievement. It is easy to get carried away by the need to drill linguistic forms. A concern for meaning must provide the motivation for our therapy.

CHAPTER 7

Augmentative and Alternative Communication

GILL WILLIAMS

Abstract

In this chapter, the use and role of augmentative and alternative communication (AAC) for the individual with learning disabilities (LD) is explored. A historical perspective from which to view current issues is provided, as is a description and classification of the different types of AAC and a rationale for the use of AAC with a range of clients. An assessment framework is described, leading to the formulation of a profile of the individual's strengths and needs which will assist the team to implement immediate and long-term intervention plans. Included are descriptions and examples of developing communicative competence through a range of augmentative modes of communication from very early responses to more sophisticated language and literacy development. Throughout the chapter the emphasis is on a co-ordinated, collaborative, multi-modal approach, integrating AAC into the whole intervention package.

Introduction

The field of augmentative and alternative communication (AAC) is still very much an emerging one, and it is only just becoming a respected science. Awareness of the historical perspective can provide a rationale for the development of AAC. Before the 1950s, although there were a few anecdotal accounts of use of non-vocal methods of communicating (e.g. Brown, 1972), very little information was available to enable the provision of advice to clients who could not use oral communication, except for persistence with articulation drill and practice, and breathing exercises (e.g. Collis, 1947; British Council for the Welfare of Spastics, 1952).

People with profound and multiple LD would have been considered 'ineducable' and therefore would not have required methods to assist them to be more effective and meaningful communicators. Medical, sociological, educational and technological developments since this time have accounted both for a more co-ordinated service for clients with LD, and for the emergence of the use of AAC as an intervention tool to be considered for a wider group of clients. Zangari et al. (1994) provided a very full review of the history of AAC up to the mid-1990s, Fawcus (1987) gave an account of the development of communication aids, and Glennen (1997a) presented a more recent historical perspective (Glennen and DeCoste, 1997:5–19).

Review of the literature

Historical perspectives

During the 1950s and 1960s, the approach towards the cognitively impaired (or people with LD) was gradually changing, particularly in the Scandinavian countries where the concept of 'normalisation' was being formulated. Nirje (1976:33   see also Chapter 1) defined normalisation as

> making available to all mentally retarded people patterns of life and conditions of everyday living which are as close as possible to the regular circumstances and ways of life of society.

During the 1970s, there were significant advances in social and educational thinking and legislation (Chronically Sick and Disabled Person's Act, 1970; The Warnock Report   DES, 1978), combined with advances in technology which enabled the emergence of AAC as a viable academic, medical and educational discipline. An emerging interest in semantics and pragmatics in the late 1970s significantly increased the body of knowledge about language and psychological development. This began to provide the background of knowledge for a more functional approach to communication which had important implications for those with multiple impairments. The Makaton Vocabulary (Walker, 1980), which employs manual signs from British Sign Language (BSL) and which was designed for deaf adults with severe LD, was later used successfully with hearing adults and children with severe communication difficulties (Grove and Walker, 1990). Primate communication research (Premack and Premack, 1974) led to a broader perspective on language and communication development and caused some professionals to consider the use of signs and graphic symbols for individuals with severe communication impairments.

In the area of cerebral palsy, although there was still a strong expectation among speech and language therapists (SLTs) that they should work on improving speech musculature, there was a growing realisation that some individuals would never develop intelligible speech (Hixson and Hardy, 1964). This led to experimentation with AAC strategies. Glennen (1997a) described the 'Non-Oral Communication Systems Project', initiated as early as 1964, which documented the use of AAC with more than 20 cerebral palsied children over a 10 year period.

In 1963, the Patient-Operated Selector Mechanism (POSSUM) was developed as a means of communication for severely disabled individuals, giving them access to a typewriter, and in 1966 it was available on prescription. In the 1970s, McNaughton (1985) introduced Blissymbolics as a graphic symbol system for cerebral palsied children unable to use traditional orthography. It was a semantically based, generative system consisting of combinations of pictographic, ideographic and arbitrary components. Through what was then called the Blissymbolics Communication Foundation, the system became internationally known, hundreds of professionals were trained in its use and many articles were written about its practical application. During the mid and late 1970s, a base of systematic research began to emerge in the field of AAC. By the 1980s, AAC was becoming a legitimate specialisation involving a wide range of disciplines (see Enderby, 1987). In the UK, six Communication Aids Centres were established in 1983, jointly funded by the Royal Association for Disability and Rehabilitation (RADAR) and the Department of Health and Social Services (DHSS). The aim was to assess individuals, advise and train professionals and become involved in research and development. This period also marked the beginnings of governmental funding for communication aids.

Lloyd et al. (1990) discussed the idea of a communication model in the absence of speech and how this related to communication use through verbal means. Light (1989) revisited the concept of 'communicative competence', as something to be aimed for in individuals using AAC. This was a sociolinguistic concept originally described by Hymes (1974) and developed by others (e.g. Savignon, 1985) in relation to second language learning. It was described by other authors in relation to the development of communication in deaf children (Greenberg, 1980) and children with LD (Donahue et al., 1983). Light defined communicative competence as

the quality or state of being functionally adequate in daily communication, or of having sufficient knowledge, judgement, and skill to communicate. (Light, 1989:138)

The four competencies she describes are:

- *linguistic competence:* 'an adequate level of mastery of the linguistic code'
- *operational competence:* 'the user must also develop the technical skills required to operate the system'
- *social competence:* 'the user of an AAC system must also possess knowledge, judgement, and skill in the social rules of communication'
- *strategic competence:* 'individuals require strategic competence to make the best of what they do know and can do. They need to develop compensatory strategies to allow them to communicate more effectively within restrictions' (Light, 1989:139–41).

The definition provided a model for discussion and research on the development of communication using AAC, and provided a framework for assessment and intervention. It is still used widely today (see MacDonald, 1998; MacDonald and Rendle, 1998), though other, more comprehensive models are being developed (Grove et al., 1996a; von Tetzchner et al., 1996).

The 1980s and 1990s witnessed several important advances in technology such as increases in computer memory, advances in synthetic speech and improved graphic capabilities, which led to the development of a wide range of portable Voice Output Communication Aids (VOCAs), although the cost of systems has remained high. Switches became more sophisticated so that even the most physically impaired clients could access devices. Communication aids could be purchased with graphic symbols already programmed in, to speed up the process of producing individualised vocabularies. Minspeak (see van Tatenhove, 1993), a method of combining multi-meaning icons on a static communication aid overlay to create an extensive vocabulary, allowed for very creative use of language by non-literate clients. During the 1990s, the development of the Windows interface for personal computers led to the development of dynamic screen systems in which the symbol vocabulary could be stored on a series of pages. This meant that systems could be set up to contain anything from one to over sixty symbols per page, thus allowing for a wide range of abilities. Clients could develop their skills through learning to use an increasingly complex vocabulary. Communication aids were becoming more like personalised computers; in fact, some systems were computers that could run programs other than a communication package, e.g. Cameleon (see appendix to this chapter for suppliers).

Alongside advances in technology and symbols, thinking in relation to LD has developed significantly during the 1980s and 1990s. The increasing move away from a medical model to a social model of disability (Swain et al., 1993; French, 1994; Barnes, 1996; Hales, 1996) has led to increased inclusion in education (Norwich, 1996; Ainscow, 1997; Florian, 1997) and a greater awareness of the issues of equality, empowerment, advocacy and independence in the wider community. This, in conjunction with huge advances in information technology and its wider availability, has caused professionals to consider AAC as a means of empowering individuals at all levels, not only those who are capable of developing language, but also for those whose communication is not yet intentional, or whose responses are not yet consistent.

AAC has widened its perspective to include not only those with physical disabilities, but also with a wide range of developmental disabilities and challenging behaviours (Mirenda, 1997) for whom symbols provide a more tangible means of conveying information than speech. Intervention methods using AAC, such as the Picture Exchange Communication System (PECS) and Facilitated Communication (FC) have been developed and researched, ensuring that AAC becomes increasingly part of the mainstream of therapeutic intervention. For those with long-term AAC needs, there is a much greater emphasis on providing a more continuous and consistent service from infancy, through school and beyond (Light, 1997). This involves careful planning and liaison between the individual's family and a number of agencies, including social services, the health authority, the local education authority, careers services and voluntary organisations. Recent British governmental initiatives, following on from the 1998 Programme of Action (DfEE, 1998b), are aiming to ensure increased partnerships during a child's education, and the emphasis on life-long learning should help to strengthen transitions.

Surprisingly, and disappointingly, despite these significant developments, the issue of funding for communication aids remains largely unresolved. In its review of the current funding situation for pupils requiring AAC in the UK, the working party producing the document *Developing Augmentative and Alternative Communication Policies in Schools: Information and Guidelines* (Chinner et al., 2001) found an inconsistency in policy and practice, lack of a national framework, inequality of opportunity and provision, and no legal entitlement to provision or identified responsibility for funding. Glennen (1997a:13–17) highlighted a similar problem in the USA. It can only be hoped that we will soon witness not only an increasing expectation of AAC use, but also a nationally co-ordinated commitment to the funding associated with it.

Definitions

The definition of augmentative and/or alternative communication (AAC) used in this chapter is 'a means by which an individual can *supplement* or *replace* spoken communication' (Chinner et al., 2001). Anything that increases the effectiveness of spoken communication, or can be used as a non-verbal means of communication, falls within this definition. Communication includes a wide range of behaviours, from any movement or behaviour which can be observed and interpreted by another person as meaningful, to the use of a code agreed upon between people where items within that code have specific meanings, i.e. a language.

AAC should be seen as part of an individual's communicative repertoire. The extent to which it is required and used will vary according to the needs and impairments of the individual and their environment. It is not something that is only considered in certain settings, or for particular age or client groups. The SLT working in the communication field should be aware of all the possible ways of using AAC as part of the whole intervention package. AAC will have different functions at different stages of life. For the infant it will be a means of developing interaction with main caregivers. In school it will be a means of accessing the educational curriculum and developing language, and throughout life it will assist in the development of emotional and social skills, independence and achieving vocational goals (Light, 1997).

AAC can be divided into 'unaided' and 'aided' communication, although most users will require a multi-modal approach encompassing both.

Unaided communication

Unaided communication has been defined as 'communication modes that use only the user's body' (Glennen and DeCoste, 1997). This includes some of the most basic and intuitive forms of communication, which may or may not be intentional. Examples of this are body language, looking, facial expression, natural gesture, use of vocalisation or intonation and touch. Signing systems such as BSL, Paget-Gorman Signed Speech (PGSS) and finger spelling, and signed vocabularies such as the Makaton Vocabulary, Sign Supported English and Signalong, are more formal modes of unaided communication. There are also signed strategies used to compensate for poor speech (for example Cued Articulation) which could be included under this heading.

Aided communication

Aided communication has been defined as 'communication modes that require equipment in addition to the communicator's body' (Glennen and DeCoste, 1997). Included here would be low-tech or 'light-tech' systems such as objects, photographs, pictures, graphic symbols (e.g. Picture Communication Symbols, Rebus, Blissymbols) or written letters of the alphabet or words, which may be organised into charts or books. High-tech systems include communication aids that produce speech or text. VOCAs (dedicated communication devices or portable computers with communication software) may use synthesised voice or digitised voice.

Aided systems require a reliable method of access. This may be by 'direct access', such as:

- fist or finger pointing to items (objects, symbols or words) in the immediate environment, on a board, in a book or on a communication aid
- eye pointing to items at a sufficient distance apart that the message can be interpreted correctly (for example, attached to a perspex frame or Velcro-compatible board, or held up by a communication partner)
- use of a computer keyboard – either standard or adapted (e.g. Big Keys, Intellikeys)
- use of an infrared or light pointer.

It may be necessary for the user to access a system by indirect access, which is usually slower than direct access, but allows for fairly sophisticated selection where movements are limited. Examples include:

- scanning with an input device such as a switch or switches
- a pointer control system such as a joystick or trackerball
- listener-mediated scanning in which the communication partner assists the user to make vocabulary selections, by verbally scanning a list of options, and waiting for the AAC user to indicate the correct selection.

Further information about different systems, access methods and devices can be found in publications such as Glennen and DeCoste (1997); Jans and Clark (1998a:37–45); Nisbet and Poon (1998); and Scott (1998:13–18).

Two important points should be noted at this stage.

- First, it is unlikely that any one mode of AAC will be used exclusively by an individual, in the same way that competent users of any language do not rely solely on one mode of communication. Rather, they tend to augment their speech with gesture and facial expression, and possibly written words, or diagrams. Therefore, a multi-modal approach should be advocated, in which users are encouraged to use all modes available to them in order to communicate most effectively.
- Second, AAC should not be considered as simply a method to be used by an individual, but also as an overall method of communication between a group of 'oral' and 'non-oral' people. As with any minority language, in order to be effectively used and developed, it needs to be part of the total communication environment. In a community where AAC users are present, there should be evidence throughout the institution of a commitment to, and a respect for, AAC, such as the use of symbols to label activity areas and notice-boards, signing in assemblies and meetings and switch access to communication and technology (see Goossens et al., 1994; Porter and Kirkland, 1995; Cottier et al., 1997).

Rationale for augmentative and alternative communication

The mission statement of the US Society for Augmentative and Alternative Communication (USSAAC) states that 'Communication is the essence of human life' (Light, 1997). Communication is the means by which the individual can express needs and wants, develop social closeness, exchange information and fulfil social etiquette routines (Light, 1988). It should be considered as a human right, and an opportunity that should be available to all individuals equally, in order that they can develop socially, emotionally and cognitively. It is important to remember, of course, that intelligible, oral speech is, where possible, the most effective form of communication. It is thus the responsibility of carers and professionals in that person's environment to ensure that an individual who is unable to communicate effectively by oral means has a means of communicating that can be interpreted by others.

In the early days of AAC intervention, there was much discussion on candidacy issues based on two main assumptions:

- AAC was only appropriate when traditional therapy had failed
- the client had to have achieved a prerequisite skill level to be a candidate for AAC.

There was also concern that the use of AAC inhibited the development of oral language (Hardy, 1983:239). Research and practice has proved, however, that AAC can successfully be used at all levels and with a wide range of clients (Kangas and Lloyd, 1988; Romski and Sevcik, 1988), that it should be commenced as early as possible, that it enhances rather than inhibits oral language (Silverman, 1980), and, additionally, that it has wider implications for independence and self advocacy. AAC should be considered at all stages and with all types of communication intervention.

Martinsen and von Tetzchner (1996) described three main groups of clients for whom AAC can be used; intervention will be different for each of these groups:

- *Alternative language group:* the members of this group are individuals who require an alternative mode for both input and output of communication. The group may include autistic clients, or people with multiple or profound impairments, who require language and communication to be introduced in a very structured and specialised way.
- *Supportive language group:* this group includes individuals who are taught an alternative language form as a temporary or augmentative measure. This may be due to delayed language development, in which case the AAC will be a 'scaffold' to the development of near-normal mastery of speech, or it may be needed because the clarity of the speech is insufficient without augmentative 'clues'. The aim in this case is to facilitate and encourage participation in conversation and other social situations.
- *Expressive language group:* in this group are individuals whose language comprehension may be good but who cannot produce verbal speech, because of physical impairment. People with cerebral palsy might be included in this group. These individuals will need AAC as a permanent means of expression, to be used in all situations. Although they may understand spoken language, they require AAC input as a model to assist them to learn how to use their system.

Different approaches will apply, depending on the group to which the client belongs (see later).

Assessment for augmentative and alternative communication

The selection of an AAC system for a client, and the intervention strategies to be used, will depend on a number of important factors relating to the individual and the environment (see Figure 7.1).

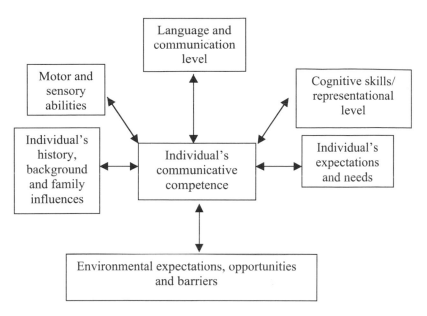

Figure 7.1 Assessment for augmentative and alternative intervention.

In order for these to be assessed in a meaningful and structured way, the assessment process should be co-ordinated by a trans-disciplinary team (i.e. 'team members from different disciplines engage in a high degree of collaboration focusing on holistic goals for the individual, rather than just discipline-specific goals' (Glennen and DeCoste, 1997:779)). The membership of the team will depend on the client's setting but will consist of some, or all, of the following staff: SLT, physiotherapist, occupational therapist, medical personnel, teaching, or other relevant staff within the client's institution. In a specialist AAC centre, there may well be additional staff including clinical engineers and information technology specialists. The assessment will involve parents and carers throughout and will involve the potential user to a greater or lesser degree. The following should be assessed.

Language and communication level

The starting point for any assessment of AAC use is to assess the client's language and communication level. There is a range of tools for this, for example, Assessing Communication Together (Bradley, 1991a, b), Assessing Communication (Latham and Miles, 1997) and some aspects of the AAC Core Curriculum (Robertson et al., 1996). The reader may be familiar with other formal and informal assessments and checklists.

The individual's language and communication level can be compared with the checklist in Table 7.1.

Table 7.1. Communication/language level

Communication/language

Pre-intentional: No consistent responses
Pre-intentional: Some consistent responses, noted on close observation

Emerging interaction skills (in response to activity)
Follow the activity
Take part in activity
Respond when it stops
Indicate that he/she's had enough

Gaining control over the interaction
Initiating an activity
Anticipating next stage
Asking for more
Taking turns
Indicating preferences

Early meanings
Recognising people, objects and routines
Anticipating activities
Requesting things
Responding to 'words'
Imitating words or actions
Making choices

First words
Using 'words' to greet, request, reject, comment
Following simple directions

Developing single-word vocabulary
Using increasing types of words, e.g. nouns, verbs, adjectives
Understanding more complex language

Early 'word' combinations
Combining ideas – with help
Understanding at 2+ word level

More spontaneous combinations
Producing novel combinations without assistance
Understanding at 3+ word level

Using syntactic structure
Using grammatical and morphological markers

Alongside this assessment, the team needs to assess the level the individual is performing at socially, by observations and questioning the individual's carers and staff. The individual's level can be compared with the checklist in Table 7.2.

Table 7.2. Social skills

Social skills
Not interested in people
Some awareness of daily routine
Prefers people to toys
Interested in particular activities
Will make eye-contact with one person
Greeting people
Actively noting activities around him/her
Making people aware of him/her
Making needs known
Noticing others in a group
Participating in a group
Making eye-contact with others in a group
Initiating conversations with more than one person present
Developing listening skills in a group setting
Awareness of others' feelings
Asking people about themselves
Able to share likes and dislikes
Able to give a talk to a group of people
Able to give and listen to opinions
Able to argue and negotiate
Other

Cognitive skills

This assessment needs to be informed by reports from a teacher or psychologist, and, for the school-aged child, much useful information may well be in the Statement of Special Educational Need (SSEN), annual reviews and Individual Education Plans (IEPs). As verbal ability is often an indicator of the level of cognitive ability, the process is more complex in the individual without intelligible oral speech. Glennen (1997b:170–3) discussed assessments of non-verbal intelligence using multiple choice which can be utilised where both expressive language and motor ability are limited. From their observations in context, parents, carers and those working regularly with the client will be able to give evidence of the client's ability for problem-solving and retaining, and for using new information, but these need to be verified by more formal observation. It may well be that as communicative competence develops, a clearer picture of cognitive ability emerges. However, it is important to be aware of the general level at which the individual is functioning in order for intervention to be commenced at the appropriate level. As part of the cognitive assessment, and on the basis of knowledge from the language and communication assessment, the team will need to ascertain the representational level at which the client can process information (i.e. can recognise and utilise concepts presented as objects, pictures or words) see Table 7.3.

Table 7.3. Representational/visual level

Representational/visual level
No consistent response
Responds to his/her environment
Responds to routines
Responds to regularly used objects (e.g. cup)
Understands the function of real objects
Responds to pretend objects (e.g. toy phone)
Responds to miniature objects (e.g. farm animals, doll's furniture)
Recognises photos of familiar items (size?)
Recognises photos of a wide range of objects (size?)
Recognises more complex photos (size?)
Recognises object pictures (size?)
Recognises more complex pictures (size?)
Recognises pictorial symbols (e.g. PCS) (size? array?)
Recognises more complex symbols
Multi-meaning icons (Minspeak, Blissymbols)
Recognises familiar words
Visual recognition of a number of whole words
Can combine letters to make words

Motor abilities

If the client is fully ambulant, with adequate gross motor skills, and able to operate a keyboard with some accuracy, an occupational therapist may be able to assist in the assessment process by looking at ways to make keyboard-type access as efficient as possible (e.g. by adding a key-guard, by providing a wrist splint, etc.). If there is significant motor impairment, the physiotherapist will need to be involved in the assessment, in order to look at range, consistency, control and strength of individual movements. Factors such as seating, positioning and splinting (for example Lycra splinting) may affect the efficiency of available movements.

The aim of motor assessment is to ascertain what movements (for example use of hands, foot, knee, head, etc.) the client can make in order to access a communication system, and whether the user will be able to access symbols directly, or by using an indirect method such as a switch. If the client is likely to use signing as a preferred means of communication (i.e. uses some natural gesture) and has shown an ability to imitate some signs, the motor assessment should concentrate on the client's ability to produce specific hand shapes and movements (see Dunn Klein, 1988; also McEwen and Lloyd, 1990). For a fuller account of the motor assessment process, consult Radell (1997) and DeCoste (1997). Details of motor assessment can be checked against the physical/operational skills checklist in Table 7.4.

Table 7.4. Physical/operational skills

Physical/operational skills
Reflex movements only
Some non-intentional but consistent movement patterns
Some discrete movements
Some gesture
Purposeful movement of one or more body part
Adequate hand (or other) function for purposeful single switch activation with prompting
Purposeful single switch activation with some ability to control timing
Sufficient switch control for automatic scanning
Able to operate 2 switches with prompting
Controlled operation of 2 switches, sufficient for step scanning
Other switch operation (accuracy)
Can eye/fist/finger point to 1 from 2 items
Can eye/fist/finger point to 1 from 4 items
Can eye/fist/finger point to 1 from 8 items
Can point to a large array of symbols/pictures (20/32/64/128)
Can operate an adapted keyboard (type)
Can operate a normal computer keyboard
Able to imitate a few manual signs (poor accuracy)
Spontaneous use of manual signs, not always intelligible
Most manual signs accurately produced, though some limit to fine motor control
Good fine motor control for manual signs

Sensory abilities

As many AAC systems will involve the use of graphic symbols or text, it is important to assess the client's visual perception and acuity (see DeCoste 1997:245–8). This will help the team to make decisions about whether the use of visual symbols is appropriate, and if so, the size, style, amount and colour of symbols that can be used. Symbols may need to have a tactile component, or an individual may need to receive auditory feedback which is available on some scanning systems. There may be visual perceptual deficits that an occupational therapist would be able to assess, in order to inform the team about physical layout of symbols. If the client requires spectacles, it is important to know whether he or she wears them and whether they are for close or distant vision. The audiologist or the client's medical notes should be consulted regarding auditory skills, as this will dictate whether a system using voice output is appropriate, and whether any alterations need to be made in the individual's environment to ensure optimum success.

History, background and family influences

As with any assessment aiming to inform the intervention process (see Bray et al., 1999, Chapter 32), it is vital to consider and analyse the client's medical, educational and social history (e.g. medical diagnosis and prognosis, have there been prolonged periods of hospitalisation, have school experiences been positive or negative, consistent or inconsistent home experiences). In addition, the amount of support and care provided by the family can make the difference between success and failure of an intervention. Cultural and religious factors may be very significant, may well affect the family's perception of disability and will need to be taken into account when selecting a system and an approach. This information will be collected from various sources, through formal and informal interviews, but it is very important to involve the client's family in this process as much as possible so that an understanding of the client's family background can be obtained. This will continue to inform practice throughout the intervention period.

Individual's expectations and needs

It is important to establish the client's self-perception in relation to others. A client may have adopted a passive or a 'challenging' role. They may be the class 'clown' or the 'sickly child', or may have become very manipulative and whiny. It is very common for teenagers to have very low self-esteem and become depressed. All these roles carry with them a series of expectations that affect communicative output. The aim of intervention is to develop positive expectations and a strong need to communicate. It is therefore important to start with a realistic baseline and a knowledge of what motivates the individual's responses.

6

The environment

Clients may well operate differently in different environments. It is important to establish the positive and negative influences within each. Beukelman and Mirenda's Participation Model (1998:148 and 153–7) explores opportunity barriers within the environment. These barriers of policy, practice, attitude, knowledge and skill need to be analysed in some detail, particularly within institutions such as schools and colleges. Chinner et al. (2001) have produced guidelines for developing AAC policies in schools in order to address the issue of AAC environments (see Table 7.5).

Table 7.5. Environmental factors

Environmental factors

Home
Little interest in or understanding of AAC, unrealistically low or high expectations
Supportive family, needs training in providing opportunities for individual
Well informed and positive family; carers have attended courses (e.g. Hanen, Makaton); use of symbols/signs at home; individual actively and appropriately involved in family life
Other comments

Institution
Little interest in or understanding of AAC; unrealistically low or high expectations of individual
Interested institution; may have some knowledge of AAC, but not in practice; staff require training in AAC basics and how to provide a positive AAC environment
Some use of AAC in the environment, but not widely used; may have AAC Policy but not implemented by all staff; knowledge of AAC basics but either unwilling or unable to implement
Very positive environment; AAC Policy in place; AAC Team or co-ordinator, evidence of a system for providing and monitoring AAC use: much evidence of AAC models and opportunities throughout the institution (e.g. symbols on notice-boards, staff and others signing to one another); individuals actively participating in activities and making relevant choices

Class/group/area
Little interest in or understanding of AAC; unrealistically low or high expectations of individual
Interested staff; may have some knowledge of AAC, but not in practice; staff required general training in AAC basics, and specific training related to the individual (e.g. access issues, vocabulary selection, creating opportunities for communication, etc.)
Very positive environment
Individual has a key worker responsible for communication; much evidence of AAC models and opportunities; individual actively involved in the group; evidence of staff understanding the individual's AAC needs and ability.

Other environments (e.g. respite/social clubs)
Little interest and/or knowledge
Interested and some awareness, but training required
Very positive and knowledgeable environment

Once all the assessment information has been collated by the AAC team, an individual profile can be created indicating the individual's strengths and needs in relevant key areas (see Table 7.6).

Table 7.6. The individual profile

Name:.. Date:..		
Key worker:..		
Communication/language	Social skills	Individual factors
Representational skills	Physical/operational skills	Environmental factors
Recommendations		

Intervention

Implementing augmentative and alternative communication

Figure 7.2 illustrates the way a profile leads to an AAC intervention plan. The first decision that needs to be considered for any one client is the starting point of the programme. Initially, with AAC intervention, it is very important to have a vision of long-term aims for a client. What are they likely to be requiring in terms of a system? Will it be low- or high-tech? Is the individual likely to be a signer, use a voice output communication aid, or use speech as the main mode of communication? Although it may be very difficult to judge during the early stages, details from the assessment will have led professionals to have fairly specific ideas about a client's potential as a communicator. It is also important to instil into parents and carers a vision for the future, as this will help to add meaning to the processes along the way.

From the funding viewpoint, it is critical to determine if the individual is likely to be requiring a voice output communication aid at some time in the future. If so, this needs to be written into a care plan as soon as possible. It may also be important from the point of view of placement; for the pre-school child, for example, it may help parents in their choice of

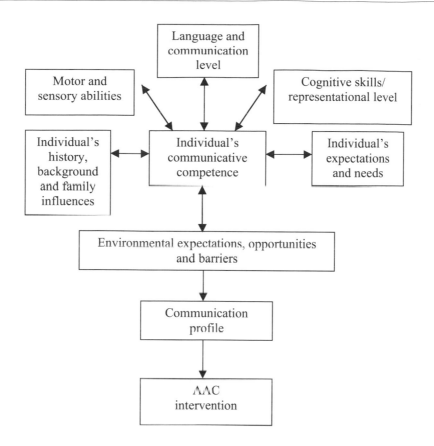

Figure 7.2. Planning augmentative and alternative intervention.

school. For the adolescent, it might help the individual and carers to focus on possible options such as further education or other adult placement.

Having considered this, a more immediate plan of action should be developed. This will include aims for the coming year, then more immediate aims, and a plan for the short term. Within the education system, this fits well into the annual review process, with immediate aims and plans being detailed on the IEP. In Health and Social Services (HSS) institutions this will fit in with 'packages of care', or 'statements of need'. At this stage, it is important to establish roles and responsibilities of key personnel. It is useful to decide on a key worker. This may be a parent, SLT, communication key worker, teacher or social worker, who will have responsibility for liaising with other professionals on the client's behalf. This is particularly important at times of transition when information needs to be transferred from one group of personnel to another.

The following sections highlight some of the principles and procedures at different levels of intervention. The starting point depends very much on the profile of the individual's strengths and needs. However, three important considerations need to be borne in mind:

- Intervention will always involve a number of personnel – roles and responsibilities for each person will need to be established (e.g. see the AAC Intervention Plan, Cottier et al., 1997:9) and there should be one person co-ordinating the work and ensuring that progress continues according to the plan.
- An AAC user cannot communicate alone – communication partners and the overall communication environment will make the difference between success and failure (Woll and Barnett, 1998).
- To become a competent AAC user, the individual will always have to develop a number of skills separately (linguistic, operational, social and strategic – see Light, 1989) and then combine them in order to achieve communicative competence. In all intervention, however, the language level is paramount. This can provide a baseline for all intervention.

In the following sections, separate aspects of working towards achieving AAC goals are discussed. The intervention with each individual will involve consideration of a number of interrelated aspects.

Getting consistent responses

With the early communicator, it is important initially to build a solid communication foundation of consistent interactive responses. The reader is referred to some of the literature on working with individuals at the earliest level of communication for guidance as to the best approach for developing early responses (see Nind and Hewitt, 1994; Ware, 1996; Lacey and Ouvry, 1998; Nafstad and Rodbroe, 1999; Coupe O'Kane and Goldbart, 2000). Beukelman and Mirenda (1998) note 'attention seeking', 'acceptance' and 'rejection' as the initial behaviours to aim for. It is quite likely that the individual already has unintentional behaviours that can be intuitively recognised by familiar carers, but unless others are attuned and responsive to them, they will not be developed into a communication system. For those individuals at the earliest stages of communication, it is vital to observe and record responses to routines and specific stimuli (the Affective Communication Assessment, Coupe O'Kane and Goldbart, 2000 is a useful tool for this). Observations at particular times of the day may highlight the fact that the client responds differentially to different stimuli. Although this can be done in real time, it is much more successful if video recorded, and then played back and analysed.

For example, the information in Table 7.7 was summarised from observations of a client named Sam.

Table 7.7. Sam – observational information

Sam's responses	Possible meanings
Stills at the sound of classical music	Like/accept
Looks at Tom when music stops	? More
Goes stiff when being put in chair	? Dislike
Shouts when Daniel comes into the room	Attention getting

These tentative observations and interpretations can form the basis of hypotheses regarding Sam's responses. Over a period of time, it will be possible to observe whether there are consistencies in responses which enable staff to understand him more systematically. A 'gesture dictionary' can be produced and added to on a regular basis, with the aim of giving unfamiliar people clues as to how to interpret and respond to his responses (see also Chapter 5 in this book). The format of this should be quite informal and personal, and written in the first person, so that it helps others to become familiar with the client as a person. This might be particularly useful with the individual with challenging behaviours which need to be responded to with very specific strategies (see Chapter 9 in this book). It is also documentation that can go with the individual at transition stages, to cue people in to the individual very quickly.

Moving on with switches

When it is felt that a client's responses have some consistent communicative meaning, the interpretation can be verbalised (e.g. 'oh you're looking at me, you want some more') and responded to. It may be that a client is assisted to press a switch attached to a tape recorder playing music, so that they can produce more music. Although it may not be intentional at this stage, it is important that the client realises that they have made something happen. A switch can be used to operate most battery-operated or simple electrical gadgets. At this stage, where the aim is to help the client to realise that they can make things happen, it is very motivating for the younger child to make toys work, or for the adolescent or adult to switch on a tape recorder, fan, bedside lamp or hairdryer. If the institution has a

Sneozelen area this can usually be operated by switches so that the client can control the different areas within it. It may be possible to gauge from these responses what motivates the client and introduce an element of choice. If the client is mobile, they may move towards certain areas and press the switch to make something happen. For less physically able individuals, another person may need to take them to different areas and then observe the levels of response. The aim is to move from an unintentional to an intentional response, and then for it to become more selective. The choice-making at this stage is relatively spontaneous and intuitive, but will become more structured as responses develop.

The next stage could be to use a switch that 'talks' and thereby add a verbal component. The AbleNet BIGmack switch (AbleNet Inc.) is a small, single-message, battery-powered communication aid that has 20 seconds of memory. When activated, it plays a recorded message. It can also activate a battery-operated device so the client could be assisted to activate the switch that would then say 'more music' and the tape recorder would play the music for 20 seconds. Other early interactional messages that can be used at this stage are 'hello', 'come here', 'more', 'go', 'stop' and 'my turn'. These are messages that can be used frequently, will always make something happen, and will provide the scaffolding for developing early social meanings. The client may not initially understand the meanings of the messages, but will learn by their outcome and effect how they can be used.

Once the client is beginning to use early interactional messages with some meaning, more purposeful choice-making can be established. This is best done in regular routines where there are definite and meaningful choices to be made, and definite consequences of making those choices: for example, drink and meal times. A client is given a choice between two drinks – milk and Coke – by being presented with them both, tasting them if necessary, and then reaching for the Coke. They are then prompted to ask for the requested item by pressing a switch that will say 'Coke, please'. Drinking the Coke will reinforce the meaning behind the message, and if they want another sip, they can press the switch again. The client learns that the picture of the Coke bottle represents Coke, so they are shown the photo while drinking; the assistant also shows the picture to another member of staff saying 'Andrew chose Coke today', and then the picture is placed on the switch to reinforce that the switch message represents Coke.

In an adult day centre, the drinks choices may be organised slightly differently and aimed at a group of people rather than an individual. The coffee jar and tea bags are placed next to each other in the kitchen and in front of each is a switch. The switch in front of the coffee jar has a pictorial symbol representing coffee, with the written word underneath it; the switch in front of the tea bags similarly represents tea. When a client comes into the kitchen, they are offered the two choices. If the tea bags are chosen, they are prompted to press the switch which then speaks the message 'tea, please'.

Developing choice-making

Once choice-making has been established, those working with the client will need to consider how to develop it. This will depend very much on the client's language, cognitive, social, representational and physical level. At its most refined, informed choice-making eventually leads to empowerment and independence for the client. Some of these choices may never be available to people with LD but it is important to understand that there is a continuum which begins with very early preferences, moves through basic choices such as what to wear, and eventually involves life decisions such as where to live and whom to vote for. Often, what is classed as choice-making may be little more than a staff member briefly holding two pictures in front of someone and, if they show any interest in either, assuming the choice has been made. This does not fit anywhere on the continuum. The aim is to develop quality choices at every level; they should be meaningful, relevant, motivating and accessible.

- *meaningful* – the individual should understand what the choice means, either because they have already experienced it, or it has been explained clearly in appropriate language
- *relevant* it should relate to what is happening in the individual's environment and have some significant effect on their situation
- *motivating* – there should be some good reason to choose one of the options, and probably to discard other options
- *accessible* – it should be possible to make the choice, both physically (for example if the client is only able to choose by eye-pointing, the choices need to be placed far enough apart to make this possible) and cognitively (the choice needs to be presented at the appropriate representational level – written words would not be accessible for someone who cannot read).

By increasing the array of choices, more options are opened to the client. For those who are cognitively able to make more choices but whose physical limitations mean they can only directly select from a choice of two, it may be possible to make choices using one or two switches. The choices can be presented as an overlay on a simple communication aid such as an ORAC (Morphonics), or on a Clicker grid (Crick Computing) on the computer. If the individual is able to use two switches, they press one switch to make a light scan each of the symbols, and the other switch to select the chosen symbol (step scanning). If the client is only able to use one switch, the light will be set up to slowly scan each of the symbols automatically and the client will press the switch to make the light stop and make the selection (automatic scanning).

Using objects

If the client is at a representational level where pictures are not yet meaningful, it may be necessary to develop early meanings and choice-making through objects (see Rowland and Schweigert, 1989). Clients may continue to use objects as their main mode of communication, either because their visual impairment is such that they will always require tactile symbols, or because cognitively they require very concrete and tangible symbols, or objects may be stepping stones towards a more representational symbol system.

The use of manual signs

If the individual has shown an ability to use natural gesture and an interest in imitating and using manual signs, this might become the main mode of communication. Although there are several other manual sign vocabularies, the one used most commonly in schools and centres for people with LD is BSL in the Makaton programme (see earlier). Key signs are used by staff alongside verbal input, to assist a client's learning of concepts and language and as a model for the user to imitate. Unlike symbols, which usually have the written word underneath so that people unfamiliar with a sign language can understand them, it may be difficult for people unfamiliar with a sign language to understand what is being communicated. It is necessary, therefore, for all those in a signing environment to learn at least the basics of the sign vocabulary being used. Another disadvantage with signs is that they are transitory and someone who is slow at processing information might forget what has been said. Also, some clients may lack the physical skills to produce good clearly articulated signs, leading to misunderstandings and frustration. However, there are some very definite advantages which make signing an AAC mode worthy of consideration at least alongside other modes of communication:

- It is an unaided mode of communication and therefore, like speech, it requires no equipment and can be used at any time.
- When signing is used well, it means that the input of the teacher closely matches the output of the user, i.e. the teacher will consider the level of the user's understanding and will present signs at that level, presenting clear input and a good model from which the user can learn. If a client is using a communication aid, and often when symbols are used, it is likely that the user will receive input verbally and be expected to produce the message using symbols. This leads to input–output asymmetries (Grove and Smith, 1997)
- Although having to train all the people associated with a signer is time consuming, it is in fact very beneficial from the signer's point of view, in that it will help others to feel more responsible for the success of the communication and feel more ownership of the system, than if the individual was using symbols that did not require any learning by the staff.

Using graphic symbols

Graphic symbols are widely used in schools, centres and colleges and they have become increasingly accessible through computer programmes such as Boardmaker and Writing with Symbols 2000. Not only can individual symbols, symbol charts and symbol communication books be produced for AAC users, but users themselves can create their own 'written' work, using computer programmes such as Writing With Symbols 2000 and Clicker. In addition, similar symbol sets can be found on communication aids allowing for compatibility across modes, and in a range of environments. It is important, therefore, to be aware of some of the issues relating to symbols which may get lost in the enthusiasm for using them as widely as possible.

Before introducing symbols to a client, it is important to ask the question, 'Does the user understand that a pictorial symbol has meaning, and represents something else?' If not, it may be necessary to teach this through exposure to symbols in the context of real experience. If symbols are considered appropriate, the next question is 'Which symbol set?' This is a very complex question and is the subject of a great deal of research in the field of AAC (see Loncke et al., 1999:157–203 for some of the recent theoretical discussion). Some of the questions that could be asked are:

- Should the institution use one symbol set for the whole institution so that there is consistency and a community of similar users, or decide on the most appropriate symbol set for each individual?

- Should the institution use a symbol set that can be easily reproduced, so that charts and displays can be made up quickly and everyone can have access to symbols?
- If most of the individuals in the institution use signs used in Makaton, should the Makaton symbol set be used for compatibility?
- Should symbols be chosen for their attractiveness?
- Should symbols be chosen because they are more guessable and more easily learned (i.e. more pictorial) (Musselwhite and Ruscello, 1984; Mizuko, 1987; Bloomberg et al., 1990), or because they are more likely to enhance language and literacy development (i.e. more representative and arbitrary but with a capacity for linguistic processing) (Schlosser, 1997a:4–13, 1997b:14–29)?
- Which symbols are more motivating and likely to start up conversations?

There is not a definitive answer to these questions. However, it is important that people who are responsible for making decisions within schools and centres ensure that they have at least considered these questions before introducing and using symbols. There are two general rules. First, when introducing symbols with young and less able users, it is important to get started quickly and ensure that symbols are used in every aspect of the environment (Elder and Goossens, 1994; Goossens et al., 1994). This can be done by, for example, ensuring that:

- there are aided language displays in all activity areas, which can be picked up and used by any member of staff
- story books are augmented by symbols
- Velcro-compatible boards are placed on the walls so that symbols can be Velcroed on to them and taken off again
- staff wear Velcro-compatible aprons when working with a group so that symbols can be easily Velcroed on to them while running an activity.

Second, if a client shows potential for developing good language and literacy skills, pictorial symbols may not provide sufficient vocabulary for developing concepts, creating new words by combining symbols or adding grammatical markers. Perhaps a more representative and arbitrary system such as Blissymbols should be considered.

For more information about symbol systems, the reader is referred to Glennen and DeCoste (1997:97–148), Beukelman and Mirenda (1998:39–88) and MacDonald (1998).

Voice output communication aids (VOCAS)

VOCAs are technologically the most sophisticated mode of AAC, and, for the able user, they provide a means of interacting more fully in the world of oral communicators. They are not without problems, however: they are expensive, they break down, their batteries need charging, their vocabularies need constant updating; they become outdated and often end up in a cupboard! The user may take a long time creating a message and then nobody listens, or the group has moved on to another topic, or the user has missed what everybody else has said. The skills involved in using a communication aid effectively are very complex, requiring years of learning by the user and everyone else in the environment.

However, a VOCA gives the client a voice and this is vitally important. It allows the user to take more responsibility for a conversation, without the need for an interpreter. It gives feedback to the user as to the appropriateness of a message. For example, if a user is unsure of a new symbol, selecting it will reveal what it means. Users who are learning how to combine words or phrases to create a sentence can hear how it sounds and whether to add extra words, or change the order around.

As with the selection of a symbol vocabulary, there are many decisions to be made when selecting a VOCA for a particular person and these relate to the individual's specific skills and needs. Some of the issues that need to be addressed are:

- Is it better for an institution to have the same type of device for all users so that there is compatibility with vocabularies and programming, and staff feel confident about working with the aid? This may be important and there are many institutions that have decided to do this, but does this limit some individuals?
- Does the user require a sophisticated expensive aid that has the capability for a vast vocabulary (for example a Dynavox, Cameleon or DeltaTalker), or are their vocabulary needs going to be limited to about 50 core phrases which could quite easily be recorded on to an ORAC, Macaw or Messagemate?
- If the user requires a more sophisticated VOCA, should it be a dedicated communication aid such as a Dynavox, or a personal computer with a vocabulary package (e.g. Cameleon), which can also be used as a computer for other work?
- Should the VOCA be a device with a dynamic screen, which allows the user to select pages for each category, and make up sentences from a number of pages (e.g. Dynavox or Cameleon) or should it have a static

taining an unchanging group of multi-meaning symbols
ɔe combined to create new utterances (e.g. DeltaTalker)? Or
ɩmbine the two methods, as with the Pathfinder?

ɪt is important to decide what vocabulary should be used with the device. Most devices have a vocabulary already programmed in, although this can be personalised for the user. This will dictate the vocabulary to a certain extent. However, some important considerations are:

- Should the vocabulary be mainly words or phrases? Phrases are quicker and more interactive, but much less flexible than words, and do not allow for creation of novel sentences.
- If the system is a dynamic screen system, how should each page be organised to allow for efficient retrieval of vocabulary?
- How can the vocabulary be both fun and interactive and yet useful in school lessons?

In addition, decisions will need to be made about how to access the device. If the user is physically able to directly select the keys by fist or finger pointing, this is by far the quickest method. If the user is less physically able, the team will need to assess the most effective method of switch access and this may change over time as skills develop.

There has been a great deal of discussion and research related to the topics above that can only be touched upon in this chapter. For a fuller discussion the reader is referred to authors such as Newell (1987); Woltosz (1988); Beukelman et al. (1991); Quist and Blischak (1992); Ratcliff (1994); Hill (1999); Romich and Spiegel (1999) and Peterson et al. (2000). For more information on types of communication aids, see Jans and Clark (1998a,b) and Rumble and Larcher (1998).

AAC and the development of language

For many AAC users the aim is 'functional' communication. However, for those individuals capable of developing language through augmented means, it is important to select vocabulary, symbols and teaching strategies that will enhance this. In order to build semantic knowledge, users should have sufficient access to an increasing and dynamic vocabulary of symbols that is appropriate to their needs and interests. It will need to be regularly updated using information gained from all those who interact with the AAC user and by careful observation of the vocabulary usage of those in the user's environment (see Yorkston et al., 1989; Beukelman et al., 1991; Fried-Oken and More, 1992; Beukelman and Mirenda, 1998; and Balandin and Ianoco, 1999). Nelson (1992) questioned how we can 'know whether a pre-literate child might actually have a variety of words in mind to express a concept or communicate a feeling, but cannot because the words are inaccessible for expression?' (Nelson, 1992:4). New vocabulary should be introduced with teaching strategies that make symbol–referent connections visually explicit – for example, by pointing to the symbol while introducing the concept. In relation to morphology and syntax, research has shown that:

- Symbol users rarely use more than one- or two-word messages (Smith, 1996; van Balkom and Welle Donker-Gimbrere, 1996).
- Symbol users and signers tend to use unusual word order (Grove et al., 1996b).
- Symbol users omit verbs and articles, preferring to use nouns as verbs (Soto and Toro-Zambrana, 1995).
- People communicating by augmentative means use a number of multi-modal combinations (e.g. combine a symbol with a gesture) and create their own sign morphology (Grove et al., 1996b and Chapter 6 in this book).
- Symbol users and signers use word overextensions (e.g. 'fish' for 'whale') and other compensatory strategies because of a lack of necessary symbols and signs.
- Symbol users rarely use plurals or tenses.

There are many possible reasons for this lack of accurate syntactic and morphological use, related to the nature of the symbols presented to the user, the situation of communicating through augmented means and the fact that the user may have specific difficulties with language processing and learning. It may be that the listener should accept a gesture as a morphological marker, or that a sentence starting with a topic marker is an efficient way of cueing the listener in to a fuller sentence. However, if the aim is for development of well-structured sentences, the type of symbols being used must be considered. For example, Smith (1996) refers to the PCS symbol for 'sit' – a line drawing of a person sitting on a chair – which was pointed to by a research participant when asked to produce the word combination *girl, sit, on, chair*). It is also important to consider the way symbols are organised in displays (i.e. if the user is expected to combine syntactic categories they should be available on one display) and how symbol use is taught (i.e. through good clear modelling).

AAC and the development of literacy

With the introduction of the National Literacy Strategy in schools (DfEE, 1998a) there has been a great interest in the development of literacy at all levels, with a resulting exploration of the ways in which literacy can be accessible to all (Detheridge and Detheridge, 1997; EQUALS, 1997; Grove, 1998; Nichol and Rendle, 1998; Berger et al., 1999; Park, 2000). Literacy can be seen on a representational continuum from very early object use to the manipulation of letters to produce words and sentences. From the earliest level, symbols can give an individual a method of accessing and recording information, and a tangible means of retaining language; story-telling using objects and symbols can develop emotional and cognitive functioning and can provide imaginative experiences for all. It is important, therefore, to consider how objects and symbols can be used to effect these ends (see B Carpenter, 1999).

In order to develop more sophisticated literacy skills through symbols, the opportunities, strategies and equipment need to be carefully structured in order to promote representational transitions. The syntactic and phonological aspects of reading and spelling require the individual to understand how words can be combined and manipulated. There is much discussion on whether and how literacy skills can develop in the absence of speech (Bishop, 1985; Bishop and Robson, 1989; Smith, 1992; Blishak, 1994; Dahlgren Sandberg and Hjelmquist, 1996) and the relationship between graphic symbols and reading (Kelford Smith et al., 1989; Bishop et al., 1994; Rankin et al., 1994; McNaughton and Lindsay, 1995). The reader is referred to these for further information.

Ensuring communicative competence in AAC throughout the environment

Woll and Barnett (1998) described the importance of looking at AAC usage from a sociolinguistic perspective, taking into account not only the communicative competence of the individual, but the competence and language use within the environment. Unless the users are in an environment that values and encourages the development of AAC as a means of communication, they are unlikely to develop full competence, and in fact may lose skills gained in a more supportive environment. This has been shown in bilingual studies, where speakers of minority languages lose fluency through lack of usage, in studies of adult AAC users who lose skills after leaving school (Barnett, personal communication, 1998; Larcher, 1998) and even within classes in special schools where AAC user loses skills gained in one classroom environment when they transfer to another type of class (Smith-Lewis, 1994). If particular systems are seen as having lower status in relation to others (e.g. AAC in relation to spoken language; signs used in Makaton in relation to a communication aid) this may lead to devaluation of a system, and therefore lack of motivation to use it. Similarly, if a system is seen to be for a particular purpose (e.g. transfer of information), it may not be encouraged in other situations (e.g. social interaction). This will affect the vocabulary that is offered to the user, and the opportunities given for communication, inhibiting growth of competence in certain areas.

If language input is predominantly in spoken English, and output is expected to be in symbols, this may lead to significant asymmetry, and an increased imbalance between the development of understanding and use of language. Studies of language acquisition in first and second languages have shown the importance of early learning of a language, and that late exposure to a second language may result in limited fluency in that language. This provides evidence for not only starting early with AAC but also providing a consistent language base from which the individual can develop communicative competence. In order to provide a consistent, positive and knowledgeable environment that values, encourages and develops communicative competence through augmented means, there needs to be an AAC policy within the institution (see Chinner et al., 2001) and the staff and carers need regular training and support from the AAC team. This will entail whole-centre awareness training for all staff, specific training for those working with particular individuals, and professional development opportunities for key personnel. There are training packages available, such as My Turn to Speak (Pennington et al., 1993) aimed at the team involved with the child communicator, and Attitudes and Strategies towards AAC (Murphy and Scott, 1995) aimed at adolescent and adult AAC users and their 'pool' of communication partners, and many useful ideas and handouts in Cottier et al. (1997) and Talking Points (Thurman et al., 1991). Regular signing classes and updates on available systems and software will help staff to feel involved and knowledgeable.

In addition to whole-centre initiatives, individual 'communication passports' (McEwen and Millar, 1993), life stories (Hamilton and McKenzie, 1999), pictorial diaries and gesture dictionaries provide a means by which important information about a non-oral person and his/her AAC system can be transferred between centres. This is an excellent way both of assisting others to communicate with the individual and keeping a record of progress. If updated regularly and used by all those who interact with the individual, it can be a very important means of ensuring that the individual is given the best possible environment in which to develop communicative competence.

Conclusion

All clients use a range of modes of communication to augment oral speech. The extent to which non-oral modes need to be developed will depend on the effectiveness of oral speech. AAC as a field has come of age; technological, social and educational advances have ensured its place in the mainstream of therapeutic intervention. AAC is not an end, but a means to an end. It is a way of enabling all individuals to have more effective access to communication. Technological advances have enabled professionals to provide better equipment for non-oral individuals, but the skill is not in the tools, rather the way they are used, and the opportunities created for their use.

Communicative competence can be viewed on a continuum from very early pre-intentional responses, to the use of sophisticated language and literacy skills; AAC is a means to increase the effectiveness of the communication at any point along the continuum. Not only do clients need to develop their communicative competence, but everyone in their environment has a responsibility to assist in this development. The more need there is for specific interpretation, or use of modes other than speech, the greater the skill and creativeness required by those in the environment. The two main groups of people who are involved in this are the professionals who have expert knowledge about 'developing communication', and the parents, or carers, who have expert knowledge about the client. It is essential that information passes freely and regularly between these two groups, and is collated and co-ordinated by one key person, especially at times of transition (e.g. starting school, changing classes, leaving school, changing residential placements).

There is still a long way to go and many attitude, knowledge and skill barriers to be broken down, in order for individuals with LD and communication impairments to receive the consistent and appropriate opportunities for developing their communication through AAC. However, there are now many examples of good practice, and technology, through software development and the internet, has provided a very effective means for these examples to be shared by a wide range of people.

Appendix: Resources and suppliers

Cambridge Adaptive Communication
The Mount, Toft, Cambridge CB3 2RU
Tel: 01223 264244
Email: david@camad.demon.co.uk
(supplier of Cameleon, MessageMate, Mayer-Johnson resources and a
wide range of switches and software including Clicker)

Communication Aids for Language and Learning (CALL Centre)
University of Edinburgh, 4 Buccleuch Place, Edinburgh EH8 9LW
Tel: 0131 667 1438
(publisher of a wide range of pamphlets and books on AAC)

Crick Software Ltd
1 The Avenue, Spinney Hill, Northampton NN3 6BA
Tel: 01604 671692
www.cricksoft.com
(supplier of Clicker software)

David Fulton Publishers
Ormond House, 26–27 Boswell Street, London WC1N 3JD
Tel: 0171 405 5606
(publisher of a range of books including special needs and PMLD)

Derbyshire Language Scheme
c/o Educational Psychological Service, Area Education Office, Market
House, Ripley, Derbyshire DE5 3BR
(supplier of Derbyshire Language Scheme resources)

Don Johnston Special Needs UK Ltd
18 Clarendon Court, Calver Road, Winwick Quay, Warrington WA2 8QP
Tel: 01925 241642
http://donjohnston.com
(supplier of Boardmaker PCS database and other special needs software
and access)

Easiaids Ltd
5 Woodcote Park Avenue, Purley, Surrey CR8 3NH
Tel: 0181 763 0203
(supplier of communication aids including Lightwriter, Fourtalk and Macaw)

Inclusive Technology
Saddleworth Business Centre, Huddersfield Road, Delph, Oldham
OL3 5DF
Tel: 01457 819790
http://www.inclusive.co.uk
(supplier of special needs software including Clicker and Writing with Symbols, and special access including AbleNet switches, Intellikeys, Concept Keyboards and Big Keys)

Liberator
Whitegates, Swinstead, Lincs NG33 4PA
Tel: 0146 550391
www.liberator.co.uk
(supplier of a range of communication aids including Chatbox, WalkerTalker, AlphaTalker, DeltaTalker, Liberator, Vanguard, Pathfinder; also Ablenet switches and simple technology, including Big Red switches, jelly bean switches and BIGmacks

Makaton Vocabulary Development Project
31 Firwood Drive, Camberley, Surrey GU15 3QD
(supplier of all Makaton sign and symbol materials)

Morphonics
5 Sharpes Hill, White Cross, Lancaster LA1 4XO
Tel: 01524 848373
Email: contact@morphonics.com

QED
Ability House, 242 Gosport, Fareham, Hampshire PO16 0SS
Tel: 01329 828444
www.qedltd.uk.com
(supplier of switches, mounting systems and a range of communication aids)

Royal National Institute for Deaf People (RNID)

105 Gower Street, London WC1E 6AH

Tel: 0171 387 8033

(supplier of information about hearing impairment and British Sign Language)

Royal National Institute for the Blind (RNIB)

National Education Centre, Garrow House, 190 Kensal Road, London W10 5BT

Tel: 0181 968 8600

(resources related to visual impairment)

SEMERC

1 Broadbent Road, Watersheddings, Oldham OL1 4LB

Tel: 0161 627 4469

www.semerc.com

(special needs software and switches)

STASS Publications

44 North Road, Ponteland, Northumberland NE20 NUR

(supplier of Cued Articulation, Cued Vowels and other language assessment and therapy materials)

Sunrise Medical

High Street, Wollaston, West Midlands DY8 4PS

Tel: 01384 446688

(supplier of Dynavox, Dynamyte and Dynamo)

Toby Churchill

10 City Business Centre, Hyde Street, Winchester SO23 7TA

Tel: 01962 842792

(supplier of Lightwriter and Macaw)

Widgit Software

102 Radford Road, Leamington Spa CV31 1LF

Tel: 01926 885303

http://www.widgit.com

(suppliers of Writing with Symbols, Boardmaker and a wide range of symbol software. They also run training courses)

Winslow Press
Telford Road, Bicester, Oxon OX6 OTS
www.winslow-press.co.uk
(supplier for Makaton and Hanen resources, and also Mayer-Johnson
materials including PCS symbol books)

CHAPTER 8

Working with Parents, Carers and Related Professions

SUE DOBSON AND ANGELA HURD

Abstract

The practice of the speech and language therapist (SLT) with individual clients is dictated by the differing aspects of their assessed communication strengths and needs. However, the style of implementation and the approaches which are acceptable to the significant others in the client's daily living patterns are open to a variety of different creative solutions. The success of these approaches is dependent on the understanding of the parents and the collaboration of the staff involved with the clients. Such interdisciplinary solutions therefore depend on the successful presentation and implementation of a challenging therapeutic role involving the SLT as a resource as well as a practitioner.

The delivery of speech and language therapy services for whole groups (i.e. parents, schools and staff teams) is discussed. The case studies presented illustrate collaborative aspects of working for the benefit of clients in the special school setting, in a residential care unit and a resource centre.

Introduction

People with learning disabilities (LD) enjoy a lifestyle that embraces a variety of activities and settings. This affects a large number of others within their local community. McConkey (1991:285–302) reasoned that it is society's response to individuals with LD which determines the degree of handicap they experience. Services to these clients must therefore place a high emphasis on encouraging participation in the care process. He concluded that it is mainly for this reason that modern

221

services place a much greater emphasis on community involvement. This suggests that the effectiveness of services can be measured by the lifestyle that they enable people with LD to experience.

The holistic care of a child or an adult with LD requires both ingenuity and creativity in implementing intervention programmes and in the establishment of appropriate and effective support systems. One of the main issues is identifying who should be involved in the therapy programme. The network of services that each individual can access and the available pathways of care can be complex. It can be hard to judge which significant others need access and to what level of information. Each SLT has to develop a working knowledge of the communication systems in their localities and ensure that there is an efficient information flow. Management strategies such as 'networking' and 'cascading' of information have therefore become a necessary part of the SLT's skills.

Clients with LD living at home, whether attending a special school and/or a day centre, may have respite residential care or a home care service, and/or attend an after-school club. An adult living in a small residential home could equally expect a wide circle of care workers and professional staff to be involved in their life. They could have up to 12 or more full- and part-time staff involved in their home environment. They could also attend a selection of daycare settings for educational, leisure or occupational activities, or they may have the option of access to other services for evening and weekend activities. There may also be visits to their family home. This means that 75 people or more could communicate and socially interact with the client in any one week.

All these scenarios would also involve people in the client's fringe who have opportunities for influencing the communication experiences and environment of this care group. Catering assistants, drivers and escorts, as well as the people within the local community such as shop assistants and staff in supermarkets, libraries, country parks, etc. also have an impact on the quality of communication environment for this client group.

Review of the literature

The literature indicates that the most successful speech and language therapy interventions for people with LD are those which take place in naturalistic environments (Owens and Rogerson, 1988; Girolametto et al., 1993; Nind and Hewett, 1994). The SLT's practice has gradually developed from the historical provision of one-to-one structured individual communication programmes (see also Chapter 3 in this book). In the past, the role of parents and carers was restricted to implementing the generalisation programmes for context-specific skills (Halle, 1988:155–86). The modern SLT's role has gradually moved away from that of someone who 'occupied' clients at certain times of the day (Brigden and Todd, 1993).

The SLT's new role with both children and adults has become that of a resource for parents and carers (Falvey et al., 1988:45–66). The design of the individual's intervention programme remains the SLT's fundamental role but practice involves more emphasis on ensuring the parents and carers are active partners and key players in the therapeutic process. The SLT is more likely to adopt the role of a consultant and trainer who supports and reviews the intervention which is delivered by the family or carers. However, this service model should not be the easier option when there is inadequate speech and language therapy provision. It requires a good deal of time and energy on the part of the SLT (Lees and Urwin, 1991). Such an approach does not reduce the therapeutic time involved in delivering each care package. McConkey (1991) stated that unless sufficiently supported by the SLT, the approach can leave the carers struggling. He also cautions that training has to break away from narrowly defined areas of skill acquisition, or attitude change, and address broader environmental issues. The SLT using this type of service model still provides a care package suitable for the needs of each individual. However, the key is in the frequency, intensity and quality of support provided for the carers. Van der Gaag and Dormandy (1993) suggested that such interventions should always be designed to improve the quality of life and provide a range of appropriate language experiences. For several years, naturalistic procedures have focused on parent–child interaction and have thus led to SLTs adopting a much more collaborative approach to language intervention (Iacono et al., 1998).

Empowering parents and giving them a key role in their child's intervention programme has several benefits. It allows parents to feel part of the team (Iacono et al., 1998). This issue sometimes gets lost, particularly when a service is expert-model driven. For example, it is not uncommon for the parents of a child attending for a set period of assessment at a Child Development Centre (CDC) to be given a diagnosis and have a detailed report to take home, but yet have inadequate support services to actually 'do' something about the concerns raised. It is impossible to get a rounded view of a child's communication skills unless the child is seen with a range of people in a range of situations. Many children are loath to 'perform' or speak to strangers in unfamiliar contexts; this is no less true of children with special needs, yet assessment based in the CDC, which often presents as an unfamiliar setting for the child, is a common model of service delivery.

There have, however, been developments since the time when all young children were seen in community clinics. Currently, many services in the UK are beginning to address the needs of the child, parents and community by taking speech and language therapy to the home, nursery and playgroup. However, this is not the case everywhere and there are areas in the UK where the community-clinic model dominates, for a number of reasons.

Therapists often wonder why some clinics have such poor attendance – looking at it from the parents' point of view, is it surprising? When asked, parents report a range of reasons including fear, family pressures and practical constraints. Tizard et al. (1981) interviewed parents and teachers about nursery activities. She found that 6 out of 14 members of staff thought the parents made no positive contribution to their children's education. However, the researchers found that between two-fifths and three-quarters of parents were in fact trying to teach their child to write, count and read.

As Fox (1975) further found, parents' failure to attend clinic does not mean they are not interested in the care and development of their child. One parent reported feeling intimidated by the SLT's knowledge level in contrast to her own. She felt that she belonged to a lower social class than the SLT and this created a barrier. This mother also felt that the SLT spoke as though she knew more about the child and the parent than the parent herself. Newson (1976), however, noted the assumption has to be made that parents are important resources in imparting information on their children about whom they are experts.

Dockrell (1989) found that parents very much wanted to be involved in their child's therapy. Her provision of groups for parents resulted in a decrease in the feelings of isolation and an increase in their feelings of competence. Not only were there benefits for the parents, but the SLTs involved reported that there was a decrease in the number of difficult parents (Dockrell, 1989). The sessions offered were attended by 65 adults, and several themes were identified:

- isolation and need for support
- difficulties in dealing with organisations/diagnosis
- the effect on other children
- marital problems
- child behaviour problems
- the future of the child and family.

Unless these issues are considered, the SLT can never gain a holistic view of the family and their needs. It is not surprising that, with all the stresses in their life, some parents can be perceived as 'difficult' by some of the professionals involved. Dockrell (1989:146–56) found that parents had needs in addition to the specific requirement of speech and language therapy for their children. Kelsey (1991) adopted the 'consumer model' of parent–professional relationship. In this model (Cunningham and Davis, 1985), unlike the 'expert' and 'transplant' models, the parent takes an equal part in the decision-making process. Kelsey (1991) investigated the way parent partnership could operate in the treatment of children with communication difficulties. All the professionals and parents responding to their initial questionnaire felt that parents needed to be more engaged in the treatment of their own children. Following implementation of their scheme, all the parents felt that they had gained useful information about the nature of their child's impairment and all felt more able to help their own child. Initially, parents favoured weekly therapy, with home-based services and some work in school or nursery with the child. However, several additional issues were highlighted at the end of the study, including a variety of models of therapy being available and the need for establishing a parent contact group. Overall, Kelsey (1991) found that parents wished to be better informed, to meet other parents and to be more involved in therapy. In our experience, this appears to be a constant need.

Iacono et al. (1998) demonstrated the potential for a collaborative model of service delivery within early intervention, and this can have long-term benefits for the child and the family. There are obviously benefits to parent empowerment for everybody involved, but it is also important not to forget that parents are first and foremost parents. If they are short of time and energy, involvement in a therapy programme may lead to stress and feelings of guilt (Tannock and Girolametto, 1992). Being the parent of a child with special needs is stressful in itself. Almond (1998) reported on what it was like to be both a SLT and a mother of a child with special needs. She felt that there was an urgent need to improve communication, time between sessions, and practical support, and to reduce the burden of empowerment because sometimes it felt as if the SLT handed over all the responsibility for the success or failure of the suggested therapy to parents and that this in turn led to tremendous guilt and frustration. Management implementation issues such as these clearly need to be addressed.

Despite the philosophical issues of turning parents into teachers, it clearly is the most effective path for the child and, arguably, for the parents. Whalley (2001:55) noted

> for those parents who do become involved in their children's learning, there are many benefits relating to both their understanding of their children and their own raised self esteem.

Research shows that the relationship between the child's linguistic behaviour and development and the parents' interaction style is reciprocal (Kelman and Schneider, 1994). The child's language output is thus affected and influenced by the mother's language input, and vice versa. This said, it is then quite difficult for the SLT to improve the parents' interaction style so that the child can gain additional communication skill. It is inevitable that some parents will feel responsible for the child's special needs in the first place, and then for the language and communication difficulties their child has. The SLT has to ensure that parents understand that they are adapting their language style because of the child's special needs and not because of anything they have or have not done (Conti-Ramsden, 1994). A number of studies have looked at parental interaction style. Kelman and Schneider (1994:93) studied the overuse of directives by parents. Their focus was on parent–child interaction patterns. They hypothesised that changing patterns in verbal and non-verbal interaction will improve the child's communicative competence without the need to focus on the child's language skills. They identified parent 'directiveness' as being important as 'parental directiveness has proven to be a key area for modification, as it has a marked influence on the child's verbal output'. Their aim was to train and encourage parents to follow the child's lead, gain and maintain the child's attention, improve their turn-taking abilities, and modify content and their linguistic input. A two-pronged approach was used. This comprised weekly sessions following video analysis, and a parent group focusing on specific exercises. The study involved 28 families with children aged 3;3 to 5;1 years of age. The study highlighted the influence on the children's language development of both verbal and non-verbal directiveness. The influence of the caregiver's relationship to the child, socio-economic background and the interaction style of the parent were also found to be important to the success of the intervention. Involving parents in the therapy was found to be beneficial in the outcome of therapy but with certain reservations, primarily addressed at the relationship between the parents and child's language behaviour.   ·

McDade (1981) followed a similar line and found that for the children's behaviour to change, the parents' must change also. Again this was done through involving the parents much more in their child's therapy. It is interesting to note that Baker (1976) made the point that most special school programmes allow the parent to assume the role of an uninformed spectator. Change in this area has been variable and seems to depend on the individual school and staff involved. This is a fair point, but how far have we come in actually solving the problem? One possible solution offered was the Hanen Parent Programme (Manolson, 1992). However, Gibbard (1998) argued that this approach is based on sparse evaluation. She argued that providing input that is frequent, familiar, repetitive and salient is not enough. This general language stimulation becomes less useful after single-word vocabulary has been established. There is a need to be more specific about language objectives. This would seem to make sense if parents are going to be motivated to carry out and continue working on intervention programmes at home. Having a child with special needs brings with it many challenges, not least the feeling of being a 'bad mother' which can be engendered when focusing on giving carers only a general indication of what they need to do rather than specific detailed objectives and activities. Fulford and Malcomess (1995) made the point that all cases are different; each behaviour and feeling, and reaction to each of these, varies from parent to child. They highlighted the need for SLTs to be more aware of the emotional relationship between the parent and child, not just the parent–child interaction. Without giving more importance to the therapeutic relationship between the parent and the therapist too, Fulford and Malcomess (1995) felt that lasting change becomes impossible. This is because the underlying emotional issues need to be addressed from a psychoanalytic and systematic thinking perspective.

Language enrichment programmes alone cannot allow for this critical emotional perspective, where exploration of the child's feelings and the parents' reaction are important to the success of the intervention. It could be argued that we are currently far from this model of 'best practice', yet, given the focus on outcomes, it has to be a critical consideration. This could indicate that rather more training for SLTs is needed in this area.

Having reviewed a range of studies, Tannock and Girolametto (1992) suggested that children's outcomes in terms of language and communication results were at best unreliable. They found several methodological weaknesses including small sample sizes, ignoring of maturation effects and general measurement difficulties. However, in studies where the parents were trained, a noticeable improvement was made in the parental interaction style subsequent to training sessions with a SLT. Simply telling parents what to do was not enough, i.e. they need to be trained. Kot and Law (1995) found significant improvements in parental interaction behaviours after these issues of training parents in how to improve their interaction were highlighted. However, there was no control group in the Kot and Law study (1995) and methodological weaknesses have been common in this type of research. Gibbard (1994:205) compared fortnightly training of mothers, over a 6 month period, with a control group. She also compared group versus individual therapy for children. From the two experiments and three groups, she found that there were 'significantly greater gains in the parental language training group and the individual speech therapy group in comparison with the non-specific training group'. She further compared groups of parents who had been trained to provide language-specific intervention and non-language-specific intervention with direct intervention from the SLT. The results clearly demonstrated that it was the group who had received language-specific intervention who produced the most improvement. It was suggested that parent-based intervention was at least as good as direct work with the SLT. However, this does not mean that working collaboratively with parents is an easy or more cost-effective option. Gibbard (1994) pointed out that specific language objectives were needed. She concluded, however, that if implemented appropriately so that SLTs give specific and appropriate advice, waiting lists could be reduced and the role of the SLT as consultant could be cost effective. Fey et al. (1993), (cited by Enderby and Emerson, 1995) found that in their study of 30 pre-school children aged between 3;8 and 5;10, all the children in the advice and intervention groups improved although those in the control group did not. However, the most improvement was seen in the children who had direct work with the SLT.

The recent literature seems to indicate that parents play a central and crucial role in the development of their children. Tannock and Girolametto (1992) noted that trained parents had numerous opportunities throughout the day to provide focused language intervention for their children, of much longer duration than any SLT can provide. Kelman and Schneider (1994) also pointed out that language improvements in the home are much more easily generalised and more resilient. However, it is clear from professional practice that parents need a detailed plan of what they should be doing. A number of parents report that general advice is just too vague and non-specific. The SLT involved needs to work in partnership but to give detailed and structured help to parents by demonstrating and encouraging parents to execute appropriate tasks in the SLT's presence. This can be followed by joint evaluation, discussion and training if necessary. Opportunities, reassurance and confidence must also be given to parents to report on and evaluate work they did outside the clinic, e.g. at home. In this way, the SLT can monitor their input, deal with any difficulties parents may have experienced in implementing the work (i.e. troubleshoot), inform, counsel, re-plan, facilitate, and so on.

Involving carers: practical issues

In order to work with parents then, there must be shifts in philosophy, as well as major changes for the service provision needed. The process must have its genesis in the first contact. Parents sometimes report that being referred at all seems to suggest to them a major questioning of their parenting skills. This, in addition to being faced with a host of professionals, each with their own priorities, with whom they have to interact, often makes life a potentially baffling and frustrating experience for the parents of a child with special needs. Parents need to be involved in the assessment process and then given the means and tools for intervention in order to deal with their child's communication needs. Being told there is a problem and given no practical help to deal with it, or come to terms with it, can destroy the parent–child relationship, and justifiably alienate parents from the process.

The partnership should therefore start from the assessment process; the parent knows what the child can do, and what is practical to expect them to do subsequently. Negotiating this from the start avoids disappointments at a later stage. Glogowska and Campbell (2000) found that initial discrepancies between parental expectations and the reality of speech and language therapy could influence the course of therapy. Parents' emotions of fear and anxiety often predominated initially, but then they really wanted action, activities and ideas, not long-drawn-out assessments. SLTs are familiar with the concept of assessment through therapy and this should really be the focus. The key to a successful partnership is dialogue and discussion. The following opening gambits should therefore be considered:

- Parents should be provided with as much information about the service as possible (leaflets, discussion, telephone contact before meeting the therapists).

- Parents' expectations of the service and their role and responsibilities in the partnership must be explored.
- Therapy options should be discussed and these need to be updated as appropriate.

Working with other professionals can be either rewarding or fraught with difficulties. Inter-professional tensions often arise. Norwich (1990) found that the tensions regarding these issues were likely to arise if the SLT was not involved in direct service delivery to the child. The benefits of good collaborative practice, for example, in a school situation, are clear. The development of communication skills transcends the curriculum and this requirement results in the formulation of joint aims and intervention between the SLT and the teacher in the classroom, or throughout the child's day. However, when collaborative practice does not work well, conflicting ideas and issues such as conflicts in timetabling may predominate and work designed to enhance a child's communication skills may be perceived as being the sole responsibility of the SLT. This may lead to resentment and distrust by both the SLT and the teaching staff. Lack of time with a client and liaison with school staff and parents is even more apparent with children attending mainstream schools, where there is perhaps even less time available for a SLT to see clients than in a special school.

One possible method for enhancing collaborative practice in schools is to use the Speaking and Listening and Reading Package (Hurd and Rowley, 1991). This package was developed in response to several needs that were identified while working in a school for children with severe learning difficulties (SLDs), although subsequent application has been much more extensive than just children in school, i.e. from birth to later adulthood. Feedback from users indicates that there were a number of potential benefits when using the package. First, users found or reported that speaking and listening skills were integrated across the curriculum. They also reported that there was a more functional emphasis than in the Derbyshire Language Scheme (Knowles and Masidlover, 1982) and that there was an equal emphasis on pragmatics (language use) as on comprehension and sentence structure. In addition, the package provided a means of assessment and profiling that could be used throughout the school and move with the child as they changed class, and the teaching staff reported that the tool that was equally useful for all children, no matter their ability. Other advantages highlighted were that the assessment format allowed identification of key teaching goals, and that parents could understand the profile and see the relationship between spoken words and pre-linguistic skills. Language and reading also went hand in hand, so that each would benefit the other. Thus, a systematic reading programme was available for a child once a basic level of symbolic understanding had been reached.

Each child is profiled during their first school term. This involves collaboration between the SLT and the classroom staff, and also the parents are seen as key members of the team. Specific aims are then drawn up collaboratively. In addition to quantified and specific individual objectives across language and literacy, the programmes of study also highlight the fact that language is a means of learning throughout the school curriculum and throughout each key stage of the National Curriculum. For example, the programmes of study highlight a variety of appropriate opportunities to encourage and facilitate language development. Feedback from users of this programme also indicates that:

- learning experiences are relevant and meaningful for the child
- the joy of language and interaction is emphasised
- equal emphasis is provided on using language as well as on understanding it and increasing complexity.

Involving carers in services for children

The parents' interaction style, preferred method of communication, and skill at interpreting their children's concerns lead the care programmes for the pre-school child. Once they understand what speech and language therapy is about and are helped to become involved, Girolametto et al. (1993) found that parents could gain considerable personal benefit by working through a speech and language therapy programme. Their anxiety is often reduced and their confidence increased. However, Lees and Urwin (1991) cautioned that it is important for the professionals to remember that parents are not part-time therapists. Once the child's educational setting is agreed, the number of people who have to be involved in the child's therapeutic intervention increases. The SLT has to include a variety of education staff in the delivery of care. This changes the direction and emphasis of school-aged children's communication programmes. The range of potential influences during assessment and intervention affects the level and frequency of contact by the SLTs with children's parents.

After the initial years of school, parents often delegate their prime role in their child's therapy intervention programme to the education staff.

This trend to a school-led service delivery by SLTs has also been determined by the series of Education Acts that began in 1981 through to the more recent 1997 Green Paper. Both school- and home-based service models of speech and language therapy need flexible responses that meet parental concerns. The priorities of the education service and the health service can be at variance. A child's Statement of Educational Need may identify speech and language therapy as an immediate priority for the school. However, the local community NHS Trust may define their priorities in different ways. Districts with low staffing, or those larger districts which are made up of scattered rural communities, may have too few therapists to provide a high profile service in local schools. Staff turnover, frozen posts and the imposition of annual cost-efficiency savings dictate the type of service each locality can provide to schools. As a result, the issue for the grass-roots clinician is often not which philosophy of care is used, but what works given their particular local conditions. Barker (1991) stated that what parents need is help through a more efficient service rather than help with the pathology of the child's disorder. A holistic approach to care planning should, therefore, provide better therapeutic outcomes and greater benefits for all those involved in providing care. The important practical issues are how to provide comparable standards of support for all parents, the educators and the paid carers: care that is satisfactory for everyone concerned with the child and is cost effective for the providers of speech and language therapy services.

Case study 8.1

This case illustrates an inclusive programme which required a variety of intervention styles that had to be interwoven and managed within the child's lifestyle and include many significant people.

Stuart was an 11 year old boy who attended a special school and had a rare syndrome. He was very active, had a visual impairment and presented with challenging behaviour. His development of comprehension and his use of non-verbal methods of communication were much better than expected for children with the same syndrome. He showed frustration at his inability to communicate his needs or make himself understood. Even his mother and teacher were often unsure what message he was trying to convey. His level of understanding of spoken language was at a level of three information-carrying words as measured with the Derbyshire Language Scheme (Knowles and Masidlover, 1982).

He used a limited number of single words and signs, all of which were very difficult to interpret and understand. Previous therapy programmes had achieved some mixed successes, but had been limited by the severe challenging nature of his behaviour. A new care package was negotiated that included both his mother and the school. Stuart's programme covered a school year. It was designed to be an integrated part of a whole-school approach. The intervention aimed to include most of the important people in his life, i.e. parents, peers and school staff. There were training packages for his parents and the school staff.

The implementation of a whole school model of service delivery (Table 8.1) involved using therapy time in a different way. It also required the school's acceptance that fewer individual appointments would be available. The school had agreed to co-operate with the flexitime use of speech and language therapy time and to support the whole care package in various ways. The speech and language therapy skill mix within the school was altered to include a speech and language therapy assistant (SLTA). Stuart began to utilise more signs to support his speech both at home and at school. His utterances were more likely to be 2–3 word phrases than single words. He made use of symbol resources if he was misunderstood. Although he continued to have outbursts of challenging behaviour, these were much less frequent. His mother stated she was now able to take him shopping, something she would not previously have considered. They were also enjoying more activities together at home, not just the limited ones on which he had previously insisted. Stuart himself became much more confident and sociable and he would eagerly approach school visitors to initiate a conversation. However, strangers continued to find him difficult to understand and he still tended to interrupt class topic groups with his preferred conversational routines.

The school evaluated this flexitime model of service very positively. They felt the SLT was more valuable to them as a consultant and trainer. The SLT ceased to need a quiet room for one-to-one therapeutic input and this eased the pressure on the school to provide accommodation for speech and language therapy one-to-one sessions, as space was at a premium. All the parents availed themselves of the easier access to the SLT and initiated contact regularly to report on their children's progress, ask for advice, etc., rather than request direct individual or intensive therapy. Many knew the therapist from the various training sessions. They were therefore more likely to telephone for informal chats or visit the therapist at the school without waiting for a special event.

Table 8.1. Provision of child's care package

Action

For the school
Presentation to senior managers
Presentation to a staff meeting
Presentation to governors

For the staff
Hanen (Manolson, 1992) course for some teachers and support assistants
Whole staff: beginners and intermediate Makaton workshops
A series of courses on feeding for lunchtime staff
SLT to plan topics for parents' weekly coffee mornings

For the classroom
Assistance in introducing symbols into the classroom
Introduction of a Social Communication Programme
SLT modelling in group activities alongside classroom staff

For other invited parents
A daytime school-based Hanen course
A matching evening Hanen course
One daytime and one evening Makaton workshop
Joint talks from SLTs and teachers for sensory impairments

For the child (Stuart)
A class based Social Communication Group
Individual signs and symbols work with SLTA
A recommended programme for use in the classroom
A symbol book for the classroom

For Stuart's mother
Attendance at parents' Hanen and Makaton courses
Symbol book to assist conversation about school activities
A symbol resource for use with home story books
Discussions, suggestions and equipment for home activities
Increased use of signs to support her own speech

For the SLT
Becoming an NVQ 3 assessor/trainer for SLT assistants
Taking a mainly training, consultative and advisory role
Working flexible hours and timetables

Services for carers of adults with learning disabilities

The main speech and language therapy contact with carers for adults with LD is with either residential or daycare workers. It is these workers from health and social services or other agencies who lead the statutory review meetings and identify clients' need for referrals to support services. A community nurse from the LD team usually mediates any referrals from parents. These two types of referral are similar in that they usually occur at a period of crisis, or a time of transition. Barker (1991) contended that these critical periods occur at times which are potentially stressful for carers, in that they arise when developmental expectations are different from what actually takes place. Van der Gaag and Dormandy (1993), on the other hand, suggested that these critical periods are the result of both positive and negative transitions which arise when adults with LD need to learn to adjust to the stages of adulthood. These authors also argue that services for adults with LD should not remain developmentally based. The planning of interventions should focus on the relevant life experiences of the adolescent and adult.

The parents of adult clients who continue to live with their family tend to have few ongoing concerns about communication. Some families have, over the years, established a common system of communication and have discovered what is successful in the home. Referrals made by family members usually arise at times of bereavement or illness, or when changes in residence may need to be arranged. These referrals are situation specific and require the SLT to work in close liaison with the LD team. In contrast, residential and daycare referrals tend to be made because there are staffing or timetable changes which have, for example, resulted in alterations in the environment. The communication support that a client has previously relied upon may have been lost, and this has highlighted the client's communication difficulties in the new situation. These referrals are therefore usually specific to a setting and most are due to changes in circumstances, or the environment, rather than because the nature of the adult's communication has altered or changed.

Residential care staff referrals for adults

Care staff who are employed in residential care settings are often eager to obtain more information about their client's communication skills and needs and have positive expectations that the adults in their care can be helped to learn to communicate more effectively. Examination of an individual's case notes will often show a recurring series of episodes of speech and language therapy. Referrals are each made by a different member of the care staff. Each referral, however, may focus on a different aspect of the client's communication. Walker et al. (1995:232–43) quoted a Rowntree Trust survey in the UK which found that care workers assume that older people with LD have the same level of need as younger ones, speech and language therapy being the most frequently identified need for this age group.

Identifying why the referral has been made is an important factor in determining whether an agreed therapeutic goal can be negotiated with the referrer, or whether a successful outcome can be achieved. There are a number of difficulties in agreeing expected service outcomes. For example, the referrer may overestimate the client's communication potential. Circumstances may mean that the intervention programme would be inappropriate because of lack of management support or staff motivation, or because of difficulties in arranging meetings (van der Gaag and Dormandy, 1993). Staffing rotas in residential daycare settings may be so complex that it is not unusual for the referrer and the SLT only to be able to agree to holding meetings infrequently. Additionally, staff in small-group homes are more likely to experience burnout and stress, which may cause lack of enthusiasm for intervention programmes (Hegarty, 1987; Cade, 1993). Low staffing levels within such units may also affect the manager's ability to introduce changes. These combined factors may result in some types of intervention models being rejected. At other times, a referral can be a reflection of a manager's need to solve staff management problems, e.g. lack of competence or deficits in staff's performance. This means that the relevant manager needs to make clear statements of the management's expected outcomes of each intervention in terms of achievement for both the clients and the staff group. Intervention input focused on a client's needs can help staff develop the necessary skills for their posts. It cannot, however, alter staff performance or compensate for inappropriate appointments of staff.

The success of speech and language therapy programmes therefore depends as much on the personality and competence of the SLT as on the pro-active nature of the intervention strategies that are offered. In order to be successful, SLTs have to establish their own *persona* and recognise their own needs and preferences within their individual professional working context (Muir et al., 1991; van der Gaag and Dormandy, 1993). These, often difficult, working circumstances demand that the SLT delivering the service feels satisfied and comfortable with the planned intervention programmes, confident about their practice, and able to own, justify and evidence their practice. The service needs clear established guidelines, both for referral and for implementation of any recommendations. Any guidelines must have been negotiated, widely circulated and accepted at all staffing levels. However, even when such policies and written contracts are standard practice they may not always be utilised. They are often forgotten or ignored when the management's immediate concerns take precedence over a client's needs.

Case study 8.2

This case study shows the need for clear definition and agreement of what outcomes can be achieved and the renegotiation of the original statement of referral.

Bernice was a 54 year old woman who had spent most of her life in a large residential hospital. Four years previously she had moved to a small bungalow. Two nurses staffed the home with 10 part-time care assistants. Bernice's referral to speech and language therapy was accompanied by the signed agreement required by local district. The agreement stated that the referrer would be willing to support and implement any suggested intervention programme. The local speech and language policy required that documentation was sent to all referrers outlining the service philosophy and policies (Figure 8.1).

These statements gave the options of a request for a service for the client or a consultancy/advisory service for the staff. It was added that any referral statement should enable a realistic description of an achievable and measurable outcome. The information sent on receipt of the referral also indicated that any assessment would involve investigation of the client's social communication environment and a high level of carer involvement. The first appointment at Bernice's home coincided with a full staff meeting. This was arranged before any client contact to agree and define a statement of the expected outcome and health benefit. The referrer was, however, not present as she had left the service. Staff said she had observed that Bernice enjoyed pressing the keys of a toy computer and that she liked to hear the animal noises it made. She had felt that Bernice should be provided with a communication aid. The home manager had felt the toy had not been an age-appropriate activity but had supported the recommendation as she felt that it was time for a further speech and language therapy referral.

None of the other care staff really believed that Bernice had the ability to use a communication aid. They felt that she had been randomly hitting the toy's keys. However, they had supported the referral as they felt that if Bernice could say five words, she ought to have an intervention programme to put them into two-word phrases. They wished her to say 'toilet, please' rather than her current use of a single word utterance, e.g. 'pee'. The SLT concluded that the staff's reasons for referral failed to offer probable achievable outcomes, but there were other reasons for the SLT accepting the referral, which were not initially presented by the staff

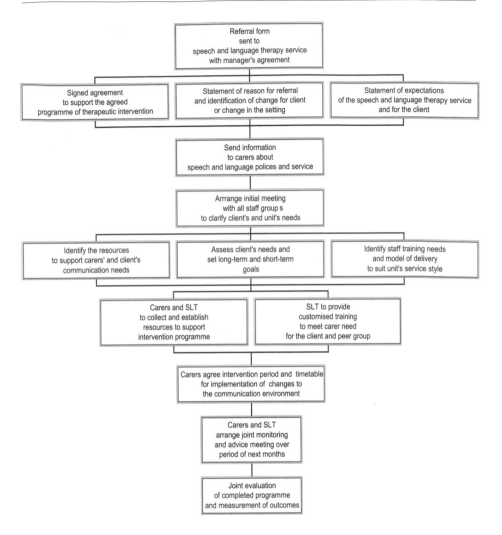

Figure 8.1. Sequence of negotiation with care staff.

group. Bernice's vision had deteriorated and she was severely visually impaired. She was easily distressed by people invading her personal space, and had become touch-defensive. She was now mainly reliant on the staff for physical movement. She spent most of her day in an armchair and occasionally moved about within the home using a walking frame. Outside the home she was pushed in a wheelchair and transported in a minibus. Some of these journeys resulted in Bernice showing outbursts of screaming and extreme distress. At these times, she would hit and scratch the care staff.

The assessment therefore focused on ways of supporting Bernice's understanding of her daily living environment rather than extending her use of communication. Ten key situations were identified; five were for events within the home to assist in the structuring of her daytime activities and the other five were for Bernice's environment outside the home. Her visits to a daycare centre, her sister's family and community outings, such as to the supermarket, were then matched to five objects of reference which she could be given before going out and to hold while on the minibus. These objects were chosen to have a high level of symbolic and contextual association with the imminent activity. For example, she held the purse she would use going shopping (Parkes, 1997). Members of staff were provided with a protocol outlining the use of these objects to support Bernice's situational understanding. The long-term aim was that Bernice should be encouraged to use the objects to communicate requests about activities, but initially they were used to enable staff to explain to her the reason for the movement, or journey. Within a fairly short period of time, this intervention resulted in a reduction of her outbursts of distress during journeys outside the unit, and thus a successful outcome.

The reason for referrals from care staff groups may sometimes initially appear to give little opportunity for success. The staff group themselves may have differing perceptions of the client's potential to communicate. However, it is always useful to explore staff's expectations of the service. A carer's stated reason for making the referral might mask a concern that they may be unable to explain without the SLT's help. Conversely, it is sometimes seen as correct procedure to request an in-depth communication assessment of the client's ability when staff may neither want nor need one. The care staff are usually the people who are most familiar with the client's level and style of communication. The SLT's role in this setting is to assist the care staff to become aware of their own knowledge and enable them to apply it in the context of the client's daily living environment. The SLT also has the further responsibility of liaising regularly with the locality's residential home managers to ensure that they are well informed about the role of the SLT and are competent to channel, monitor and focus the referrals made by their staff groups.

Daycare centre referrals for adults

SLTs working in daycare settings need to establish ownership and responsibility for the client's communication problem in large fluctuating care staff groups. The medical employment base of speech and language therapy has in the past fostered an 'expert' model of service with the responsibility for care owned by the specialist services rather than the users of the service. This allows carers little feeling of responsibility for communication within their own environment (Dobson, 1995). Speech and language therapy input for adults with LD most often concentrates on the quality of the communication environment that supports the adult's existing level of competence. This functional approach requires the staff teams to implement the changes recommended by the SLT. It concentrates on restructuring staff and peer group social interactions. The day centres require communication intervention programmes that foster those client's skills required for the client's independence in community placements. The SLT needs to successfully interweave both these differing expectations and co-ordinate the appropriate input with other supporting services.

A difficulty for SLTs can be a staff group's decision to make a simultaneous block of referrals for all types of intervention input for one individual. Differing waiting list times and priorities may then mean the client and staff then experience 'serial therapy' from different clinical specialisms over an extended period of time. The resulting variety of professional recommendations may not be linked to, or integrated into, a complete care plan. The direct care staff often lack, and cannot be expected to have, the necessary skills to integrate the fragmented information they receive from each separate profession's reports. This type of problem can only be addressed by adopting an inter-disciplinary approach using the concept of a 'core team' for each referral. In this way, an identified lead clinician provides the referrers with an integrated care package that is designed to include all the different recommendations for a management plan.

The underlying philosophy of care and the legislation involved in the provision of adult daycare has evolved from sheltered work environments, to social and leisure activity centres, and more recently, to fostering real employment. These various changes have had considerable influence on the parents and care staffs' expectation of the speech and language therapy services. The speech and language referrals received from daycare services may therefore often be defined as an expectation of the development of communication skills to enable participation and the potential access to a wider variety of community services.

Case study 8.3

This referral from a day centre demonstrates how a co-ordinated team response by an identified lead SLT can support an intervention for an existing communication problem which is triggered by a change in the client's social environment.

Michael was a quiet 36 year old man who was considered by staff to be polite, well-behaved and retiring. Nine months after Michael's only brother died of cancer, his centre keyworker sought advice about how to help him with his bereavement. Michael had gradually become less sociable and was at the time of referral refusing to join in his keygroup's social activities or outings. Care staff asked for advice on the language level and usage of communication that they should use to facilitate discussions on Michael's feelings and emotions about his brother's death. A clinical team consisting of a clinical psychologist, an occupational therapist and a SLT subsequently discussed the referral. The therapists believed Raghavan's (1998) view that a cognitive behavioural approach was more appropriate. This method suggested that the appropriate action was an intervention which aimed to improve social competency, rather than to facilitate discussions on grief and its processes. The SLT led the clinical team's response to the referral. All her actions were informed by regular discussions with the other members of the core team for this case. This involved the team sharing knowledge and skills about suitable activities, group dynamics and meta-cognitive approaches.

Assessment showed that Michael's 'quiet, shy manner' was masking a previously unidentified expressive communication problem. The staff's difficulty in understanding his use of extremely quiet, single-word answers and occasional use of a short phrase was not only due to inaudibility, or his reluctance to communicate. In addition, it was felt that he might have a degree of both verbal and manual dyspraxia. It was further apparent that Michael found one-to-one interactions distressing and preferred a very large social distance between himself and the speaker. His expression of emotions was limited to smiling when amused, or becoming physically agitated when distressed. His understanding of emotions in others was limited to the extremes of the 'happy/sad' parameter with some confused perceptions of 'fear/surprise' and 'anger'. This reflected the findings of Gray et al. (1983), who observed an inability in people with LD to cope with high-intensity emotions. Buitelaar et al. (1999) noted that inability to verbalise emotions effectively was linked to working memory skills and social and communication impairment.

It seemed that Michael's social withdrawal as an expression of grief for his brother had merely emphasised an existing long-term social communication problem. It was felt that Michael needed to be provided with a symbolic means of supporting and augmenting his existing verbal communication and to be encouraged to participate in small social groups. The core team's discussions with Michael's key care group about the assessment and recommendations resulted in a plan for change. The next time the day centre's timetables were reviewed, Michael was offered a greater number of centre-based activities. Two of these groups were specifically designed to support his social communication. The intention was to provide a routine with cognitive and verbal scripts with certain peers acting as role models (Volden and Johnston, 1999). Other of Michael's peers were involved with him in creating symbolic resources and games to support the work on understanding and expressing emotions. The groups stressed co-operative learning, achievement and constructive feedback. The aim was to use collaborative learning strategies to foster self-esteem (Goodwin, 1999).

The intervention programme targeted 'happiness/pleasure' and 'anger' and 'sadness', and was designed to include situations, actions, people and objects that triggered such emotions (see Table 8.2). Shades of differing emotions were represented by emotion thermometers which were both symbolic representations and had standard language scripts.

Michael's widowed father, who had chosen not to be involved with his son's intervention programme, was fully informed by the day centre and was provided with a copy of the assessment report and recommendations.

Michael's episodes of agitated behaviour became less frequent and he was active in choosing his timetable activities. The groups proved very

Table 8.2. Staff's action plan for Michael

Action

Formation of core team
OT, SLT, psychology and referrer
Identify lead clinician
Set meeting schedule

Preparation
Staff training about expressing emotions
Staff training about emotion and single-word use
Timetable and group composition discussions
Presentation to parent group about symbols and funding for software and laminator
Plan 8 weeks' theme and topic work
Modify software package for resources

Two groups' activities and organisation
Choose and make games and resources for 'Emotions' group
Allocate weekly topics to team members

For Michael's communication use
To create a small filofax of symbols

popular with both staff and day centre users. Michael enjoyed these centre-based activities and began to participate in them when specifically told that it was his turn, and there were several notable occasions when he actually forced a turn for himself within the activities. He enjoyed the use of symbols and the scripts. He was particularly proud of his personal filofax of symbols. There were continuing benefits when the day centre staff persuaded Michael's father to use symbols to correspond in the centre's home message book. It is of course difficult to attribute changes in his behaviour to the intervention programme, but it was thought that the programme had contributed to these changes, at least in some way. Staff felt he was more content, settled and socially active. The centre staff decided not to make any direct attempts at counselling Michael about his bereavement. The focus on social skills and the change in activities were seen as resolving the staff's original concerns. The provision and acceptance of symbolic communication to augment his interactions had extended his ability to communicate.

The problems that the care staff at day centres present to SLTs may be their personal view of a possible solution to an obvious problem. Staff may lack the knowledge or skill to identify the underlying cause of the presenting communication difficulty. The SLTs need to exercise skill and tact in order to negotiate an achievable and an agreed, realistic solution. When the problem is complex, it may involve the active co-operation of more than one profession. This does not mean all the core team members need to be involved in the direct management of the case. It may be difficult to gain the involvement of the parents of the people who attend day centres in the implementation of the care package. Older parents sometimes feel that their own involvement in any programme is no longer relevant. They may only occasionally be involved with the daycare service provision through social events or fundraising activities. Other parents may decline any involvement at all and require only that they are fully informed of their son's or daughter's care package. Referrals to other support services, which involve increasing their son's or daughter's social skills, may be seen as unnecessary. The parents may be pensioners and feel their son or daughter should share their own preference for quiet social activities. Alternatively, daycare can be viewed by carers as a benefit for themselves, rather than as a development opportunity for their son or daughter. Parental involvement with the care package for an adult with LD needs to be on the family's own terms. If successful changes in the method or style of communication can be achieved in the day centre, parents may become involved at a later stage in the intervention programme.

The key to successful programmes in a daycare centre is choosing a centre-based project that will show initial success and involve all the relevant professional groups. The involvement of key day centre staff who already have a positive attitude to the therapy services is more likely to foster achievement. It is easier to persuade other staff who might have had initial reservations to become involved, or to initiate other new projects, if a joint care programme is seen to offer positive results. When the clients feel less distress and show an increased enjoyment in their daycare setting, the staff who care for them often experience a correspondingly positive improvement in their work environment. Success in an approach with a group of clients, or a particular service area, is a key factor in demonstrating the benefits of speech and language therapy and is likely to encourage all the staff and clients in larger establishments to value the support and advice of the SLT and their joint collaborative role with the other support services. However, no intervention can be isolated from the skill base and knowledge held by other professions. The day centre's activities must be designed to meet the different levels of cognitive, motor and sensory needs of all the clients involved. Communication always takes place within a defined social context and this is influenced by the values and attitudes of the group members and the activity the centre encompasses.

Conclusions

A successful speech and language therapy programme for the client who is referred to the service can only be achieved by involving everyone: the parents, peers, education and day care staff, residential care staff and other professions. The client's speech and language therapy intervention therefore needs to take account of both the clients' individual communication needs and the wishes and expectations of those who provide all the direct care.

The SLT needs to be aware that the problems or solutions that the carers initially present may need to be re-negotiated, discussed and agreed. The final care package should take into account not only the communication needs of the individual, but also the unique daily living environment of those who will implement the speech and language therapy intervention. There should also be a clear contract with the referrer to support and lead the care package. The intervention programme should be supported by, and provided with, appropriate resources and materials. An intervention can only occur if an agreed contract of this type is available to all concerned. The successful programme involves carers, thereby enabling them to feel ownership of the design of the programme, the methods of implementation and the resources that support it. The major role of the SLT is to act as a facilitator who enables the carers to identify and manage a solution which suits their own circumstances.

It is only by including wider aspects of care into the design and planning of the client's individual speech and language therapy programme that successful outcomes for clients and carers can hope to be achieved.

CHAPTER 9

The Management of Challenging Behaviour within a Communication Framework

JILL BRADSHAW

Abstract

This chapter begins with an overview of the definitions and prevalence of challenging behaviour (CB), including the ways in which it is defined in practice. Secondly, a review of the literature on the functional analysis approach focuses on the ways in which communication issues are currently addressed. Thirdly, possible ways in which communication could be included are suggested.

The need to consider all aspects of communication is discussed, highlighting the importance of considering the communication used by both people in the communication partnership. This includes examples of the ways in which communication breakdown may lead to CB.

Finally, communication interventions are considered within a framework of current approaches. These aim to modify the environment and teach the individual skills in order to effect a reduction in their CB. Practical approaches to developing communication within the partnership are suggested and illustrated using case studies.

Introduction

Much of the research around CB identifies the communicative competence of the individual as a factor that is influential in the ways in which CB develops and is maintained. Although relatively little is known about the precise nature of the relationship between communication and CB (Bunning and Bradshaw, in submission), interventions which target the communication skills of an individual have been shown to be effective (Carr and Durand, 1985; Durand, 1990; Carr et al., 1993, 1994; Emerson, 1995; O'Neill et al., 1997; Thurman, 1997).

Review of the literature

Definitions of challenging behaviour

'The presence of challenging behaviour in people with learning disability (LD) has serious consequences for their quality of life' (Lowe et al., 1995:595). It can be defined as

> behaviour of such an intensity, frequency or duration that the physical safety of the person, or others, is likely to be placed in serious jeopardy, or behaviour which is likely to seriously limit or deny access to, and use of, ordinary community facilities. (Emerson et al., 1987b:8).

Emerson (1995:4) amended this definition to include 'culturally abnormal behaviour(s)' to highlight the importance of considering social and cultural norms. CB is not defined in terms of its form in this statement but by its consequences (Lowe and Felce, 1995).

The concept of CB is socially defined and 'does not just refer to the person's behaviour but also to the impact that behaviour has on their lifestyle' (McGill et al., 1996:10). Adopting this term (rather than 'problem behaviour' or 'behaviour disorders') implies that the nature of the challenge is a 'shared, or mutual, responsibility' (Lowe and Felce, 1995:118), with the challenge being in providing support and services. Emerson (1995) proposed that by viewing the situation rather than the behaviour as a challenge, responses will be more constructive. The ways in which services are designed and in which the individual is supported will be a factor in determining whether or not the behaviour is perceived as presenting a challenge.

> The same person, showing the same behaviour, may be seen as challenging by members of staff in one setting and not by those in another (Qureshi, 1994:17).

Prevalence of challenging behaviour

Prevalence figures are dependent on the definitions used and on the ways in which the data is collected (Qureshi, 1994; Emerson, 1995; McGill et al., 1996).

> Few, if any, studies directly address the issue of incidence of challenging behaviour among people with learning disabilities and only a limited number of studies address the issue of the duration or persistence of challenging behaviour. (Emerson, 1995:20)

The Mansell Report (Department of Health, 1993) estimated that over the whole of the UK, 20 adults with a mild, moderate or severe LD per

100,000 total population present a significant challenge at any one time. McGill et al. (1996) reviewed the recent British literature and found prevalence rates of between 7 and 18%.

Prevalence of challenging behaviour in children with learning disabilities

There are similar difficulties in ascertaining the prevalence in children with LD. Kiernan and Kiernan (1994) gave figures of 8% of children in schools for severe LD in England and Wales who were identified as being 'extremely challenging' or 'very difficult to manage', and a further 14% presented demonstrated challenges of a lesser nature. Kiernan and Qureshi (1993) estimated that 10 children per total population of 220,000, (that of an average English NHS district) presented with severe CB. A report by the Mental Health Foundation (1997), using the data gathered from a number of studies in England and Wales, estimated 25 children per total population of 250,000.

Types of challenging behaviour

CB may be loosely divided into those behaviours which are 'outer directed' (e.g. aggression to other people) and those which are 'inner directed' (e.g. self-injury). By definition, CB encompasses both types of behaviour (as they are defined by 'consequences' rather than 'form'), but there is evidence that referrals for specialist treatment (assuming that these represent individuals whose behaviour poses the most challenges) are for people presenting with behaviours which disrupt the environment, rather than those which interfere with the learning of the individual (Lowe et al., 1995). In a study carried out by Lowe and Felce (1995), behaviours presenting the most serious management problems included aggression, wandering away, disturbing noises, temper tantrums and sexual delinquency. Withdrawal, inactivity or stereotypical behaviours were not rated as posing equivalent challenges. These ratings and referrals may not be a good indication of severity, as in, for example, the dangers to the person's own safety when considering self-injurious behaviour (SIB).

Causes

Behaviour which challenges service delivery can be seen as

> the outcome of complex interactions amongst a range of factors – organic, psychiatric, environmental, ecological, historical – some of which will be more important than others in individual cases. (Emerson et al., 1994:6)

A number of biological and organic factors, including autism, vision and hearing difficulties and epilepsy, have been linked to behaviour which challenges services. With the exception of Lesch–Nyhan syndrome and Prader–Willi syndrome, studies of biological or organic factors have been unable to provide evidence of a causal link (Murphy, 1994).

The dominant causal framework adopted has been that of functional analysis. This aims to analyse the relationships between behaviours and the context in which they occur (Emerson, 1995). McGill (1993) high-lighted the importance of considering both the individual and their environment and discussed possible interactions between challenging needs (those features of individuals which are associated with a higher probability of CB) and challenging environments (those features of the social and physical environment which are known to be associated with an increased probability of CB).

Services

The Mansell Report (Department of Health, 1993) identified three different approaches to the development of services:

- *Removers* frequently place people in out-of-area placements rather than attempting to develop local services.
- *Containers* provide services locally which are of poor quality and focus on containing the behaviour rather than on skills development.
- *Developers* seek to provide services locally which address individual needs.

The Mansell Report acknowledges that the development of quality services for people with CB is more expensive than ordinary community services because of the increased staffing costs (including training) and management input. People with CB are more likely to be placed in institutionalised services (Emerson et al., 1994) and to move between institutions.

The 1997 Mental Health Foundation report of children with learning disabilities and severe challenging behaviour highlighted the shortage of LD and mental health services in the UK which specialise in working with children. It pointed out that those children who are able to access such services are often offered one-off interventions, usually in response to a crisis situation. The report states the need for 'long-term preventative and continuing input' (p. 69).

Specialist support services

Many services have aimed to develop local competence in this field by setting up 'challenging needs teams' which provide support to people in both community and hospital settings. The professional backgrounds of staff employed by such teams rarely include specialist communication knowledge (Emerson et al., 1996) and until the importance of considering communication can be shown, this situation is unlikely to change to one where teams comprise members of staff with specialist communication knowledge. This deficiency needs also to be considered in the light of evidence of the proportion of people with LD who experience communication difficulties. There is little information available in the UK regarding the number of speech and language therapists (SLTs) who work with people who present challenges. In a survey of SLTs in the UK, Stansfield and Cheseldine (1996) found that 33% of generalists and 85.5% of specialist therapists working in the field of learning disability had come into contact with people with CB.

A survey of eight undergraduate training establishments in the UK carried out by the specific interest group (SIG) for adults with LD and CB in 1995 (SIG, 1995), found that only three of these included CB as a lecture topic and that the maximum amount of time allocated was three hours. Stansfield and Cheseldine (1994) recommended that SLTs working in this field need to develop skills in the management of CB and background knowledge of intervention techniques.

SLTs with a specific interest in CB attending a post qualification course were surveyed by Bradshaw and Baker (1996, 1997) regarding the number of clients on their caseload and the length of involvement. SLTs who specialised in CB had fewer clients on their caseload and had an increased length of involvement, but there did not appear to be major differences in the actual communication assessments and interventions implemented (see Table 9.1).

The relationship between communication and challenging behaviour

Prevalence of communication difficulties

It is widely acknowledged that CB is associated with communication difficulties (Richman et al., 1982; Ceci, 1986; Blunden and Allen, 1987; Murphy, 1994). This includes difficulties with understanding, expression and using language functionally. Prevalence figures are difficult to estimate

Table 9.1. Differences in caseload between speech and language therapists working with people with challenging behaviour

	Percentage of time spent with adults with challenging behaviour	
	Less than 50%	More than 50%
Number of clients with challenging behaviour on caseload per session*	9	2
Range	1.5–50	0.5–3
Average length of time on caseload	15 months	22 months
Range	3–24 months	12–30 months
Average length of time for assessment	2 months	4 months
Range	3 hours–6 months	2–6 months
Average length of time for intervention	13 months	18 months
Range	2–23 months	9–26 months
Number	27	12

*A session was defined as 0.5 days

because they depend initially on the operational definition of CB used in any particular study.

Language is essential for internalising social codes and for the self-regulation of behaviour. It is used to express emotions and feelings and to influence the behaviour of other people (Gordon, 1991). Difficulties with understanding and expression have been noted to be a contributory factor in the behaviours exhibited by children with language difficulties (Brownlee and Bakeman, 1981; Caulfield et al., 1989). Chamberlain et al. (1993) used the results of assessments of the communication skills of 64 clients living on a ward and categorised communication skills into profound multiple LD, pre-verbal and verbal. Those clients who were less able in terms of communication skills showed the most behavioural problems. There is clearly a need for more detailed research into the nature of communication difficulties, the role of the communication partner and the relationship between communication and CB throughout the assessment and intervention process.

Communication-based approaches

Carr and Durand (1985) discussed the application of a communication hypothesis to CB and suggested that as behaviours may be seen as non-verbal communication, development of communication skills may result in a reduction in CB (as the individual acquires more effective ways of communicating). Communication interventions which aim to reduce CB have typically focused on the message-sending skills of the individual with a LD (Remington, 1997). If such an approach is taken, the opportunities for producing durable changes within the communication partnership may be limited: for example, using functional communication training to introduce a communicative form to replace the CB while giving little consideration to the mismatches in the communication partnerships between the significant others and person with a LD. Such a narrow focus may lead to communication interventions implemented around an incident of CB with no attention given to the overall communication needs of the individual.

In this chapter, we discuss behavioural approaches to assessment and intervention with individuals who present challenges to services and highlight where communication interventions may fit within this approach. The approaches suggested are not intended to replace a detailed communication assessment and intervention. A detailed communication assessment is needed to gain information about the individual's communication skills set (the range of communication skills available to them) and the ways in which these skills are utilised within the settings that are part of the individual's daily life. This assessment is, in essence, no different from conducting a detailed assessment of communication with any individual with a LD. Any difficulties which do arise during the course of this communication assessment are often as a result of the practical difficulties in obtaining this information. Examples of this are attempting to observe communication within an impoverished communication environment, or interacting with the individual to gain information on communication skills while being unsure of what are the possible triggers to an incident of CB (and where social interaction may be a trigger for the behaviour).

Assessment

Assessment of challenging behaviour: a functional analysis approach

Behavioural approaches currently in use such as 'functional analysis' of the behaviour, aim to assess the function that the behaviour serves for the individual and to intervene by modifying the environment and teaching the individual skills (LaVigna et al., 1989) in order to create situations whereby:

- either the behaviour no longer serves a useful purpose for the individual (as the environment provides the necessary reinforcement), or
- the individual is able to achieve the function of the behaviour using socially appropriate and valued means rather than the behaviour which is perceived as challenging (Carr et al., 1994).

There is a range of assessment tools which can be used to conduct an analysis of the function a behaviour serves. However, Toogood and Timlin (1996) found that the level of agreement between the different assessment methods was poor. Assessment methods include questionnaires such as the Motivation Assessment Scale (Durand, 1990), semi-structured interviews such as the Functional Analysis Interview Form (O'Neill et al., 1990; 1997), direct observation (including momentary time sampling, continuous event recording, recording the antecedents and consequences of the behaviour) and the use of analogue conditions which aim to test the probability of the behaviour occurring under a set of experimental conditions in order to further clarify the functions of the behaviour (see Emerson, 1995 for a review of assessment approaches).

For example, use of the Motivation Assessment Scale (Durand, 1990) may indicate that the behaviour is more likely to occur in those situations where requests are made of the individual. Direct observations may reveal a high rate of behaviour when the individual is engaged in activities; and an analysis of antecedents and consequences may show a high rate of behaviour when an individual is given an instruction to complete a task. The interpretation of the assessments may lead to the hypothesis that the behaviour serves the function of escape from demands.

Analogue assessments may include a condition where the number of demands and the complexity of the tasks are controlled and the resulting CB observed. For example, if high rates of behaviours occur in conditions where the task demands are high, and if low rates are seen in conditions where task demands are low, the hypothesis would be supported.

Consideration of communication within a functional analysis approach

Within a 'functional analysis' approach, communication is usually considered in terms of the individual's skills set (skills are seen as present or absent and the influence of the environment or situation is rarely considered). Emphasis is also given to expressive skills (Remington, 1997). Assessments invariably assume intentional communication status and consider interventions which use referential means of communicating (e.g. the use of objects or photographs). Consideration is often not given to the implications of sensory or physical impairments for current communication skills, or communication skills development.

For example, the Motivation Assessment Scale (Durand, 1990) is a rating scale comprising 16 questions designed to assess the functional significance of a specified behaviour, in a specified setting, in order to determine the probable function that the behaviour serves. The assessment does not refer to the individual's communication skills, or the communication used by other people. Analysis of the antecedents and consequences of the CB does not include information on communication acts: for example, questions concerning requests to the individual do not probe the ways in which requests are made and whether these are within an individual's understanding skills set.

The Functional Analysis Interview (O'Neill et al., 1997) aims to review any potential variables such as time of the day, contexts, etc., and to enable assessors to focus on those aspects that are particularly important. This is followed by an observation of the individual in which setting events (events likely to result in CB), perceived functions and consequences of the target behaviour are recorded, using the information gathered during the interview. The questionnaire gathers a range of information including the client's behaviour, the antecedent and consequences, daily routine events, etc. It also includes a section on communication, but this is limited in a number of ways:

- There is a focus on the individual's expressive rather than receptive communication skills; this includes the form and function of communicative acts.
- Little consideration is given to the communication used by communication partners and whether or not there is a match between interaction from other people and the individual's communication skills set.
- There is an assumption that the individual will have intentional communication skills, this being 'the concept that you can affect other people's behaviour by your own actions, or vocalisations' (Coupe O'Kane and Goldbart, 1998:7), and therefore the role of inference and the ways in which intentions are inferred by the communication partner (Sperber and Wilson, 1995) are not assessed.
- Reference is not made to the influence communication skills have within the context of the individual's daily life (e.g. ability to predict events, make choices, etc.).

- Environmental influences on communication skills are not considered.

Both assessments are concerned with identifying the events that reinforce, or maintain, the likelihood of behaviours occurring again given the same set of circumstances. The Motivation Assessment Scale does not request information regarding the communication status of the person; the Functional Analysis Interview requests limited information on the expressive communication skills of the individual and less on understanding skills; neither assessment considers communication as a partnership.

Possible influences of communication

Communication assessments based on a continuous processing model (Fogel, 1993) aim to acknowledge the contributions of all parties involved in the communication event. By using a transactional model, the analysis of antecedents and consequences of an episode of CB would also include an evaluation of the communication acts used within the communication partnership. This would enable assessment of the impact of any communication breakdown on the episode of CB.

This information could then be included in a formulation of the influencing factors in the development and maintenance of the CB (for example, the impact of being in an environment where information is not adapted to the individual's understanding skills set). This information is vital to understanding the way in which the CB functions for the individual and the options for intervention. Presenting this information on a flow chart allows a large amount of information to be presented at once (Mattaini, 1995). A visual presentation may also make it easier for people with LD and their carers to understand the factors contributing to the development and maintenance of CB and allows the impact of specific interventions to be easily represented (Clare, 1996).

McGill et al. (1996) acknowledged the limitations of using an antecedent–behaviour–consequence (ABC) model of assessment and extend this model to include the actions of significant others, the thoughts and feelings of the people involved and the events prior to the immediate antecedent. It also places these thoughts, feelings, actions and events within the personal and environmental context (both temporary and persistent) for both individuals (see Figure 9.1).

Persistent environmental contexts might include a climate of social control; temporary environmental contexts might include temperature,

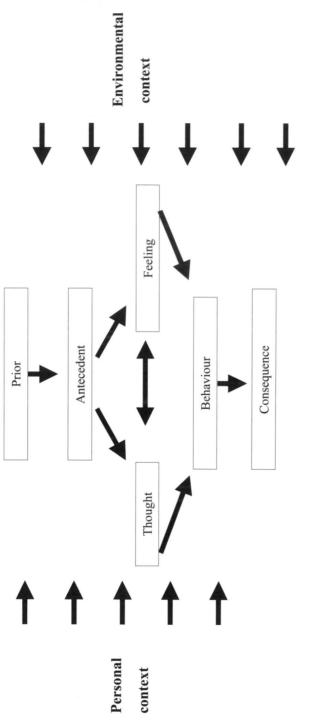

Figure 9.1. The environmental and personal context of challenging behaviour. From McGill et al. (1996). Reproduced with permission.

crowded environment, etc. Examples of factors in the persistent personal context include epilepsy, communication difficulties and sensory impairments. Factors in the personal and environmental context described in this model will also influence how individuals are able to use their communication skills. Table 9.2 includes examples of this.

Table 9.2. The personal context in relation to communication

Temporary	Persistent
Hearing loss*	Hearing loss
Understanding skills*	Understanding skills
Expressive skills*	Expressive skills
Emotional state	Repeated experiences of unsuccessful
Physical health	communication acts
Relationship to speaker	Lack of information given in a
etc.	meaningful way
	etc.

*These are classified as both temporary and persistent as an individual may have a persistent difficulty which is affected by numerous environmental and personal factors.

Communication needs to be represented as an interactive process which is affected by numerous factors (see Figure 9.2).

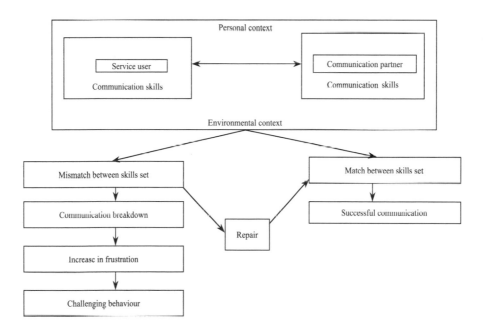

Figure 9.2. Process of communication.

Communication factors within the communication partnership need to be considered as an overall influence, as well as assessing the impact of communication breakdown around an incident of behaviour. A mismatch between the communication used by the member of staff and the individual with LD may lead to an increase in frustration. Although it is possible to repair this breakdown at a number of stages within the process, it may be more difficult to do so once frustration occurs, as this may have a negative impact on communication skills.

For example, Jane is asked to do the washing up. She hits the member of staff and goes into the other room to watch television. This is a typical pattern of the antecedents and consequences around Jane's behaviour, and a simple analysis might lead to the conclusion that Jane's behaviour is maintained by 'escape from demands'. Jane has communication difficulties and it is possible that she would be willing to take part in the task, but does not understand what she is being asked to do. It is essential that communication is considered within this process; people with communication difficulties may not have the skills to request clarification. The following are examples of some aspects of communication that may need to be considered:

Communications from other people, e.g. demands

- Does the person understand the communication – form/number of ideas, language used, attention gained first, processing time given?
- Has the person been given information about how long the activity will last?
- Was the person told what would be happening afterwards, e.g. do they know that they will be having a break?

Communications by the individual

- Did the person intentionally communicate, e.g. did they say no?
- Were there any signals given that others could have interpreted, e.g. a change in facial expression?
- Does the person have any other means of obtaining the consequence of the behaviour, e.g. by accessing the item directly?
- If so, why was this not employed? (e.g. past experience shows communication not as successful as the behaviour, or the environmental support needed to enable communication was not present).

By analysing these situations over time, a clearer picture can develop of the ways in which communication may contribute to the development and maintenance of the behaviour. An example framework is given in Table 9.3 (see p. 260).

Interventions

The communication hypothesis – implications for intervention

Assigning a function to a behaviour is insufficient to determine that the behaviour is a communication act. Although behaviours may be considered as being similar to non-verbal forms of communication (Donnellan et al., 1984) and problem behaviour may have similarities with some definitions of communication, particularly of non-verbal communication, it is impossible to make a definitive statement about its relationship to communication (Durand, 1986).

Cipani (1990) hypothesised that behaviours which may be communicative are those which are socially mediated and require the action of another person to achieve the intended effect. However, caution should be applied before it is assumed that a behaviour is a conscious attempt to influence the behaviour of another person (see Stamp and Knapp, 1990 for a discussion of the role of conscious intent). Meaning may be ascribed to the act by the significant other, and the act may be interpreted as having meaning, but the behaviour may not be intended as a communication. These issues are also present when interpreting the meaning of communication by people with severe and profound LD (Grove et al., 1999). For individuals who have non- or pre-intentional communication skills, the level of conscious communicative intent to send a message may be low, and therefore the behaviour may be unlikely to represent a conscious intention to affect the behaviour of another person.

In giving consideration to the communicative properties of the CB, the following issues may be important (Cipani, 1990):

- Does the behaviour represent a communication by non-standard means? For example, an individual who always receives a drink in response to hitting their head may use this as a non-standard gesture to inform the communication partner that s/he is thirsty.
- Is the behaviour an intentional attempt to influence the other person's behaviour?

Table 9.3. Evaluation of communication breakdown

Situation	People present	Communication	Response	Attempt at repair	Breakdown resulted from
Where did the exchange take place and what was happening?	*Who was present?*	*What was the communication? Who communicated? How did they do this? Who was it directed towards?*	*What was the response? Who responded? How did they do this? Who was it directed towards?*	*Was there an attempted repair? Who attempted the repair? What was the repair? Was this successful?*	*Inappropriate form? Too complex? Attention not gained? Not understood?*
Kitchen, making drinks, high level of background noise	Support worker (SW), Rehana, Bill	SW – 'what time are you going to your class?'	Bill – 'I want to phone my sister' (directed towards SW)	No attempt to repair	Difficulties understanding use of time resulted in use of repetitive theme
Coming down the stairs after getting ready to go out	Support worker, Tom	SW – 'Let's go and make a shopping list. I think we need to get some more biscuits'	Tom went into the kitchen, sat at the table and said 'biscuit', directed towards SW	SW showed Tom the empty biscuit tin and gave him the shopping bag	Difficulties understanding the complex instruction, also associated with transition difficulties.

- Is the behaviour a reaction to an internal state? This hypothesis may be applied to an individual who spits out food as a reaction to the unpleasant taste. This may result in the individual being removed from the table and incorrectly interpreted as having the 'communication function' of 'escape'.
- Is the behaviour an attempt to access the reinforcer directly?

Carr et al. (1994:23) stated that 'the communication hypothesis does not state that individuals systematically and intentionally use their problem behaviour to influence others' and 'the communication hypothesis is not useful because it tells us what people with disabilities are thinking but rather because it suggests a constructive and educational way of addressing problem behaviour'.

Although assigning a level of conscious communicative intent can be seen as an academic debate because in reality it may be difficult to determine conscious intention, it does have possible implications for the way in which interventions are applied and for the causal interpretations given by caregivers. This has been shown to influence caregivers' responses to the behaviour (Hastings et al., 1997).

Implications of assigning communicative intent to a behaviour which is seen as challenging

Assigning meaning to a behaviour and therefore consistently responding to that behaviour as if it were a communication, in theory means that behaviour may become an intentional communication. It is known that this is an important process in the development of intentional communication in young infants. Communication partners' ascription of meaning contributes to this development (Gibb Harding, 1983). An aim of any intervention should be to develop and respond to more standard (or less challenging) means of communication.

Interpreting the behaviour as having conscious communicative intent may lead to an overestimation of the communication skills. Caregivers frequently begin to report that children understand speech as they begin to show communicative intent (Chapman, 1978). Carers' overestimation of the comprehension skills of people with LD is a key factor in understanding CB. For example, some behaviours may occur as a result of the client's misunderstanding about what they have been asked to do (Clarke-Kehoe and Harris, 1992). Overestimation of skills may also lead to additional difficulties in the diminished opportunities provided to the individual (Barlett and Bunning, 1997). Overestimating abilities may also lead to interventions with demands which are not within the skills set of the service user. An example of this is when staff members try to introduce photographs to use as an expressive form of communication for a service user with LD although the client has pre-intentional communication skills.

If behaviour is interpreted and communicative intent assumed, the obvious response to a CB by the carer or SLT would be to introduce functional communication training, to replace a behaviour with an equivalent communication response; for example, to teach a client to produce a sign for drink rather than hitting their head (see Durand, 1990; Carr et al., 1993, 1994; Mirenda, 1997). However, it is essential that this includes accurate communication and sensory information upon which to base decision-making, in order to design an appropriate intervention. If we assume that the client is able to communicate intentionally, does this give staff the impression that the behaviour is being used to manipulate them, i.e. 'they only do that because they want to get out of here/want attention?' Again this may lead to the assumption that this client could use more standard means for communicating this message (e.g. functional communication training) but is not doing so (on purpose?).

> The notion of intent, however, can be rather unhelpful in understanding challenging behaviours as it can all too readily support an attitude which characterises the user as manipulative and, in effect, blames them for their behavioural disabilities. It is also clear that, however intent is defined, many CBs shown by people with severe or profound learning difficulties cannot be thought of as intentional in any useful sense. (Brown et al., 1989:4)

A multi-component approach

A multi-component intervention approach is described by LaVigna et al. (1989). It involves both intervening within the environment and developing the skills of the individual. It includes both proactive strategies which develop the skills of the individual and others, and reactive strategies which aim to develop a safe response and gain rapid control over the behaviour, should the behaviour occur (LaVigna et al., 1989). A number of elements are described within the approach, including implementing changes within the environment (i.e. ecological manipulation), teaching the individual skills (i.e. positive programming), and direct treatment strategies (including behavioural and pharmacological interventions).

Considering communication within a multi-component approach

A communication-based approach to intervention may include developing the individual's communication skills, for example by implementing functional communication training. This aims to replace the individual's CB with a communication response, e.g. teaching the individual to use a symbol to request attention as a replacement for self-injurious behaviour (SIB), which serves the function of gaining attention from staff. Mirenda (1997) reviewed 21 studies (involving 52 participants) where functional communication training was employed. Information was not always available regarding the selection of an augmentative and alternative communication technique and in some cases was determined by equipment availability (see also Chapter 7 in this book). Functional communication training mainly considers the 'form' of communication and may fail to take into account the 'range' of communication issues, e.g. how significant others communicate with the client with a LD, the client's pragmatic skills, etc.

Because of the limitations of the ways in which communication is assessed during the functional analysis, the interventions may not be tailored to meet the individual's communication needs. For example, functional communication training may be attempted with an individual who is unable to communicate intentionally. The response may be learnt by operant conditioning but not used as a way of communicating. If this response is under the same stimulus control as the behaviour, however, and is produced under the condition where another person is present and it is directed towards this person, it would be difficult to prove the client's level of conscious intent. Similarly, the support given to an individual to increase participation may not be adapted to meet the individual's communication needs.

Significant others have a vital role in the communication partnership. Interventions should always consider their communication, and frequently this is the starting point of interventions. After assessing their communication and how this impacts on the communication of the client, the following may be possible targets for intervention; within such an approach, the following communication issues listed in Table 9.4 need to be considered.

Case study 9.1

Sam was referred at age 39. As a child, he displayed aggressive outbursts which were often directed towards his younger sister or other children. He lived at home until he was 16 and attended a specialist behavioural support unit. He was given a diagnosis of autism during his childhood. At 16, he was admitted to a long-stay institution where his range of behaviours included smearing faeces, and verbal and physical aggression. The likelihood of these behaviours increased at times of anxiety.

Table 9.4. Speech and language therapy interventions within a multi-component approach

Ecological manipulations	Positive programming	Direct treatment	Reactive strategies
Increase levels of meaningful stimulation	Increase/maintain existing communication skills	Medication effects on communication	Language used
Increase levels of social contact	Increase/maintain vocabulary, options for form of communication, consistency and clarity of form, range of functions within vocabulary	Language used in direct treatment strategy	Repair strategies for communication breakdown
Alter the communications of other people (range of functions/match understanding skills/ proportion of communications staff–client etc.)			
Increase predictability	Choice of strategy used for teaching skills		
Increase levels of purposeful engagement	Functional communication training		
Increase consistency of staff responses to communication and shaping communication	Choice making Schedule building		
Creating situations where the individual has opportunities, a reason and a need to communicate	Self management strategy chosen and form of introduction		

During Sam's first community placement five years earlier, staff experienced great difficulties in understanding and managing his behaviours. The initial move into the community had caused him great distress but he settled down after a year. As he was the only verbal client in the environment he received a lot of staff attention, often higher during the night, when there were two night-shift staff.

When Sam's mother died, he was not informed as his sister did not want to cause him distress. He had been in regular contact with his mother and his challenging behaviours increased in frequency and intensity after her death. He would often continue to talk about her in the present tense and would often tell members of staff that she was coming to see him. Sam's service was also under review and he was due to move into a smaller community group home in the coming months. The service users had a leaving party months before the move actually took place and Sam did not have any real understanding of what was happening, as staff members had not been preparing him for the move because they did not want to upset him.

Sam eventually moved into his new home and, though the first month was trouble free, a gradual deterioration in behaviour began to show. He was not sleeping, would get up at night and eat large quantities of bread or breakfast cereal, was tearful at times and made frequent references to his mother. He was being excluded from community activities as he would become verbally abusive upon entering the group or activity. Staff would remove him before his behaviours could escalate in these settings and would often take him out to the café, the pub or their own homes, as an alternative. His verbal abuse was on the increase both inside and outside his new home and he was becoming increasingly anxious, and difficult to engage in activities. The staff were either ignoring the verbal abuse, or reacting back with equally emotional responses which could prolong the behaviour for hours, often resulting in physical aggression directed at the member of staff. Sam's sleep pattern grew very erratic and he could go for several nights without having slept. At these times, he was engaging in intense anal poking and faecal smearing and could well be very agitated from shift to shift over a number of days. It was also at this time that he became diurnally urine-incontinent.

Assessment results of his general skills showed Sam to be very distracted by both visual and auditory stimuli in the environment. People were the main source of distraction. He found it extremely difficult to concentrate on tasks. Sam had tardive dyskinesia, which means that his fine motor skills were rather shaky, and he often required physical prompts for some elements of tasks. If he was unable to complete a task successfully, he became frustrated. Assessment of his communication skills indicated that Sam was able to communicate using speech, though this was difficult to understand as he had no teeth. Much of his communication was echoed. He understood one or two ideas in an utterance without situational cues. His understanding was greater for concrete language. He demonstrated many repetitive themes in his communication, e.g. cars, road names, directions, and he had difficulties starting and stopping conversations.

Sam had several communication strategies which he used to gain and maintain members of staff's attention. He could be continuously verbal, following staff from room to room. His speech consisted of strings of repeated phrases. Most of this was relevant to the situation though difficult to understand, and did not necessarily use language which he understood. He often repeated what other people said to him and had learned many strategies for responding to questions, e.g. using stereotypical phrases such as 'did he' or 'is it', which he used to maintain staff attention. Staff perceived Sam as being more able than the two people with whom he shared. He was also currently seen as the problem person. Sam's staff team overestimated his skills, including his communication skills. They also had a perception that normalisation meant that people were treated 'normally', so that if Sam yelled abuse, it was appropriate to yell back.

Sam had mental health difficulties. He was diagnosed as having a bipolar affective mood disorder. The cyclical changes in mood could be rapid, going between the two extremes within a few days. When he was at the top of his cycle, Sam's speech was constant, rapid, increased in volume and very difficult to understand. He was very distracted by other people in the environment and aggression could be triggered by the slightest indication that he was not accessing staff attention at a level he needed. He attempted to engage his preferred member of staff continuously, had great difficulties in attending to tasks, or to the communication of other people, though sometimes understood and processed a key word in something they said. He was not able to follow gestures, e.g. pointing.

When at the bottom of the cycle, Sam's speech was reduced in volume and in amount. It was often very difficult to engage him in a conversation though sometimes he gave 'yes/no' answers. His motivation was greatly reduced for all activities. It was unclear whether he was able to process the communication of other people at the time as his responses were minimal. He had extreme difficulties in carrying out any tasks then, and often spent his time lying on the settee. It was difficult to motivate him to eat or drink.

The functional analysis included a detailed communication assessment and indicated that his behaviours were attention maintained.

Staff's responses were reinforcing this function. Communication (both verbal and non-verbal) maintained a central role in the development and maintenance of his behaviour as can be seen in the formulation in Figure 9.3. An overview of the intervention plan for Sam appears in Table 9.5.

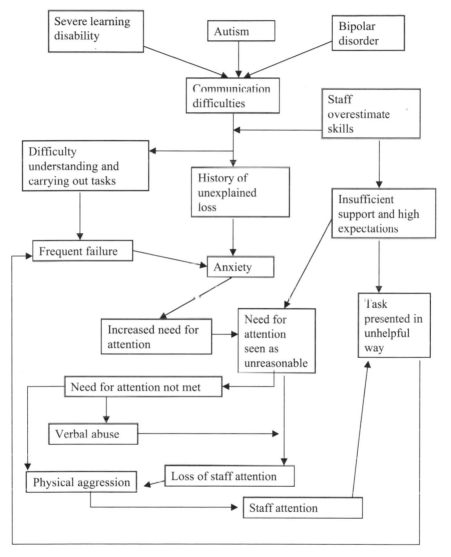

Figure 9.3. Sam – pre-intervention formulation.

Members of staff were observed supporting Sam throughout the day in a variety of activities using suggested intervention strategies. These were used to analyse the support given, the effect on Sam's behaviours, and the communication used. Videos were also used for the purposes of staff training. Numerous strategies were implemented with the staff team over a number of months (see Table 9.5).

Table 9.5: Interventions for Sam

Ecological manipulations

Modification of communication used by staff to include use of photographs to plan future activities (sequence of three activities with Sam choosing the order, limited to the next activity in times of anxiety) and who will be on shift

Staff use of language within communication skills set (gaining attention, reduced complexity and amount of language, reference to situational and visual cues)

One member of staff allocated to support for one hour (with direct treatment strategy used)

Staff not to work with Sam in the hour before they end the shift

Increase in materials and activities available for self occupation

Set strategy to terminate all conversations

Set strategy to assist termination of repetitive themes

Limit of visual and auditory distractions

Increased range of communication functions, including positive feedback

Increased sensitivity to Sam's mood and providing additional support as necessary – use of physical prompts and making sure he is successful

Consistent staff response to talking about mum

Introduction of activities to increase socially valued role

Frequent tasks throughout the day, with frequent breaks

Consistent bedtime routine

Direct treatment

Attention given at set intervals (maximum of ten minutes between intervals but with decrease in length of interval in times of anxiety), with procedure followed for terminating all interactions

Conversation and attention following engagement in activity

Termination of interaction only when Sam engaged in activity

Recognition that at times of great anxiety, attention may need to be constant

---

Positive programming

Teaching Sam to request attention by using people's names (by modelling)

Reactive strategies

Blocking, moving slowly away, early recognition of triggers and increased support at these times.

Taking care not to match Sam's style of communication in times of increased anxiety – use reduced volume and amount of speech

---

Following the intervention, Sam's challenging behaviour reduced in frequency and intensity (see Figure 9.4). The communication used by staff was modified (including the use of photographs, clear ways of introducing and terminating conversations, etc.) so that Sam was able to gain a greater understanding of what was expected of him and have greater opportunities to be involved in communication acts. His community participation also increased.

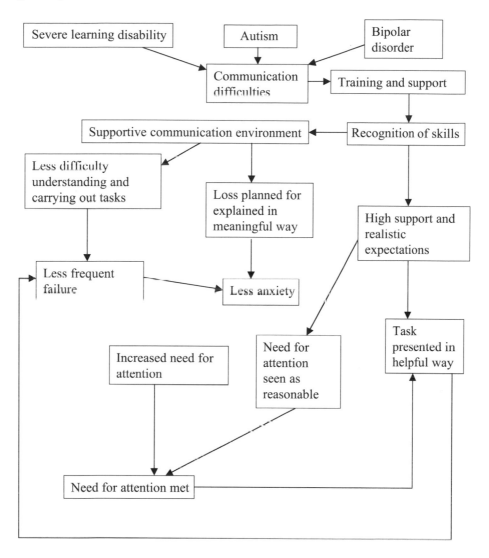

Figure 9.4. Sam – post-intervention formulation.

Case study 9.2

Sharon was 34 with a severe LD and autism. She lived in a small house with four other people with LD. The staff team had limited understanding of her support needs. Sharon spent much of her time standing and rocking to and fro. It was very difficult to interrupt this activity, but members of staff became increasingly concerned about the amount of time she was spending doing this. Staff had attempted to engage her in household activities, but this often resulted in Sharon hitting herself. When she engaged in SIB, this usually resulted in the removal of the demand. Sharon also had difficulties in moving between environments and activities, partly as a result of her autism, but also as a consequence of the chaotic and unpredictable environment. Sharon had difficulties in communicating her needs, though she did have a small vocabulary of signs. Her understanding of information was in the here and now. Staff wanted to be able to give her prior warning of activities, but found it difficult to identify successful ways of communicating this to her.

Staff had difficulties in communicating with Sharon as they tended to overestimate her communication skills, in particular her ability to understand abstract information. They would frequently give her more information than she could process, or use language that was too complex. As they assumed that Sharon could understand this complex language, they did not routinely provide additional contextual and situational support. This resulted in frequent confusion and communication breakdown for both people in the communication partnership. Observations of her communication skills showed that Sharon was able to understand a key word in what other people said but when she was engaged in rocking, she found it much more difficult to attend to, and process, speech. Her understanding was dependent on having the item being communicated about either in view, or nearby. Staff communicated using short sentences and phrases.

Sharon had a small vocabulary of single signs. These included signs used in the Makaton language programme (Walker, 1980) such as '*BED*', '*HELLO*', '*BISCUIT*', '*TEA*' and '*GOOD MORNING*'. She also had a speech sound that was an approximation to 'tea'. This was not always used with communicative intent. She was able to fulfil her basic needs, engage in social exchanges and regulate the behaviour of other people using the communication skills mentioned above, and via a range of informal gestures, use of objects, taking people to the item, or to the area where an activity usually took place, or going and standing near an item and waiting for staff to intervene.

Other skills were difficult to assess, as any request to carry out a task resulted in SIB.

As part of the SLT's assessment, Sharon was observed on a number of occasions in a range of environments. Naturally occurring situations were used as analogue conditions. These included presentation of request:

- when Sharon was engaged/not engaged in rocking
- using verbal/signed/pictorial/object communication
- followed by withdrawal, followed by presentation of the same request.

Also,

- 'momentary time sampling' of levels of engagement (as defined in the Individualised Sensory Environment Assessment Schedule; Bunning, 1996)
- varying length of activity
- varying support given within activity.

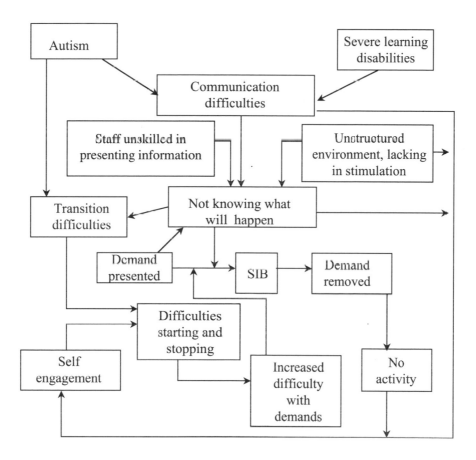

Figure 9.5. Sharon — pre-intervention formulation.

The results of initial assessments found that Sharon was spending 79% of the time in self-engagement activities (rocking). The analogue conditions not only provided information to add to the formulation but also highlighted a number of areas for intervention. The central difficulty seemed to lie in increasing her level of purposeful interaction whilst minimising the SIB which often resulted from the presentation of a demand.

The formulation in Figure 9.5 illustrates her needs and the inter-relation between such needs. An intervention plan was formulated, an overview of which appears in Table 9.6.

Table 9.6. Interventions for Sharon

Ecological manipulation

Modification of communication used by staff to include use of objects to communicate the next activity

Staff use of language within communication skills set (gaining attention, reduced complexity and amount of language, reference to situational and object cues, use of signed communication)

Limit visual and auditory distractions

Increased range of communication functions, including positive feedback

Consistent response to Sharon's communications

Frequent tasks throughout the day, with frequent breaks

Increased support to complete activities with focus on task sharing

Tasks introduced using object cues. Task presented enthusiastically. Sharon presented with object cue and then staff withdrew for a few minutes before re-presenting the task. There was no expectation from the staff that Sharon would become involved in the task on the first presentation of the activity

Consistent daily routine

Direct treatment

Positive attention when Sharon was not engaging in rocking

Positive programming

Introduction of object and signed communication for Sharon to use

Introduction of a sign for requesting a break from task. This was modelled by staff initially, after one minute of starting the task, Sharon was given a short break before being supported to continue

Reactive strategies

Supporting Sharon to complete a minimal task, followed by staff modelling the sign for break and leaving Sharon for five minutes before re-presenting the task

Alterations in the communication environment, the development of Sharon's communication skills, altering the way in which tasks were presented and support provided led to greater opportunities for involvement in purposeful interactions. By carrying out analogue conditions, it was clear that Sharon was usually able to carry out a task for up to one minute before self-injuring (and sometimes for longer than this). Members of staff were able to ensure that no task lasted for longer than this time and modelled the sign for 'break'. They were able to gradually increase this time period over the months and to begin to teach Sharon to use the sign for 'break' in these situations. Her self-engagement decreased to 52%. An overview of the results of the intervention are illustrated in Figure 9.6.

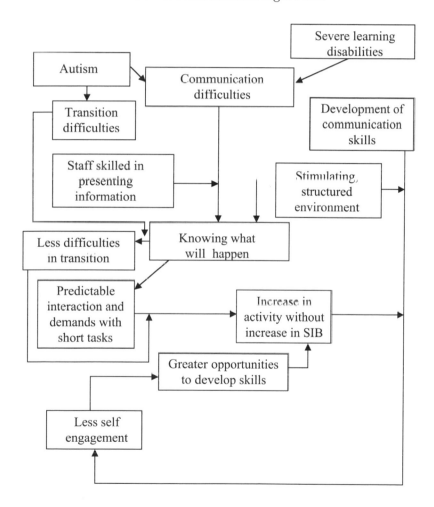

Figure 9.6. Sharon – post-intervention formulation.

Factors to consider in prioritisation

The issue of prioritisation is sometimes a complex one. The following is a list of factors which should be considered when prioritising clients who challenge services. It was developed by a UK specific interest group (SIG, 1996) for adults with LD and CB. As SLTs are working within differing frameworks and teams, it is not possible to write definitive guidelines. Prioritisation may be needed at all levels of intervention. Baker (1994) suggested the use of a matrix to determine priority.

The greatest influencing factors are usually service issues. When intervention is not possible because of the inability of the service or environment to change, SLTs (as part of a team approach) should continue to advocate for the client's needs and state clearly what needs to happen before interventions will be possible. Factors can be considered according to the client, service and environmental needs. These include those factors that increase the likelihood of the breakdown of the placement or indicate risks to the safety or quality of life of the person or others. In general, the greater the risk factors, the greater the need to consider intervening in some way. Presence of communication issues will also increase the priority for SLT intervention. Additional consideration will need to be given to the service and skills of the staff. This is not to suggest that this information would be used to decide whether or not a service would be offered, but may well influence the type and nature of assessment and intervention.

Examples of these factors are given below:

Individual priorities

- Risk of placement breakdown e.g. service is considering an out of borough placement
- Frequency, intensity and duration of behaviour perceived to be challenging.
- Client experiencing acute, recurrent levels of distress
- Risk of harm to self/others
- Legal requirements
- Effect on quality of life (e.g. access to community facilities)
- Degree of isolation
- Prevention of crisis/deterioration
- Frustrations in communicative acts
- Mismatch between client's communicative skills and significant other's interactions

- Communicative needs not being met by current skills
- Life events/personal circumstances/physical well being
- Awareness of difficulties
- Consent/motivation/co-operation

Service priorities

- More than one client in the same service experiencing acute, recurrent levels of distress
- Commitment of service managers to implement change
- Request for intervention
- Involvement of Challenging Needs Team/MDT.

Environmental priorities

- Ability of environment to change
- Staff skills (including understanding/perceptions of the behaviour perceived as challenging)
- Ability of environment to change.

Other considerations include

- Involvement of other professionals (N.B. The SIG in the UK advise that SLTs should not be working with clients who challenge services unless as part of a co-ordinated multi-disciplinary team)
- Skills of the speech and language therapist (including confidence).

Conclusion

Successful communication interventions must take into account the skills of both the sender and the receiver and aim to facilitate successful message sending and therefore, receiving in both the sender and the receiver. Interventions should focus on what is functional in the environments in which clients are supported and on the significant other people within these environments. Interventions should aim to increase the opportunities for successful communication to take place and for these communications to be motivating and rewarding for all those involved. They should focus on increasing communicative competence in all situations and not just in those situations where communication breakdown contributes to CB.

CHAPTER 10
Dual Diagnosis

SUE DOBSON

Abstract

In this chapter, assessment and management issues related to clients with dual diagnosis (DD) are discussed. The term is defined and a brief review of the literature on this subject is presented. Through case studies, assessment and therapy strategies which a speech and language therapist (SLT) can use, are illustrated. The importance of teamwork is stressed and discussed.

Introduction

Staff who work with adults with learning disabilities (LDs) sometimes refer clients for speech and language therapy who have both LD and a psychiatric disorder. Diagnosis of a mental illness usually relies on what the client is able to explain about their feelings, symptoms and experiences, as well as any observations of alterations in their communication and non-verbal behaviours. Those people with LD who develop an additional psychiatric disorder may have existing handicaps in their communication and social interaction skills. It is therefore often difficult to determine the relationship with, and interaction between, the original LD and the mental illness. An additional problem is that many of the behaviours that are associated with LD are similar to those social difficulties which contribute towards a diagnosis of a psychiatric disorder.

Referrals for speech and language therapy for people with DD can vary from requests for assistance with alterations in speech clarity and fluency through to assistance with re-establishing social communication skills. SLTs who work with adults with LD have a caseload of people who exhibit a wide spectrum of communication disorders. The inclusion of people with a DD within an already diverse caseload is a challenge that demands the development of a new therapeutic role. The role applies previous skills and experience but requires the development of an additional knowledge base.

Review of the literature

The main suggestion in the literature is that the population of adults with LD have a greater incidence of psychiatric problems (Corbett, 1979; Rutter et al., 1970). The term 'DD' has arisen because of the need to provide individual care for each client's unique needs rather than classify which is the primary or secondary need. In a DD, both the LD and the emotional disorder are considered primary healthcare needs which have equal importance. The estimates of the incidence of DD for people with LD varies from 16 to 60% depending on the population studied (Zarkowska and Clements, 1988; Gravestock and Bouras, 1997).

Leudar and Fraser (1985a) noted that there was often no clear diagnostic distinction between behaviour disturbance and mental handicap. In these cases the problems with diagnosis of a mental illness are confounded because both disorders are recognised by their behavioural symptoms. Qureshi (1994) noted that 12–16% of people with LD have a mental illness and that 52% of people with a challenging behaviour diagnosis take antipsychotic drugs. The distinction between those with challenging behaviours and those with a behavioural disorder is therefore not always clear-cut. For example, a comparison of the descriptions of behaviour for people with LD and the emotional presentations of mental illnesses from Qureshi (1994) and Gravestock and Bouras (1997) showed a similar list of behavioural realisations such as social withdrawal, agitation, ritual behaviours, non-compliance, self-injury and inappropriate language use.

People with LD can suffer from the same range of mental illnesses as the rest of the population, including psychoses, schizophrenia, manic depression, neuroses and personality and behavioural disorders. Gravell and France (1991a) stated that certain symptoms which are highly important in other people may have little or no psychiatric significance for people with LD. The underlying developmental delay has, therefore, to be separated from factors such as disorientation, echolalia, behaviour, mannerisms, repetitive movements and healthy but aberrant responses to life stress. Fraser (1991) suggested that if a person has a LD, the usual clusters of clinical features are less significant than for the normal population, particularly for schizophrenia and psychoses. He stated that differentiation between schizophrenia and depression is extremely difficult in people with LD, but that diagnoses of manic depression are slightly easier because of the possibility of observations of sleep patterns, weight loss and behaviour. For people with a DD of LD and personality disorder or neurotic disorder, the symptoms are not exclusive to each disorder. People with LD may actually experience more educational failure, discrimination, family disruption and disappointments in life than the normal population. This greater level of life stress leads to higher incidence of personality disorders and neurosis. Their limited communication skills means this is mediated by behavioural outbursts and repetitive ritualistic behaviours, self-injury, insomnia, aggression and restlessness.

Speech and language therapy and Dual Diagnosis

Nursing staff who are members of LD teams often hold qualifications for both LD and psychiatry. The need for both qualifications arises because of the percentage of people on their caseload who have a DD. SLTs have historically worked with people with LD. In recent years, an increasing number have begun to specialise in working with people with psychiatric disorders. However, there are few SLTs who would describe themselves as specialising in both LD and psychiatry. It does appear that the changing pattern of referrals to SLTs who work with adults with LD is leading to the profession evolving its own body of knowledge. LD posts, by their very nature, serve a wide and mixed caseload of clients in terms both of the variety of presenting communication disorders and of the degree and severity of the clients' LD. Often, a SLT's caseload will cover service provision to people with challenging behaviours, autism, hearing loss, visual impairment and physical handicaps. There is almost a tendency to become a generalist within the specialism of speech and language therapy services for people with LD. Some localities have therefore begun to appoint separate speech and language therapy posts for challenging behaviour, autism, sensory impairment and multiple and profound LD.

There is a growing expectancy of an additional service provision to people with DD. This further extends the existing speech and language service. The skills that a SLT uses are adaptable and can accommodate different caseloads. However, working with people with a DD adds new and unique problems of case management. A diagnosis of mental illness is usually made on the basis of detailed interviews with the patient. The patient's descriptions of his/her feelings, emotions and cognitive experiences enable the examining psychiatrist to make a differential diagnosis. This is supported by evidence from observations of the client's current use of verbal and non-verbal communication, social interactions and behaviour. All of these may already be disordered in people with LD. The development of a mental illness therefore imposes further disabilities on already disordered communication, social interactions and behaviours. This leads to diagnostic overshadowing (Reiss and Sysko, 1993). The availability of detailed historical records about all these factors is therefore important to nurses and therapists. Unfortunately, this kind of information is often not available for people with LD. It has either not been recorded in sufficient detail to be useful, or has been mislaid in the moves from one kind of residence, or style of care, to another. Staff who have known the clients from childhood may recall some information, but this is often anecdotal and of questionable reliability or value.

The functional areas affected by the development of a psychiatric, behavioural or emotional disorder in addition to an existing LD are, according to Gravestock and Bouras (1997):

- physical appearance: health and hygiene
- biological functions: sleep, feeding, bowels, bladder
- activity: energy and movements
- verbal and non-verbal communication
- mood and emotional reactions
- perceptions of others, objects and environments
- relationships and sexuality
- self perception, insight and esteem
- repertoire of adaptive and maladaptive behaviours
- attention, thinking and learning
- memory and adaptation
- attitudes to health and support needs.

Some of these functional changes associated with the various types and subtypes of psychiatric disorders affect spoken language and communication as well as non-verbal communication and social behaviour. It is these functional changes which will often lead to the LD team, or care workers, to make a request for speech and language therapy involvement (see Table 10.1).

In particular, referrals to speech and language therapy usually relate to changes in the client's social use of communication or appropriate social behaviours (see Table 10.2).

Referrals and changes in social behaviour

Most referrals occur at a time of crisis or transition when outbursts of aggression or a behavioural change has put clients themselves and/or

Table 10.1. Types of referrals to speech and language therapy for clients with dual diagnosis

Because of changes in:

Levels of verbal and non-verbal communication
Frequency of use of communication
Understanding or language processing
Tolerance of alterations in daily routines
Behaviour: sexual, social and feeding

Table 10.2. Requests for assistance made on referral

Management of language development for clients

Discussions about sexual changes and behaviour
Including clients in social interactions and groups
Establishing social programmes for self development
Developing awareness of social relationships
Developing educational programmes
Assistance with feeding difficulties

others at risk, either physically or socially. The referrals occur because the multi-disciplinary team invites the SLT to join the core team of the client concerned. The SLT's membership of this team is typically short-term and time-limited. The SLT acts as an advisor/consultant and perhaps demonstrates, or trials, an intervention, but the resulting care package is managed and supported by the core team leader.

Case study 10.1

In this case study, the SLT supports the work of other professionals and informs their care planning.

Kieron was a very happy, well-built, sociable man, 39 years old, who had no verbal communication. He was thought to have some form of auditory processing deficit that had affected his language development and severely limited his social functioning. He was able to communicate with staff with limited success by the use of signs, symbols, body language and actions, and could easily follow instructions in and around the centre. Kieron lived with his sister and her young family and travelled independently within his local community. At 39 years of age, Kieron's sexual behaviour had altered. He had begun to expose himself to children in the local community and this had resulted in his arrest. It was felt that he could have developed a behavioural/personality disorder, but that there may also have been an underlying psychosis.

Kieron's appearance had changed. He looked a lot older than his age. He had lost nearly 13 kg in weight, and looked haggard, drawn and unkempt. He shook visibly, sweated excessively and was very anxious. He was also unusually passive and agreed with whatever was said, or actively altered his response to suit his listener's view. He was very responsive and perceptive of his communication partner's slight alterations in facial expression or gesture.

The social worker required that Kieron develop an awareness of his actions and their effect on his future. Assessment of his level of understanding of communication showed that this was unchanged. He was able to understand 5+ information-carrying words in a signed and spoken sentence and could read and understand symbol sentences of the same length, but had little or no understanding of speech unless in a very familiar context. Kieron could still use symbols from the Makaton vocabulary to communicate and arrange them into short phrases but remained unable to read written script.

The Makaton Vocabulary Development Project team (Walker, 1980) was approached for assistance and they offered copies of the signs and symbols that were requested for the situation. Kieron then attended a two month period of twice weekly speech and language therapy sessions. During these sessions, he used Makaton symbols to discuss separate topics, physically handling symbol sentences to accept or reject the statements about behaviour. The language used for his behaviour was colloquial and was checked with Kieron for usage before each session. For example, a pack of symbol sentences was used each session to address either the time, the place or the people for whom sexual exposure was appropriate, or inappropriate. A sentence, supported by symbols, such as 'When the doctor tells me, I can show my penis', was presented with other sentences where the behaviour was inappropriate. Each sentence was then:

- discussed in isolation from other situations
- discussed and compared with other situations.

Work continued as follows:

- single symbols were sorted to people and appropriate behaviour
- completion of symbol sentences from a selection of symbol options

- composition of whole sentences appropriate to a situation/person using photographs
- completion of a worksheet (unsupported).

When all the topics were completed, the final sessions addressed all the settings, situations and people likely to be involved. A month later, all the worksheets were presented to Kieron again and a report was written for the social worker's use. This stated that Kieron had only a limited awareness of the consequences of his actions for other people. He knew which were appropriate times and places for the behaviour he had used. However, he was more worried about the present consequences for himself than about the effects of his behaviour on others. The social worker successfully used this information to negotiate a care package that maintained Kieron in his sister's home.

Referral and changes in social communication

People with LD often have poor abilities to recognise and understand emotions in others or to effectively express their own emotions either verbally or non-verbally. Those individuals who can communicate about emotions may only be able to do so in a very restricted form and make little distinction between shades of emotion, such as slight dissatisfaction or extreme displeasure. Their perceptions of emotions in others, such as fear, anger and surprise, may be confused (Leudar and Fraser, 1985a). Conversely, those with a mild or moderate LD and a mental illness may be able to communicate effectively about their emotional state but fail to draw attention to, or communicate, their signs and symptoms. It is only their change in social functioning that alerts staff to their altered mental state.

Identification of possible change in emotional state and the onset of mental illness therefore has to rely on the skill of care staff in observing emotional changes, or on accurate records of a client's affective state. If the client is at a pre-intentional stage of communication, the client's emotional state is interpreted by the care staff's use of their personal knowledge to determine the meaning of each behaviour – the type of 'Simon always touches his hair if he's very anxious' knowledge of which a person who was unfamiliar with the client would be unaware. This subjective interpretation of emotional states may vary from one individual care staff member to another, depending on their sensitivity and emotional set. A person who is pale and shaking can be perceived as either very worried or extremely angry (Bailey et al., 1986), depending on the observer's perception of the situation. Collection of all the staff's observations of body language, facial expression, gestures and the non-verbal aspects of communication is required. If the client uses verbal communication as well, additional information is needed about the non-verbal aspects of speech (e.g. pitch, tone of voice, volume and intonation and rate of utterance). This information is then supplemented and supported by observational assessments by the SLT.

Case study 10.2

The intervention described in this case study led to a slight improvement in the client's communication but the main outcome was the staff's improved understanding of the social changes which had led to the altered behaviour.

Michelle had attended the same day centre for 15 years. The SLT was consulted when, 6 months previously, Michelle had stopped speaking with peers and staff but continued to communicate at home. This was linked to the centre's reorganisation of activity groups. The initial interview between the referrer and the SLT suggested that she had been an effective communicator who had used clear telegrammatic speech. A diagnosis of 'selective mutism' had been suggested by the clinical psychology service. No neurological or progressive deterioration was involved. The request for a communication assessment and social management programme by the day centre staff showed they were, as is common, ignoring the significance of her symptoms in terms of an emotional disorder (Raghavan, 1996). The SLT undertook a series of observations of the whole client group's activities and social communication structure to determine the function of Michelle's communication withdrawal. Leudar and Fraser (1985b) suggested that withdrawal from communication is usually active and complex. Withdrawal may be an attempt to gain control of an interaction but silence can mean passive compliance, fury, and resentment, or have no actual pragmatic communicative meaning at all.

In the new group settings, Michelle's daycare worker's time was being more dominated by her verbal peers. It was felt that Michelle was responding to this social change by actively withholding communication. Her strategy of silence seemed to be aimed at gaining and maintaining attention. When it was her turn in a group activity, the momentum of the whole group ceased while everybody, staff and peers, waited for her response and persuaded her to take part. It was felt that Michelle's withdrawal of communication was a sign of stress but she was also using it to show her resentment about the changes. However, it also seemed to be an attention-gaining strategy since it successfully maintained the focus of attention on herself in a way she could not achieve with her speech and language skills.

These findings were discussed and accepted by the unit's staff, and it was suggested that one of the group activities could be altered to give increased status to non-verbal communication within the whole day centre. Michelle's key group was therefore asked to develop the use of symbols within the centre and to be advocates for a 'total communication' environment. They became responsible for the production of symbol materials and games to enable the teaching of manual signs.

The care staff were encouraged to reflect on the way their management of Michelle's silence could reinforce her use of withholding co-operation. The room's physical arrangement was changed and the seating of the group members was altered. One staff member took responsibility for maintaining the momentum of the group activity and Michelle was placed directly in her eye line. The co-worker praised Michelle for any non-verbal interaction and co-operation. No demands for verbal interactions were made. Once the project was operating successfully, the SLT withdrew and had contact only as and when requested by the client group for support with their activity project. Michelle continued to remain mostly silent but she had begun to participate a little more in the group's activities.

New referrals to speech and language services for people with a DD tend to be relatively infrequent – about 1–2 per year for each 100 000 of the total local community population. These can be from community-based services or from secure accommodation services which cater for those people with LD who are also sectioned under the Mental Health Act. The most common requests for assistance are from specialised community residential or specialised daycare services. These daycare unit referrals usually take the form of requests for assistance with group activities or input into educational projects (Dobson et al., 1999). The staff have an idea which they wish to implement but feel that they need support in establishing social and communication targets within their care plan. Community LD teams, or the behavioural nurse therapists who may be attached to clinical psychology departments, also make referrals. The requests are for both assessment and intervention but occasionally they may be to assist with a differential diagnosis.

Case study 10.3

Improved services and staff development projects may trigger referrals for clients who may have previously been misdiagnosed. However, new awareness of the characteristics of particular 'fashionable' disorders may require therapists to present clear arguments to support their clinical judgements.

Paul was a 32 year old man who had a history of many alterations in his care patterns. Paul's outbursts of verbal abuse and his self-injurious behaviour had recently become more frequent and severe. They were associated with an increase in self-imposed isolation and avoidance of company. He reinforced his distress and heightened his anxiety by the use of ritual phrases referring to past events. He was prescribed both tran-quillisers and antipsychotic drugs and had recently been re-referred to a psychiatrist. The referral to the SLT indicated that there was a discussion about Paul having high-functioning autism/Asperger's syndrome as well as psychosis and mild LD. This opinion was derived from the staff's recent completion of a behaviour screening checklist.

On the initial visit, Paul appeared to be listening and responding to voices, turning to look over his shoulder and comment. He was able to report what the voices he heard were saying, was very distracted and there was a marked time delay before he responded to questions or remarks. His speech was noted to be slow and disjointed. His conversa-tional style lacked coherence. Assessments demonstrated his comprehen-sion and expression of language was at the average age level of 10 years 2 months. There was no evidence of 'computer-like impassivity' associ-ated with Asperger's syndrome but he did appear to have some pragmatic deficits which impeded social synchronisation (Berney, 1997).

The early case history that was available failed to suggest that Paul had exhibited the traits associated with autism in early childhood. The SLT needed to consider Paul's realisation of the three aspects of social communication (Bradshaw et al., 1997) in relation to the triad of impair-ments for autism spectrum disorders as described by Wing (1996). Some of Paul's functional use of language and elements of his style of social interaction were compatible with descriptions of Asperger's syndrome in adults. This syndrome and psychosis have other features besides commu-nication styles and patterns of social interaction which are common to both disorders:

- lack of empathy
- dislike of changes in structure and routine
- special or unusual interests
- the tendency to be a loner
- poor motor co-ordination
- possible self-injury.

A small number of people with autism spectrum disorders, particularly those with Asperger's syndrome, are known to develop psychoses as adults (Szatmari et al., 1989). The SLT's report regarding his use of social communication was therefore a necessary contribution to inform the core team's future case management. Paul's current social behaviour appeared to give little support for the diagnosis of autism or Asperger's syndrome. It was felt that the screening checklist used prior to the referral had given a false positive result. The section about communication had lacked sufficient discrimination to take account of his mild LD and its effect on Paul's ability to use language in social interactions.

The voices Paul talked about appeared to be beyond his control. They were not the result of him considering his internal thought processes as not belonging to him (P Carpenter, 1999), as can occur with autism. Nor did the voices appear to be delayed reactions to previous events, rehearsals or replays of previous conversations. It was also reported that his behaviour was similar in all settings. It did not vary to any great degree depending on the circumstances or with the social partners involved, as described with Asperger's syndrome by Attwood (1998).

The report that the SLT presented to the referring team described and discussed this evidence of his social use of communication. It acknowledged that adults with high-functioning autism and Asperger's syndrome are prone to develop secondary mood disorders (Clarke, 1996). The conclusion was that Paul did not appear to show the communication disabilities that are associated with adults with autism spectrum disorders. However, it was felt that the use of social stories (Gray, 1994), as used with people with autism, might enable Paul to develop control of his own behaviour. The SLT's recommendations also outlined staff's best style of responses and language use when Paul was becoming distressed. The aim was to define a structure so that language use enabled the achievement of control rather than imposing control through language in an attempt to attain structure.

The action plan outlined a collaborative working strategy with a behavioural nurse therapist:

- improving the quality of Paul's social communication environment
- helping Paul develop cognitive and visual scripts to control his own behaviour.

The final package of intervention offered training, resources, support and development to the work of the care staff at both Paul's residential and daycare units.

Referral for alterations in speech clarity or fluency

When working with clients with a DD, the SLT has to be aware that prescribed medication may be a factor in some of the presenting speech problems of some clients. The case history prior to assessment and any proposed treatment must always include such factors as the type and number of different medications, the length of time they have been prescribed and any recent alterations in the levels of dosage. This is particularly important in those referrals that occur because of a change in the client's speech clarity or fluency. It is not uncommon for a referral to be made because a person with a DD has developed a dysarthria. If, on examination and assessment, the SLT can find no evidence of an under-lying neurological cause and there is no evidence of a deteriorating disorder, the client's drug therapy programme has to be considered as a causal factor. Some anti-psychotic agents that are used in both schizophrenia and mania have a tendency to produce extrapyramidal movement disorders. For some clients, these drugs have side effects which result in a slowing of control over the speech musculature. The symptoms may be jerky speech, dysrhythmic phonation, poor articulation, monotonous intonation and a soft voice (Muir et al., 1991). These types of side effects can be managed, or relieved, by the prescription of anti-parkinsonian agents.

Long-term high dosage of neuroleptic medication may lead to 'tardive dyskinesia' (Tyrer and Dunstan, 1997). This can also result in articulation difficulties, but differs in that phonation tends to be loud with a dysarthria which may appear more like a stutter. Lowering or stopping of the original level of drug dosage may cause a worsening in these dysarthric symptoms. The medical team may consider that none of the medication management solutions are appropriate, given the nature of the client's disorder. The SLT then has to assist with the management of the client's speech clarity by traditional therapeutic methods using an individual one-to-one approach (Muir et al., 1991). This would involve work on posture, breathing exercises, tongue, lip and palate exercises and vocal training. The success of this type of intervention depends on the client's level of co-operation, understanding of the listener's needs in a conversation and being motivated to maintain a level of easily understood speech clarity. The client needs to develop self-awareness of head and neck posture, breathing, voice levels and rate of speech. There is also a need for a willingness to accept and implement feedback about speech clarity both within the therapeutic situation and in general conversation. The client's ability to accept and maintain the use of such strategies is therefore the most important factor in obtaining a successful therapeutic outcome.

This type of presentation of dysarthria due to the prescribed medication often occurs in those clients whose second diagnosis is schizophrenia. They may already have other existing conversational and linguistic features that alter their speech patterns. The success of any such intervention is therefore difficult to predict and the SLT has to be aware that fluctuations in the presenting emotional disorder will also be a criterion for continuing treatment. It is not unusual for a client to incorporate the reason for their speech problem into their hallucinations, or delusions. For example, one man explained at length, to anyone who would listen, that his Parkinson-like festinating speech pattern was due to the Earth spinning out of its orbit because of Russian nuclear bomb testing.

Some patients who present with a stutter may have had a well-recorded history of non-fluent speech which ceased on the introduction of antipsychotic medication in late adolescence. The stutter only reoccurs in later life when drug therapy has been reduced or withdrawn. It is then difficult to judge whether the client has a recurrence of their original problem with fluency, or whether it is due to issues relating to drugs. Such clients respond best to the introduction of one of the techniques, such as prolonged speech, which aim to teach the control of the non-fluency. However, this very much depends on the attitude and support provided by the client's immediate care team.

Forensic cases

Forensic cases involving offenders with a DD usually involve the SLT assisting the clinical psychologist, or the psychiatrist, after the behavioural assessments have been completed. Their role is to assess the client's levels of verbal and non-verbal communication comprehension and expression. They may also give opinions about comparisons between clients' perceived competence and their actual performance in different activities and settings, and with various people. The lead member of the forensic team will also require the SLT to give details of any additional disabilities such as language disorders, word-finding difficulties or specific deficits in understanding and recognising emotions, social use of communication and social interaction skills. Once the assessment is complete the SLT supports the multi-disciplinary team in their work on behavioural interventions by advising on levels of language use by staff and the methods of supporting the interventions used by other professions.

The information collected by the team may be used in pending court cases and is most often presented by the consultant leading the team. However, there are occasions when a SLT is required to present evidence as well. This task cannot be undertaken unless the SLT concerned has had additional relevant training in this type of presentation. The questions addressed in court may relate to whether the patient is fit to plead, whether treatment is necessary and where it can be delivered. A description of an individual's communication skills is also needed because a precondition for successful participation in particular types of treatment groups is good verbal communication skills (Gravell and France, 1991b). Because the assessment of clients with a DD is often an informal one, the analysis of observations, the use of carer narratives and subjective judgements based on knowledge and experience may not be easily accepted by the court as defensible documentation.

The problem for the SLT is that there is a limited number of reliable and valid assessments available for this group of service users. The clinician may have to use a range of paediatric and adult communication assessments, only some of which are designed for people with LD. The Test of Reception of Grammar (TROG; Bishop, 1989), for example, supplies one useful type of information, but the materials are child orientated and it is inappropriate to give the age range of the ceiling items achieved. The British Picture Vocabulary Scales (BPVS; Dunn et al., 1982) do have an adult version, but most of the patient group would need to access the children's levels of the assessment. In addition, knowledge of the level of vocabulary and grammar understood does not give information about the number of key words which can be understood and processed at any one time, nor does it account for varied performance in differing settings, or responses to different use of language by carers. At present, there is no accredited formal assessment for adults with LD which would provide this type of information.

The range of assessments that are specifically designed for adults with LD include formal assessments but also rely heavily on checklists completed by those who are currently in daily contact with them. The analysis of results may therefore be subjective due to the knowledge of past events, attitude, value systems and bias due to the cultural and social behavioural viewpoints of those supplying the information. Other assessments, such as the Communication Assessment Profile (van der Gaag, 1988), supply the required detailed information about the client's whole system of communication through both assessment and carer input, but the charting of performance of individuals on the assessment is against the performance of other people within the LD population.

A creative approach to using the information gathered can assist the SLT; for example, plotting the results of a Personal Communication Plan

(Hitchings and Spence, 1991) from various care groups on to acetates so that overlays from different settings can be compared may assist analysis of the data. However, the resulting reports drawing together the holistic picture of each individual's communication strengths can never be in a standard format. The headings used, and the description of results, have to be in text form and detailed explanations which are free of medical terms are used. These explanations may need to be supported by scenarios or descriptions of the client's interaction style and actual quotations of responses to different types of carer language scripts. The report needs to define when alternative methods of communication were used to support a client's understanding and the effect this had on the client's responses. Pragmatic skills also have to be included. Comments on the understanding and expression of emotions must of necessity be included as well.

Once the assessment is complete, the SLT's role depends on the agreement reached by the multi-disciplinary team. Communication interventions are most often integrated within a planned group activity such as assertiveness skills, exercise programmes, personal and social skills, or sex education sessions. The SLT may be required to provide indirect input in the form of:

- identifying and prioritising the individual patient's communication goals
- advising on the level and type of language used in the activity
- advising on the seating plan relevant to the patients' social interaction styles
- defining staff's social roles for the activity
- providing alternative methods of communication to support staff and patient's communication
- planning the structure and defining the routine of the group
- modifying the activity so that it provides support for understanding
- integrating a social use of communication intervention into a daily activity
- evaluating the learning outcomes in terms of communication.

The SLT may also be directly involved in other professions' interventions which use cognitive or behaviour therapy, or psychotherapy, to facilitate change in the patient. The SLT would take a supportive role in relation to the group leader who may be a behaviour nurse therapist, a psychologist or a social worker. This is an important role because the area of greatest difficulty for many clients is their lack of vocabulary or communication skills about feelings (France, 1991) and, without support, it may limit their ability to successfully participate in treatment. The clinical emphasis is most commonly one of underlining the fact that communication is not a separate ring-fenced activity but one in which everybody has an equally important therapeutic role. It is not owned by one profession and it cannot be separated or isolated from other parts of a client's care plan.

Conclusion

SLTs who work with clients with a DD need to utilise all the more traditional therapeutic methods employed in working with people with LD. The ability to introduce intervention programmes that use alternative and augmentative communication techniques and foster the development of social skills are, therefore, essential professional skills. They also need to be able to work as part of a varied selection of multi-disciplinary teams, utilise and adapt to a range of differing service models.

The additional and equally important diagnosis of a psychiatric illness for an individual with LD, however, means that the SLT also needs to develop a further knowledge base. They need to know about working with clients with psychotic, behavioural and emotional disorders. There is a growing body of literature to help SLTs who choose to work with people with a DD. There is certainly an increasing clinical demand for this kind of specialist SLT input to clients' care plans.

Working with clients with a DD mainly involves integrating group intervention packages which focus on facilitating social interactions and foster effective communication within existing social activities and care settings. The outcomes for the individuals who attend the groups are usually successful, in that they foster all the clients' well-being, develop the use of effective communication strategies and reduce the degree of social handicap that the clients may experience in group settings. They can also reduce the level of distress the care staff express about their own inability to interact because of their clients' communication difficulties. A smaller number of referrals require an individual approach with one-to-one therapy. This type of referral often demands the use of more traditional therapeutic approaches. Therapy outcomes for these clients are more variable because of the level of co-operation and motivation that is required from the individuals involved.

It also has to be borne in mind that fluctuations in the individual client's mental state, levels of medication and other behavioural or emotional factors may interrupt or lead to the cessation of any current speech and language therapy intervention. Most episodes of therapy are short and time-limited to the specific current reason for the referral. However, like other interventions involving clients with LD, re-referral for any other further period of therapy at a later date is quite common.

References

Abbeduto L, Furnan L, Davies B (1989) Relation between the receptive language and mental age of persons with mental retardation. American Journal on Mental Retardation 93: 535–43.

Abramson L, Jarvis C (1993) Kindergarten parent participation. Head Start influences. Paper presented at the Second National Head Start Research Conference, 1993, Washington, DC.

Abudarham S (ed) (1987) Bilingualism and the Bilingual, Chapter 6. NFER-Nelson, Windsor.

Abudarham, S (1996) The receptive lexicon of Dual Language Gibraltarian primary school children. PhD Thesis. Collected Original Resources in Education 20(3) Fiche 1 A04, Carfax Publishing Co., Abingdon.

Abudarham S (1998) Working in collaboration with 'bilingual' co-workers. Proceedings of the IALP 24th International Conference, 1998, Amsterdam. Folia Phoniatrica 1: 439–41.

Adamson L, Bakeman R (1997) The development of shared attention during infancy. In: Vasta R (ed) Annals of Child Development, 8. Jessica Kingsley Publishers, London, pp. 1–41.

Adamson LB, McArthur D (1995) Joint attention, affect and culture. In: Moore C, Dunham P (eds) Joint Attention: its origin and role in development. Laurence Erlbaum Associates, Hillsdale, NJ, pp. 205–21.

Ainscow M (1997) Towards inclusive schooling. British Journal of Special Education 24(1): 3–6.

Almond K (1998) Failing to live up to its promise? Royal College of Speech and Language Therapists Bulletin (August): 10–11.

Anisfield M (1984) Language Development From Birth to Three. Lawrence Erlbaum Associates, Hillsdale, NJ.

APA (1994) Diagnostic and Statistical Manual of Mental Disorders, 4th edn. American Psychiatric Association, Washington, DC.

Appleton M, Buckley SJ, MacDonald J (2000) A three-year longitudinal study of reading development among pre-school children with Down syndrome and pre-school typically developing children. Down Syndrome Research and Practice 7: 1.

Ara F, Thompson C (1989) Intervention with bilingual pre-school children. In: Duncan DM (ed) Working with Bilingual Language Disability, Chapter 9. Chapman & Hall, London.

ASHA (1993) Guidelines for Caseload Size and Speech and Language Service Delivery in Schools 35 (supplement 10). American Speech and Hearing Association, USA, pp. 33–9.

Atherton K, Lindsay A, Richards I, Spring K (1999) How I work with assistants. Speech and Language Therapy in Practice (Spring): 25–8.

293

Attwood T (1998) Asperger's Syndrome: A guide for parents and professionals. Jessica
    Kingsley Publishers, London.
Awcock C, Habgood N (1998) Early intervention project: Evaluation of WILSTAAR, Hanen
    and specialist playgroup. International Journal of Language Communication Disorders
    Supplement 33: 500–5.
Bailey R, Matthews F, Leckie C (1986) Feeling – the way ahead in mental handicap. Mental
    Handicap (14 June): 65–8.
Baker B (1976) Parent involvement in programming for developmentally disabled children. In:
    Lloyd LL (ed) Communication Assessment and Intervention Strategies. University Park
    Press, Baltimore, MD.
Baker P (1994) Detecting needs: The challenging needs matrix. Pavilion/Tizard Centre
    Seminar on Designing and Delivering Services for People with Challenging Behaviour,
    1994, King's Fund Centre, London.
Balandin S, Ianoco T (1999) Crews, wusses, and whoppas: Core and fringe vocabularies of
    Australian meal-break conversations in the workplace. Augmentative and Alternative
    Communication 15(2): 95–109.
Barblan I, Chipman H (1978) Temporal relationships in language: A comparison between
    normal and language retarded children. In: Drachman G (ed) Salzburger Beitrage zur
    Linguistik. Neugenbauer, Salzburg, pp. 3–32.
Barclay J (1998) People, plans and possibilities. Community Living (October/November) 9–10.
Barker P (1991) Parents' problems and perspectives. In: Fraser WI, McGillivray RC, Green
    AM (eds) Hallas' Caring for People with Mental Handicaps. 8th edn. Butterworth-
    Heinemann, Oxford, pp. 244–57.
Barlett C, Bunning K (1997) The importance of communication partnerships: A study to
    investigate the communicative exchanges between staff and adults with learning disabili-
    ties. British Journal of Learning Disabilities 25: 148–53.
Barnes C (1996) Theories of disability and the origins of the oppression of disabled people in
    western society. In: Barton L (ed) Disability and Society: Emerging issues and insights.
    Longman, Harlow. Chapter 3.
Barnett S (1998) Personal communication.
Barrett M, Diniz F (1989) Lexical development in mentally handicapped children. In:
    Beveridge M, Conti-Ramsden G, Leudar I (eds) Language and Communication in
    Mentally Handicapped People. Chapman & Hall, London, pp. 3–32.
Bartel N, Bryen D, Keehn S (1973) Language comprehension in the moderately retarded
    child. Exceptional Children 39: 379–82.
Barton L (ed) (1996) Disability and Society: Emerging issues and insights. Longman, Harlow.
Batchelor ES, Dean RS (1991) Neuropsychological assessment of learning disorders in children.
    In: Ohrzut JE, Hynd GW (eds) Neuropsychological Foundations of Learning Disabilities –
    a handbook of issues, methods, and practice, Chapter 4. Academic Press, London.
Bates E, Benigni L, Bretherton I, Cameioni L, Volterra V (1979) The Emergence of Symbols,
    Cognition and Communication in Infancy. Academic Press, New York.
Bates E, Bretherton I, Snyder L (1988) From First Words to Grammar: Individual differences
    and dissociable mechanisms. Cambridge University Press, Cambridge.
Baxendale J, Frankham J, Hesketh A (2001) The Hanen Parent Programme: A parent's per-
    spective. RCSLT National Conference – Sharing Communication, April 2001,
    Birmingham. International Journal of Language and Communication Disorders –
    Supplement. Taylor & Francis, London, pp. 511–16.
Bedrosian JL, Calculator SN (1988) Introduction: A misunderstood population. In: Calculator
    SN, Bedrosian JL (eds) Communication Assessment and Intervention for Adults with
    Mental Retardation. Taylor & Francis, London. Chapter 1.

Bee H (1981) The Developing Child, 3rd edn. Harper and Row, New York.

Beech J, Harding L, Hilton-Jones D (1993) Assessment in Speech and Language. Routledge, London.

Bellugi U, O'Grady L, Lillo-Martin D, O'Grady Hynes M, van Hoek K, Cortina D (1990a) Enhancement of spatial cognition in deaf children. In: Volterra V, Erting C (eds) From Gesture to Language in Hearing and Deaf Children. Springer-Verlag, Berlin, pp. 278–98.

Bellugi U, Birhle A, Jernigan T, Trauner D, Doherty S (1990b) Neuropsychological, neurological and neuroanatomical profile of Williams syndrome. American Journal of Medical Genetics Supplement 6: 115–25.

Berger A, Henderson J, Morris D (1999) Implementing the Literacy Hour for Pupils with Learning Difficulties. David Fulton, London.

Berney TP (1997) Autism and Asperger's syndrome. In: Read SG (ed) Psychiatry and Learning Disability. W.B. Saunders, London, pp. 151–84.

Berrueta-Clement JR, Schweinhart LJ, Barnett C, Epstein S, Weikart DP (1984) Changed Lives: the effects of the Perry Preschool Project on youths through age 19. High/Scope Educational Research Foundation, Ypsilanti, MI.

Beukelman D, McGinnis J, Morrow D (1991) Vocabulary selection in augmentative and alternative communication. Augmentative and Alternative Communication 7(3): 171–85.

Beukelman D, Mirenda P (1998) Augmentative and Alternative Communication Management of Severe Communication Disorders in Children and Adults, 2nd edn. Paul H. Brookes, Baltimore.

Bishop DVM (1985) Spelling ability in congenital dysarthria: Evidence against articulatory coding in translating between phonemes and graphemes. Cognitive Neuropsychology 2(3): 229–51.

Bishop DVM (1989) Test of Reception of Grammar (TROG). Dr D. Bishop, University of Manchester, Manchester, UK.

Bishop DVM (1992) The underlying nature of specific language impairment. Journal of Child Psychology and Psychiatry 33: 3–66.

Bishop DVM, Robson J (1989) Unimpaired short-term memory and rhyme judgement in congenitally speechless individuals: Implications for the notion of 'articulatory coding'. Quarterly Journal of Experimental Psychology 41A(1): 123–40.

Bishop K, Rankin J, Mirenda P (1994) Impact of graphic symbol use on reading acquisition. Augmentative and Alternative Communication 10(2): 113–25.

Blackwell CL, Hulbert CM, Bell J, Elston L, Morgan W, Robertshaw BA, Thomas C (1989) A survey of the communication abilities of people with a mental handicap. British Journal of Mental Subnormality 35. 63–71.

Blishak D (1994) Phonological awareness: Implications for individuals with little or no functional speech. Augmentative and Alternative Communication 10(4): 245–54.

Bloom L, Capatides JB (1991) Language Development From 2 to 3. Cambridge University Press, Cambridge.

Bloom L, Lahey M (1978) Language Development and Language Disorders. John Wiley & Son, New York.

Bloomberg K, Karlan G, Lloyd LL (1990) The comparative translucency of initial lexical items represented in five graphic symbol systems and sets. Journal of Speech and Hearing Research (December) 33: 717–25.

Bluma S, Shearer M, Froham A, Hilliard J (1976) Portage Guide to Early Education. Cooperative Educational Services, Portage, WI.

Blunden R, Allen D (1987) Facing the Challenge: An ordinary life for people with learning difficulties and challenging behaviours. King's Fund, London.

Bol G, Kuiken F (1990) Grammatical analysis of developmental langauge disorders: A study of the morphosyntax of children with specific language disorders, with hearing impairment and with Down's syndrome. Clinical Linguistics and Phonetics 4: 77–86.

Bondy A, Frost L (1986) The Picture Exchange Communication System. Pyramid Educational Consultants, Brighton.

Bondy A, Frost L (1994) The picture exchange communication system. Focus on Autistic Behavior 9: 1–19.

Borghi R (1990) Consonant phoneme and distinctive feature error patterns in speech. In: Van Dyke D, Lang D, Heide F, Van Duyne S, Soucek M (eds) Clinical Perspectives in the Management of Down's Syndrome. Springer, New York, pp. 147–52.

Bowler DM, Lister Brook S (1997) From general impairment to behavioural phenotypes: Psychological approaches to learning difficulties. In: Fawcus M (ed) Children With Learning Difficulties: a collaborative approach to their management. Whurr Publishers, London, pp. 1–17.

Bradley H (1991a) Assessing Communication Together: A systematic approach to assessing and developing early communication skills in children and adults with multi-sensory impairments. Penarth Mental Handicap Nurses Association.

Bradley H (1991b) ACT – Assessing Communication Together. APLD Working for People with Learning Disabilities, Nottingham.

Bradley H (1998) Assessing and developing successful communication. In: Lacey P, Ouvry C (eds) People with Profound and Multiple Learning Disabilities – a collaborative approach to meet complex needs, Chapter 5. David Fulton Publishers, London.

Bradshaw J (1998) Assessing and intervening in the communication environment. British Journal of Learning Disabilities 26: 62–6.

Bradshaw J, Baker V (1996;1997) Short Course for Speech and Language Therapists Working with Adults with Learning Disabilities who Challenge Services. Tizard Centre, University of Kent, Canterbury.

Bradshaw J, Brent E, Macdonald S (1997) Disentangling the nature of autism. In: Holt G, Bouras N (eds) Mental Health and Learning Disability. Pavilion Publishing, Brighton, pp. 143–56.

Braine M (1976) Children's first word combinations. Monographs of the Society for Research in Child Development 41(164): 1–96.

Branigan G (1979) Some reasons why successive single word utterances are not. Journal of Child Language 6: 411–21.

Bray M, Ross A, Todd C (1999) Speech and Language Clinical Process and Practice. Whurr Publishers, London.

Brewer N (1987) Processing speed, efficiency and intelligence. In: Borkowski JG, Day JD (eds) Cognition in Special Children: Comparative approaches to retardation, learning disabilities and giftedness. Ablex, Norwood, NJ.

Bricker D, Squires J (1989) The effectiveness of parental screening of at-risk infants. Topics in Early Childhood Special Education 9(3): 67–85.

Bridges A, Smith J (1984) Syntactic comprehension in Down's syndrome. British Journal of Psychology 75: 187–96.

Brigden P, Todd M (1993) Concepts in Community Care for People with a Learning Difficulty. Macmillan, London.

Brinkworth R (1983) Personal communication.

Brinkworth R, Abudarham S (1984) The development of communicative skills in a group of 12 Down's syndrome children aged 3 months and 5 years. International Association of Logopedists and Phoniatrists Conference, Edinburgh, 1983, 328–33.

British Council for the Welfare of Spastics (1952) Notes for Parents on the Home Care of Children Handicapped by Cerebral Palsy, 4th edn. British Council for the Welfare of Spastics, London.

Broadley I, MacDonald J, Buckley S (1993) Working memory in children with DS. Down's Syndrome: Research and Practice 3: 3–8.

Brown C (1972) The Childhood Story of Christy Brown. Pan Books, London.

Brown H, Emerson E, Barrett S, Cummings R (1989) Using Analogue Assessments. Centre for the Applied Psychology of Social Care, University of Kent, Canterbury.

Brown R (1973) A First Language: The early stages. Harvard University Press, Cambridge, MA.

Brownlee JR, Bakeman R (1981) Hitting in toddler–peer interaction. Child Development 52: 1076–9.

Brownlee KT (1996) Development of an individualised sensory environment for adults with learning disabilities and an evaluation of its effects on their interactive behaviours. Unpublished PhD Thesis. City University, London.

Bryan T (1998) Social competence of students with learning disabilities. In: Wong B (ed) Learning about Learning Disabilities, 2nd edn, Chapter 7. Academic Press, London.

Bryen D, Goldman A, Quinlisk-Gill S (1988) Sign language with students with SPMR: How effective is it? Education and Training of the Mentally Retarded 23: 129–37.

Buckley S (1992) The development of the child with Down's syndrome: Implications for effective education. In: Rogers P, Coleman M (eds) Medical Care in Down's Syndrome: a preventive medicine approach. Dekker, New York: pp. 29–67.

Buckley S (1993) Developing the speech and language skills of teenagers with Down's Syndrome. Down's Syndrome Research and Practice 1: 34–9.

Buckley S (1999) Promoting the cognitive development of children with Down syndrome: The practical implications of recent psychological research. In: Rondal JA, Perera J, Nadel L (eds) Down Syndrome – a review of current knowledge. Whurr Publishers, London. Chapter 9.

Buitelaar JK, van der Wees M, Swaab-Barneveld H, van der Gaag RJ (1999) Verbal memory and performance IQ predict theory of mind and emotion recognition ability in children with autistic spectrum disorders and in psychiatric control children. Journal of Child Psychology and Psychiatry 40(6): 869–81.

Bulpitt D (1989) Means, reasons, and opportunities model: Training material. Leicester Health Authority & Central Nottinghamshire Health Authority, Nottingham.

Bunning KT (1996) The principles of an 'individualised sensory environment'. RCSLT Bulletin 525: 9–10.

Bunning KT, Bradshaw J (in submission) The importance of communication skills to people who challenge services: Defining the role of the speech and language therapist.

Burford B (1989) Action cycles: Rhythmic actions for engagement with children and young adults with profound mental handicap. European Journal of Special Needs Education 3: 189–206.

Burke GM (1990) Unconventional behaviour: A communicative interpretation in individuals with severe disabilities. Topics in Language Disabilities 10: 75–8.

Burke P, Cigno K (eds) (2000) Learning Disabilities in Children. Blackwell Science, Oxford.

Butterfield N, Arthur M, Sigafoos J (1995) Partners in Everyday Communicative Exchanges. Maclellan & Petty, Sydney, Australia.

Bzoch K, League R (1971) The Receptive and Expressive Emergent Language Scales (REEL). NFER, Windsor.

Cade BW (1993) Burnout: Snuffed out fire within. Social Work Today 14(18): 8–10.

Calculator SN (1988) Exploring the language of adults with mental retardation. In: Calculator SN, Bedrosian JL (eds) Communication Assessment and Intervention for Adults with Mental Retardation. Taylor & Francis, London. Chapter 4.

Calculator SN, Jorgensen C (1991) Integrating AAC instruction into regular education settings: Expounding on best practices. Augmentative and Alternative Communication 7(3): 204–12.

Cameron RJ, White M (1987) The Portage Early Education Programme. NFER-Nelson, Windsor.

Cardoso-Martin C, Mervis CB, Mervis CA (1985) Early vocabulary acquisition by children with Down syndrome. American Journal of Mental Deficiency 90: 177–84.

Carpenter B (1987) A formative evaluation of a Makaton-based reading programme. Unpublished MPhil thesis. University of Nottingham.

Carpenter B (1999) A multi-modal approach to literacy. The SLD Experience 23 (Spring): 10–13.

Carpenter P (1999) The use of medication to treat mental illness in adults with Autism Spectrum disorders. Autism 99 Internet Conference.

Carr EG, Durand M (1985) The social-communicative basis of severe behaviour problems in children. In: Reiss S, Bootzin RR (eds) Theoretical Issues in Behaviour Therapy. Academic Press, New York, pp. 219–54.

Carr EG, McConnachie G, Levin L, Kemp DC (1993) Communication based treatment and severe behaviour problems. In: Van Houten R, Axelrod S (eds) Behavioural Analysis and Treatment. Plenum Press, London, pp. 231–67.

Carr EG, McConnachie G, Levin L, Kemp DC (1994) Communication-Based Intervention for Problem Behaviour. Paul H. Brookes, Baltimore.

Caulfield MB, Fischel JE, DeBaryshe BD, Whitehurst GJ (1989) Behavioral correlates of developmental expressive language disorder. Journal of Abnormal Child Psychology 17: 187–201.

Ceci J (1986) Handbook of Cognitive, Social-Neuropsychological Aspects of Learning Disabilities. Erlbaum, Hillsdale, NJ.

Chamberlain L, Cheung Chung M, Jenner L (1993) Preliminary findings on communication and challenging behaviour in learning difficulty. British Journal of Learning Disabilities XXXIX, 2(77): 118–25.

Chapman RS (1978) Comprehension strategies in children. In: Kuranagh JF, Strange W (eds) Speech and Language Learning in the Laboratory, School and Clinic. MIT Press, Cambridge, MA, pp. 308–30.

Chapman RS (1995) Language development in children and adolescents with Down Syndrome. In: Fletcher P, MacWhinney B (eds) Handbook of Child Language. Blackwell, Oxford, pp. 641–63.

Chapman RS, Schwartz SE, Kay-Raining Bird E (1991) Language skills of children and adolescents with Down Syndrome 1. Comprehension. Journal of Speech and Hearing Research 34: 1106–20.

Chiat S (2000) Understanding Children with Language Problems. Cambridge University Press, Cambridge.

Chinner S, Hazell G, Skinner P, Thomas P, Williams G (2001) Developing Augmentative and Alternative Communication Policies in Schools: Information and Guidelines. ACE Centre Advisory Trust, Oxford.

Cholmain C (1994) Working on phonology with young children with Down's syndrome: A pilot study. Journal of Clinical Speech and Language Studies 1: 14–35.

Chronically Sick and Disabled Person's Act (1970) Her Majesty's Stationery Office, London.

Cipani E (1990) The communicative function hypothesis: An operant behaviour perspective. Journal of Behaviour Therapy and Experimental Psychiatry 21(4): 239–47.

Clare I (1996) Working with an individual. Pavilion Conference: Understanding and Responding to Challenging Behaviour, King's Fund, London.

Clarke DJ (1996) Psychiatric and behavioural problems and pharmacological treatments. In: Morgan H (ed) Adults with Autism. Cambridge University Press, Cambridge, pp. 197–230.

Clarke-Kehoe A, Harris P (1992) It's the way that you say it. Community Care (9 July): 21–22.

Coggins TE (1979) Relational meaning encoded in the two-word utterances of Stage 1 Down's Syndrome children. Journal of Speech and Hearing Research 22: 166–78.

Cole KN, Harris SR, Eland SF, Mills P (1989) A comparison of two service delivery models: in class and out of class therapy approaches. Paediatric Physical Therapy 1: 49–54.

Collis E (1947) A Way of Life for the Handicapped Child: A new approach to cerebral palsy. Faber, London.

Comblain A (1994) Working memory in Down's Syndrome. Down's Syndrome: Training Rehearsal Strategies 2: 123–6.

Connell P (1987) Teaching language, form, meaning and function to specific-language-impaired children. In: Rosenberg S (ed) Advances in Applied Psycholinguistics, Vol. 1. Disorders of First Language Development. Cambridge University Press, Cambridge, pp. 40–76.

Conners FA (1992) Reading instruction for students with moderate mental retardation: Review and analysis of research. American Journal on Mental Retardation 96(6): 577–97.

Conti-Ramsden G (1994) Language interaction with atypical language learners. In: Gallaway C, Richards B (eds) Input and Interaction in Language Acquisition. Cambridge University Press, Cambridge, pp. 183–96.

Cooper J, Moodley M, Reynell J (1978) Helping Language Development. Edward Arnold, London.

Cooper JH (1981) An Early Childhood Special Education Primer. Technical Assistance Development System (TADS), Chapel Hill, NC.

Corbett J (1979) Psychiatric morbidity and mental retardation. In: Snaith P, James FE (eds) Psychiatric Illness and Mental Handicap. Headly Brothers, Ashford, pp. 11–25.

Cottam PJ (1986) Speech therapy service provision and management of mentally handicapped adults: the results of a questionnaire survey. British Journal of Mental Subnormality 32: 108–13.

Cottier C, Doyle M, Gilworth K (1997) Functional AAC Intervention: A team approach. Imaginart International, Inc, Arizona.

Coulter L, Gallagher C (2001a) Piloting new ways of working: Evaluation of the WILSTAAR programme. RCSLT National Conference – Sharing Communication, April 2001, Birmingham, UK. International Journal of Language and Communication Disorders – Supplement. Taylor & Francis, London 36, 270–5.

Coulter L, Gallagher C (2001b) Evaluation of the Hanen early Childhood Educators Programme. In: RCSLT National Conference – Sharing Communication, April 2001, Birmingham, UK. International Journal of Language and Communication Disorders – Supplement. Taylor & Francis, London 36, 264–9.

Coupe O'Kane J, Goldbart J (2000) Communication Before Speech: Development and assessment, 2nd edn. David Fulton Publishers, London.

Cross A, Park K (2000) Whose needs come first? The use of objects of reference with people who have severe and profound learning disability. Communication Matters 14(1): 25–6.

Crystal D (1982) Profiling Linguistic Ability. Edward Arnold, London.

Cullen C (1987) Nurse training and institutional constraints. In: Hogg J, Mittler P (eds) Staff Training in Mental Handicap. Croom Helm, London, pp. 335–71.

Cullen C (1988) A review of staff training: The emperor's old clothes. Irish Journal of Psychology, 9, 309–23.

Cunningham CC (1987) Early intervention in Down's syndrome. In: Hoskins G, Murphy G (eds) Prevention of Mental Handicap: a world view. Royal Society of Medicine Services, London, pp. 169–82.

Cunningham CC, Davis H (1985) Working with Parents – frameworks for collaboration. Open University Press, Buckingham.

Curtiss S (1988) The special talent of grammar acquisition. In: Obler L, Fein D (eds) The Exceptional Brain. Guilford, New York, pp. 364–86.

Dahlgren Sandberg A, Hjelmquist E (1996) Phonologic awareness and literacy abilities in non-speaking preschool children. Augmentative and Alternative Communication 12(3): 138–53.

Dale P (1991) The validity of a parent report measure of vocabulary and syntax at 24 months. Journal of Speech Hearing Research 34: 565–71.

de Graaf E (1995) Early intervention for children with Down's Syndrome. In: Vermeer A, Davis W (eds) Physical and Motor Development in Mental Retardation. Karger, Basel, pp. 120–43.

Dean E, Howell J, Hill A, Waters D (1990) Metaphon Resource Pack. NFER-Nelson, Windsor.

DeCoste DC (1997) Augmentative and alternative communication assessment strategies: motor access and visual considerations. In: Glennen SL, DeCoste DC (eds) Handbook of Augmentative and Alternative Communication. Singular, London, pp. 243–82.

Department of Health (1993) Services for People with Learning Disabilities and Challenging Behaviour or Mental Health Needs: report of a project group. HMSO, London.

DES (1978) Special Educational Needs: Report of the Committee of Enquiry into the education of handicapped children and young people (The Warnock Report). HMSO, London.

DES (1981) Education Act. HMSO, London.

Detheridge T (1998) Personal communication.

Detheridge T, Detheridge M (1997) Literacy through Symbols. David Fulton Publishers, London.

Devaney BL, Ellwood MR, Love JM (1997) Programs that mitigate the effects of poverty on children. Future of Children 7(2): 88–112.

Dewart H, Summers S (1997) The Pragmatics Profile of Everyday Communication Skills in Children. NFER-Nelson, Windsor.

Dewart H, Summers S (1997) The Pragmatics Profile of Everyday Communication Skills in Adults. NFER-Nelson, Windsor.

DfE (1994) Code of Practice on the Identification and Assessment of Special Educational Needs. Central Office of Information, London; EDUC JO22465NJ 5/94.

DfEE (1997) Excellence for all Children: Meeting Special Educational Needs. Department for Employment and Education. Stationery Office, London.

DfEE (1998a) The National Literacy Strategy: Framework for teaching. Department for Education and Employment, London.

DfEE (1998b) Meeting Special Educational Needs: A programme of action. Department for Education and Employment, London.

DfEE (1998c) Learning and Working Together for the Future: Aims and objectives. Department for Employment and Education. Stationery Office, London.

DfEE (2000a) Framework for the Assessment of Children in Need and their Families (SEN Update, March). HMSO, London.

DfEE (2000b) Special Educational Needs – special edition (December). HMSO, London.

DfEE (2000c) National Curriculum Handbook for Secondary Teachers in England. Key Stages 3 and 4. Department for Employment and Education. Stationery Office, London.

Dobson S (1990) Report on Speech Therapy Services to adults with learning difficulties. Huddersfield Health Authority, Huddersfield.

Dobson S (1995) Together we can talk. Community Care 1091 (19–25 October): 19–25.

Dobson S, Stanley B, Maley M (1999) A communication and integrated exercise programme in a day centre for adults with challenging behaviours. British Journal of Learning Disability 27(1): 20–2.

Dockrell J (1989) Meeting the needs of the parents with speech and language difficulties. Child Language Teaching and Therapy 5(2): 146–56.

Dockrell J, McShane J (1993) Children's Learning Difficulties – a cognitive approach. Blackwell Publishers, Oxford.

Donahue M, Pearl R, Bryan T (1983) Communicative competence in learning disabled children. Advances in Learning and Behavioural Disabilities 2: 49–84.

Donaldson ML (1995) Children with Language Impairments – an introduction. Jessica Kingsley Publishers, London.

Donnellan AM, Mirenda PL, Mesaros RA, Fassbender LL (1984) Analysing the communicative functions of aberrant behaviour. Journal of the Association of Persons with Severe Handicaps 9(3): 201–12.

Dooley J (1976) Language acquisition and Down's syndrome: A study of early semantics and syntax. Unpublished doctoral dissertation, Harvard University.

Dore J (1975) Holophrases, speech acts and language universals. Journal of Child Language 2: 21–40.

Duchan J, Erickson J (1976) Normal and non-retarded children's understanding of semantic relations in different verbal contexts. Journal of Speech and Hearing Research 19: 767–76.

Dunn LM, Dunn LM, Whetton C, Pintillie D (1982) British Picture Vocabulary Scale (BPVS). NFER-Nelson, Windsor.

Dunn Klein M (1988) Pre-Sign Language Motor Skills: Skill starters for motor development. Communication Skill Builders, Arizona.

Dunst C (1978) A cognitive-social approach to assessment of early non-verbal behaviour. Journal of Communication Disorders 2: 110–23.

Dunst C (1981) Infant Learning. DLM Teaching Resources, Texas.

Dunst C, Lowe L, Bartholomew P (1990) Contingent social responsiveness, family ecology and infant communicative competence. National Students Speech, Language, Hearing Association Journal 17: 39–49.

Durand VM (1986) Self-injurious behaviour as an intentional communication. In: Gadow KD (ed) Advances in Learning and Behavioural Disabilities, 5. JAI Press, Greenwich, Conn., pp. 141–55.

Durand VM (1990) Severe Behavior Problems: A functional training approach. Guildford, New York.

Eisenberg RB (1976) Auditory Competence in Early Life. University Park Press, Baltimore, MD.

Elder P, Goossens C (1994) Engineering Training Environments for Interactive Augmentative Communication: Strategies for Adolescents and Adults who are Moderately/Severely Developmentally Delayed. Southeast Augmentative Communication Conference Publications, Birmingham, AL.

Elksnin LK (1997) Collaborative speech and language services for students with learning disabilities. Journal of Learning Disabilities 30(4): 414–26.

Elksnin LK, Capilouto J (1994) Speech and language pathologists' perceptions of integrated services in school settings. Speech and Hearing Services in the Schools 25: 258–67.

Emerson E (1995) Challenging Behaviour: analysis and intervention in people with learning difficulties. Cambridge University Press, Cambridge.

Emerson E, Barrett S, Bell T, Cummings R, McCool T (1987a) Developing services for people with challenging behaviour. Journal of Behaviour and Cognitive Psychotherapy 21: 171–98.

Emerson E, Barrett S, Bell C, Cummings R, Hughes H, McCool C, Toogood A, Mansell J (1987b) The Special Development Team: Developing services for people with severe learning difficulties and challenging behaviours. Institute of Social and Applied Psychology, University of Kent, Canterbury.

Emerson E, Felce D, McGill P, Mansell J (1994) Introduction. In: Emerson E, McGill P, Mansell J (eds) Severe Learning Disabilities and Challenging Behaviours. Chapman & Hall, London, pp. 3–16.

Emerson E, Forrest J, Cambridge P, Mansell J (1996) Community support teams for people with learning disabilities and challenging behaviours: Results of a National Survey. Journal of Mental Health 5(4): 395–406.

Enderby P (ed) (1987) Assistive Communication Aids for the Speech Impaired. Churchill Livingstone, London.

Enderby P (1997) Therapy Outcome Measure (TOM): User Manual. Singular Publishing Group, London, pp. 40–1.

Enderby P, Davies P (1989) Communication disorders: planning a service to meet the needs. British Journal of Disorders of Communication 24: 301–31.

Enderby P, Emerson J (1995) Does Speech and Language Therapy Work? Whurr Publishers, London.

Enderby P, John A (1999) Therapy outcome measures in speech and language therapy: comparing performance between providers. International Journal of Language and Communication Disorders 34(4): 417–29.

Enderby P, Simpson M, Wheeler P (1992) A review of therapy services for adults with learning difficulties in South West Regional Health Authority. Report to SWRHA.

EQUALS (1997) Access to the Whole Curriculum for Pupils with Learning Difficulties: language and literacy. EQUALS , Newcastle.

Evans C (2000) Home benefits. Royal College of Speech and Language Therapists Bulletin (December): 6–7.

Evans C (2001) The Kenilworth WILSTAAR project – a randomised controlled trial. RCSLT National Conference – Sharing Communication, Abstracts of the College' Conference in Birmingham, April 2001. Royal College of Speech and Language Therapists, London, p. 21.

Falvey MA, Bishop KB, Greno-Scheyer M, Coots J (1988) Issues and trends in mental retardation. In: Calculator SN, Bedrosian JI (eds) Communication Assessment and Intervention for Adults with Mental Retardation. Taylor & Francis, London, pp. 45–66.

Fantz RL (1963) Pattern vision in newborn infants. Science, London, pp. 296–7.

Fawcus M (ed) (1997) Children with Learning Difficulties – a collaborative approach to their educational management. Whurr Publishers, London.

Fawcus R (1987) Communication aids: past, present and future. In: Enderby P (ed) Assistive Communication Aids for the Speech Impaired. Churchill Livingstone, London, pp. 4–11.

Feldman M (1997) The effectiveness of early intervention for children of parents with mental retardation. In: Guralnick MJ (ed) The Effectiveness of Early Intervention. Paul H Brookes Publishing Co., London, pp. 171–91.

Fenn G, Rowe J (1975) An experiment in manual communication. British Journal of Disorders of Communication 10: 3–16.

Fewell R, Kaminski R (1988) Play skills development and early instruction for young children with handicaps. In: Odom SL, Karnes MB (eds) Early Intervention for Infants and Children with Handicaps: An empirical base, Paul H Brookes Publishing Co., London, pp. 145–58.

Fey ME, Cleaves PL, Long SH, Hughes DL (1993) Two approaches to the facilitation of grammar in children with language impairment: An experimental evaluation. Journal of Speech and Hearing Research 36: 141–59.

Fischer MA (1983) An Analysis of Pre-verbal Communication behaviors in Down's Syndrome and Non-Retarded Children. Unpublished PhD Thesis. University of Oregon.

Fish D, Coles C (1998) Developing Professional Judgement in Health Care. Butterworth-Heinemann, Oxford.

Florian L (1997) 'Inclusive Learning': The reform initiative of the Tomlinson Committee. British Journal of Special Education 24(1): 7–11.

Fogel A (1993) Two principles of communication: Co-regulation and framing. In: Nadel J, Camaioni L (eds) New Perspectives in Communication Development. Routledge, London, pp. 8–22.

Fonagy I (1972) A propos de la genèse de la phrase enfantine. Lingua 30: 31–71.

Fowler AE (1998) Language in mental retardation. In: Burack J, Hodapp R, Zigler E (eds) Handbook of Mental Retardation and Development. Cambridge University Press, Cambridge, pp. 290–333.

Fowler A, Gelman R, Gleitman L (1994) The course of language learning in children with Down's syndrome: Longitudinal language level comparisons with young normally developing children. In: Tager-Flusberg H (ed) Constraints on Language Acquisition: studies of atypical children. Erlbaum, Hillsdale, NJ, pp. 91–140.

Fox M (1975) They Get this Training but They Don't Really Know How You Feel. National Fund for Research into Crippling Diseases, Horsham.

France J (1991) Psychoses. In: Gravell R, France J (eds) Speech and Communication Problems in Psychiatry. Chapman & Hall, London, pp. 113–55.

Fraser B (1991) Psychiatry. In: Fraser WI, MacGillivray RC, Green AM (eds) Hallas' Caring for People with Mental Handicaps. Butterworth-Heineman, Oxford, pp. 188–201.

French S (1994) On Equal Terms: Working with disabled people. Butterworth-Heinemann, Oxford.

Fried-Oken M, More L (1992) An initial vocabulary for nonspeaking preschool children based on developmental and environmental language sources. Augmentative and Alternative Communication 8(1): 41–56.

Fulford D, Malcomess K (1995) Reflecting on the links between the earliest mother-infant relationship and communication difficulties. In: 'Caring to Communicate': Royal College of Speech and Language Therapists Conference, 1995, York, pp. 213–22.

Garber HL (1988) The Milwaukee Project: Preventing mental retardation in children at risk. American Association of Mental Retardation, Washington, DC.

Garber HL, Hodge JD, Rynders J, Dever R, Velu R (1991) The Milwaukee Project: Setting the record straight. American Journal of Mental Retardation 95: 493–525.

Garcia Pastor C (1999) Inclusion: a committed form of working in school. In: Rondal J, Perera J, Nadel L (eds) Down Syndrome – a review of current knowledge. Whurr Publishers, London.

Garland C, Stone NW, Swanson J, Woodruff G (eds) (1981) Early Intervention for Children with Special Needs and their Families: findings and recommendations. Westar Series Paper No. 11. ED 207 78. University of Washington, Seattle, WA.

Gathercole SE, Baddeley AD (1990) Phonological memory deficits in language disordered children. Is there a causal connection? Journal of Memory and Language 29: 336–60.

Gibb Harding C (1983) Setting the stage for language acquisition: communication development in the first year. In: Golinkoff R (ed) The Transition from Prelinguistic to Linguistic Communication. Laurence Erlbaum, Hillsdale, NJ, pp. 93–113.

Gibbard D (1994) Parent based intervention with pre-school language delayed children. European Journal of Disorders of Communication 29(2): 131.

Gibbard D (1998) Parent based approaches – the case for language goals. Speech and Language Therapy in Practice (Summer): 11–13.

Gill S, Ridley J (2000) Reshaping opportunities, sharing good practice. Speech and Language Therapy in Practice (Summer): 14–17.

Girolametto LE (1988) Improving the social-conversation skills of developmentally delayed children: an intervention study. Journal of Speech and Hearing Disorders 53: 156–67.

Girolametto LE (1999) Interactive Focused Stimulation for Toddlers with Expressive Vocabulary Delays. Hanen website, http://www.hanen.org; retrieved on 11 January 2001.

Girolametto LE (2000) Directiveness in Teachers' Language Input to Toddlers and Pre-schoolers in Day Care. Hanen website, http://www.hanen.org; retrieved on 11 January 2001.

Girolametto LE, Tannock R, Siegal L (1993) Consumer-orientated evaluation of interactive language intervention. American Journal of Speech and Language Pathology, September 3: 41–51.

Girolametto LE, Verbey M, Tannock R (1994) Improving joint engagement in parent–child interaction: an intervention study. Journal of Early Intervention 18(2): 155–67.

Girolametto LE, Steig Pearce P, Weitzman E (1996) Interactive focused stimulation for toddlers with expressive vocabulary delays. Journal of Speech and Hearing Research 39: 1274–83.

Glennen SL (1997a) Introduction to augmentative and alternative communication. In: Glennen SL, DeCoste DC (eds) Handbook of Augmentative and Alternative Communication, Chapter 1. Singular Publishing, London, pp. 3–20.

Glennen SL (1997b) Augmentative and alternative communication assessment strategies. In: Glennen SL, DeCoste DC (eds) Handbook of Augmentative and Alternative Communication. Singular Publishing, London, pp. 170–73.

Glennen SL, DeCoste DC (eds) (1997) Handbook of Augmentative and Alternative Communication. Singular Publishing, London.

Glogowska M, Campbell R (2000) Investigating parental views of involvement in pre-school speech and language therapy. International Journal of Language and Communication Disorders 35(3): 391–407.

Goals 2000 (1994) Educate America Act. US Government Printing Office, Washington, DC.

Goldin-Meadow S, Mylander C (1990) Beyond the input given: The child's role in the acquisition of language. Language 66: 323–55.

Goldstein H, Angelo D, Mousetis L (1987) Acquisition and extension of syntactic repertoires by severely mentally retarded youth. Research in Developmental Disabilities 8: 549–74.

Gompertz J (1997) Developing communication: Early intervention and augmentative signing from birth to five years. In: Fawcus M (ed) Children with Learning Difficulties – a collaborative approach to their education and management, Chapter 4. Whurr Publishers, London.

Goodwin MW (1999) Cooperative learning skills: What skills to teach and how to teach them. Intervention in School and Clinic 35(1): 29–33.

Goossens C, Crain S, Elder, P (1994) Engineering the Preschool Environment for Interactive Symbolic Communication: 18 months to 5 years developmentally, 2nd edn. Southeast Augmentative Communication Conferencee Publications, Birmingham, AL.

Gordon N (1991) The relationship between language and behaviour. Developmental Medicine and Child Neurology 33: 86–9.

Gratch G (1979) On levels of awareness of objects in infants and students. In: Oates J (ed) Early Cognitive Development, Chapter 14, Croom Helm, London

Gravell R, France J (1991a) Mental disorders and speech therapy: An introduction. In: Gravell R, France J (eds) Speech and Communication Problems in Psychiatry. Chapman & Hall, London, pp. 1–21.

Gravell R, France J (1991b) Hearing loss, mental, handicap, acquired brain damage and forensic psychiatry. In: Gravell R, France J (eds) Speech and Communication Problems in Psychiatry. Chapman & Hall, London, pp. 56–91.

Gravestock S, Bouras N (1997) Emotional disorders. In: Holt G, Bouras N (eds) Mental Health in Learning Disability. Pavilion Publishing, Brighton, pp. 17–26.

Gray CA (eds) (1994) The New Social Story Book. Jenison Public Schools. Future Horizons, Arlington, Michigan.

Gray JM, Fraser WL, Leudar I (1983) Recognition of emotion from facial expression in mental handicap. British Journal of Psychiatry 142: 566–71.

Greenbaum CW, Auerbach JC (1998) The environment of the child with mental retardation: risk, vulnerability and resilience. In: Burack J, Hodapp R, Zigler E (eds) Handbook of Mental Retardation and Development. Cambridge University Press, Cambridge, pp. 583–605.

Greenberg M (1980) Social interaction between deaf preschoolers and their mothers: the effects of communication method and communication competence. Developmental Psychology 16(5): 465–74.

Greenfield P, Reilly J, Leaper C, Baker N (1985) The structural and functional status of single word utterances and their relationship to early multi-word speech. In: Barrett M (ed) Children's Single Word Speech. John Wiley & Sons, New York, pp. 233–68.

Groome D, Dewart H, Esgate A, Gurney K, Kemp R, Towell N (1999) An Introduction to Cognitive Psychology – processes and disorders. Taylor & Francis, London.

Grossman H (ed) (1983) Classification in Mental Retardation. American Association of Mental Deficiency, Washington, DC.

Grove N (1995) An analysis of the linguistic skills of signers with learning disabilities. PhD thesis, London University.

Grove N (1998) Literature for All: Developing literature in the curriculum for pupils with special educational needs. David Fulton Publishers, London.

Grove N, Dockrell J (2000) Multi-sign combinations by children with intellectual impairments: An analysis of language skills. Journal of Language, Speech and Hearing Research 43: 309–23.

Grove N, McDougall S (1991) Exploring sign use in two settings. British Journal of Special Education 18: 149–56.

Grove N, Norwich B (1997) Children Using AAC in London Schools: Estimates of prevalence and profiles of use. London University Institute of Education/The Mercers Company, London.

Grove N, Smith M (1997) Input-output assymetries: Language development in AAC. ISAAC Bulletin 50 (November): 1–3.

Grove N, Walker M (1990) The Makaton vocabulary: Using manual signs and graphic symbols to develop interpersonal communication. Augmentative and Alternative Communication 6: 15–28.

Grove N, Dockrell J, Woll B (1996a) The two-word stage in manual signs: language development in signers with intellectual impairments. In: von Tetzchner S, Jensen MH (eds) Augmentative and Alternative Communication: European perspectives. Whurr Publishers, London, pp. 101–18.

Grove N, Clibbens J, Barnett S, Loncke F (1996b) Constructing theoretical models of augmentative and alternative communication. In: Bjorck-Akesson E, Lindsay P (eds) Communication ... Naturally: theoretical and methodological issues in augmentative and alternative communication. Proceedings of the Fourth ISAAC Research Symposium, 1996, Vancouver, Canada.

Grove N, Bunning K, Porter J, Olsson C (1999) See what I mean: Interpreting the meaning of communication by people with severe and profound intellectual disabilities. Journal of Applied Research in Intellectual Disabilities 12(3): 190–203.

Grunwell P (1985) Phonological Assessment of Child Speech (PACS). NFER-Nelson, Windsor.

Gunzburg HC (1977) Progress Assessment Chart, 5th edn. SEFA (Publications), Stratford-upon-Avon, Warwickshire.

Guralnick MJ (1999) Developmental and systems linkages in early intervention for children with Down's syndrome. In: Rondal J, Perera J, Nadel L (eds) Down Syndrome – a review of current knowledge, Chapter 5. Whurr Publishers, London.

Hales G (ed) (1996) Beyond Disability: Towards an enabling society. Sage, London.

Halle J (1988) Adapting the natural environment in the context of training. In: Calculator SN, Bedrosian JL (eds) Communication Assessment and Intervention for Adults with Mental Retardation. Taylor & Francis, London, pp. 155–86.

Hamilton L, McKenzie K (1999) Moving on: life stories. Speech and Language Therapy in Practice (Winter): 4–7.

Haney JI, Wilson JW, Halle J (1988) Adults with mental retardation: Who they are, where they are, and how their communicative needs can be met. In: Calculator SN, Bedrosian JL (eds) Communication Assessment and Intervention for Adults with Mental Retardation. Taylor & Francis, London. Chapter 3.

Hardy J (1983) Cerebral Palsy. Prentice Hall, Englewood Cliffs, NJ.

Haring N, Bricker D (1976) Overview of comprehensive services for the severely and profoundly handicapped. In: Haring N, Brown L (eds) Teaching the Severely Handicapped. Grune and Stratton, New York, pp. 17–32.

Hart B, Risley TR (1980) In vivo language intervention: Unanticipated general effects. Journal of Applied Behavior Analysis 13: 407–32.

Hart B, Risley TR (1995) Meaningful Differences in the Everyday Experience of Young American Children. Paul H. Brookes, Baltimore.

Harvey J (1998) Clinical Governance: guidance for nurses. Royal College of Nursing, London.

Hastings RP, Reed TS, Watts MJ (1997) Community staff causal attributions about challenging behaviours in people with intellectual disabilities. Journal of Applied Research in Intellectual Disabilities 10(3): 238–49.

Hegarty JR (1987) Staff burnout. Mental Handicap (September): 93–5.

Heim MJM, Baker-Mills A (1996) Early development of symbolic communication and linguistic complexity through augmentative and alternative communication. In: von Tetzchner S, Hygum Jensen M (eds) Augmentative and Alternative Communication: European perspectives. Whurr Publishers, London, pp. 232–48.

Hewlett N (1990) Process of development and production. In: Grunwell P (ed) Developmental Speech Disorders – clinical issues and practical implications, Chapter 2. Whurr Publishers, London.

Hill K (1999) Assessment, intervention and resources. Exceptional Parent (December): 45–8.

Hitchings A, Spence R (1991) The Personal Communication Plan for People with a Learning Disability. NFER-Nelson, Windsor.

Hixson J, Hardy J (1964) Restricted mobility of the speech articulators in cerebral palsy. Journal of Speech and Hearing Disorders 29: 293–306.

Hodapp R, Leckman J, Dykens E, Sparrow S, Zelinsky D, Ort S (1992) K-ABC profiles in children with fragile X syndrome, Down syndrome, and nonspecific mental retardation. American Journal on Mental Retardation 97: 39–46.

Hodgkinson P (1998) Communication in ALD – what do carers think? Speech and Language Therapy in Practice (Spring): 4–7.

Houghton J, Bronicki B, Guess D (1987) Opportunities to express preferences and make choices among students and severe disabilities in classroom setting. Journal of the Association for Persons with Severe Handicaps 12: 18–27.

Hughes S (2000) The application of CHILDES for multi-modal transcription: a case study. 6th ISAAC Research Symposium, 7–8 August 2000, Washington DC.

Hulme C, Mackenzie S (1992) Working Memory and Severe Learning Difficulties. Erlbaum, Hove.

Hunt-Berg M (2000) Exploring CHILDES for multimodal transcription in AAC. 6th ISAAC Research Symposium, 7–8 August 2000, Washington DC.

Hurd A (1991) The Speaking and Listening Package. Far Horizons, Mill Lane, Cleeve Prior Worcestershire, UK.

Hurd A, Rowley C (1991) Speaking and Listening and Reading Package. Far Horizons, Mill Lane, Cleeve Prior, Worcestershire, UK.

Hurst-Brown L, Keens A (1990) E.N.A.B.L.E.: Encouraging a natural and better life experience. Forum Consultancy, London.

Hymes D (1974) On communicative competence. In: Pride JB, Holmes J (eds) Sociolinguistics. Penguin, London, pp. 269–93.

Hyvärinen L (1995) Considerations in the evaluation and treatment of the child with low vision. American Journal of Occupational Therapy 49(9): 891–7.

Iacono T, Chan J, Waring R (1998) Efficacy of a parent-implemented early language intervention-based collaborative consultation. International Journal of Language and Communication Disorders 33(3): 281–304.

Idol L (1997) Key questions related to building collaborative and inclusive schools. Journal of Learning Disabilities 30(4): 384–94.

Jans D, Clark S (1998a) High technology aids to communication. In: Wilson E (ed) Augmentative Communication in Practice: An introduction. Call Centre, Edinburgh, pp. 37–45.

Jans D, Clark S (1998b) Alternative access to communication aids. In: Wilson E (ed) Augmentative Communication in Practice: An introduction. Call Centre, Edinburgh, pp. 46–50.

Jeffree D (1997) Observation of play in the early assessment and development of children with severe learning difficulties. In: Fawcus M (ed) Children with Learning Difficulties – a collaborative approach to their educational management, Chapter 3. Whurr Publishers, London.

Jeffree D, McConkey R (1996) PIP Developmental Charts. Hodder and Stoughton Educational, London.

Johansson I (1990) Early Intervention in Down's Syndrome. Jessica Kingsley Publishers, London.

Johansson I (1994) Language Development in Children with Special Needs: Performative communication. Translated by Eva Thomas. Jessica Kingsley Publishers, London.

John A, Enderby P (2000) Reliability of speech and language therapists using therapy outcome measures. International Journal of Language and Communication Disorders 35(2): 287–302.

Johnson M (1997) Outcome measurement: towards an interdisciplinary approach. British Journal of Therapy Rehabilitation 4(9): 472–7.

Jones J (2000) A total communication approach towards meeting the needs of people with learning disabilities. Tizard Learning Disability Review 5(1): 20–6.

Jones J, Turner J, Heard A (1992) Making communication a priority. Bulletin of the College of Speech and Language Therapists 478: 6–7.

Jones OHM (1977) Mother child communication with pre-linguistic Down's syndrome and normal infants. In: Schaffer H (ed) Studies in Mother–Infant Interaction. Academic Press, New York, pp. 379–401.

Jones S (1990) INTECOM: a package designed to integrate carers into assessing and developing the communication skills of people with learning difficulties. NFER-Nelson, Windsor.

Kahn J (1982) Cognitive training and its relationship to language of profoundly retarded children. American Association on Mental Deficiency Annual Convention, Boston, 1982.

Kaiser AP (1993) Functional language. In: Snell ME (ed) Instruction of Student with Severe Disabilities, 4th edn. Macmillan, London, pp. 347–79.

Kaiser AP, Yoder PJ, Keetz A (1992) Evaluating milieu teaching. In: Warren SF, Reichle J (eds) Communication and Language Intervention. Paul H. Brookes, Baltimore, pp. 9–47.

Kaiser AP, Yoder PJ, Fischer R, Keefer M, Hemmeter M, Ostrosky M (1997a) A Comparison of Milieu Teaching and Responsive Interaction Implemented by Parents. Vanderbilt University, Nashville, TN 37203.

Kaiser AP, Hemmeter M, Hester P (1997b) The facilitative effects of input on children's language development: Contributions from studies of enhanced milieu teaching. In: Adamson L, Romski M (eds) Communication and Language Acquisition: discoveries from atypical development. Paul H Brookes, Baltimore, pp. 267–94.

Kamhi AG, Masterson JJ (1989) Language and cognition in mentally handicapped people: Last rites for the difference-delay controversy. In: Beveridge M, Conti-Ramsden G, Leudar I (eds) Language and Communication in Mentally Handicapped People. Chapman & Hall, London. Chapter 4.

Kangas KA, Lloyd L (1988) Early cognitive skills as prerequisites to augmentative and alternative communication use: What are we waiting for? Augmentative and Alternative Communication 4(4): 211–21.

Karlan GR, Brenn-White B, Lentz A, Hodur P, Egger D, Frankoff D (1982) Establishing generalised productive verb-noun phrase usage in a manual language system with mentally handicapped children. Journal of Speech and Hearing Disorders 47: 431–42.

Karnes MB (ed) (1983) The Undeserved: Our young gifted children. Council for Exceptional Children, Reston, VA.

Karnes MB, Lee RC (1978) Early Childhood. Council for Exceptional Children, Reston, VA.

Kaye K, Fogel A (1980) The temporal structure of face to face communication between mothers and infants. Developmental Psychology 16: 454–64.

Kelford Smith A, Thurston S, Light J, Parnes P, O'Keefe B (1989) The form and use of written communication produced by physically disabled individuals using microcomputers. Augmentative and Alternative Communication 5(2): 115–24.

Kelly A (1996) Talkabout: A social communication skills package. Winslow Press, Bicester.

Kelly A (1997) Social skills training for adolescents with a learning disability. In: Fawcus M (ed) Children with Learning Difficulties – a collaborative approach to their educational management, Chapter 6. Whurr Publishers, London.

Kelman E, Schneider C (1994) Parent–child interaction: An alternative approach to the management of children's language difficulties. Journal of Child Language Teaching and Therapy 1: 81–96.

Kelsey E (1991) Parent partnership in the treatment of communication-impaired children. Journal of Child Language Teaching and Therapy 7(2): 167–78.

Kernan K (1990) Comprehension of syntactically indicated sequence by Down's syndrome and other mentally retarded adults. Journal of Mental Deficiency Research 34: 169–78.

Kersner M (1992) Tests of Voice, Speech and Language. Whurr Publishers, London.

Kiernan C, Kiernan D (1994) Challenging behaviour in schools for pupils with severe learning difficulties. Mental Handicap Research 7: 117–201.

Kiernan C, Qureshi H (1993) Challenging behaviour. In: Kiernan C (ed) Research to Practice? Implications of research on the challenging behaviour of people with learning disabilities. BILD Publications, Clevedon, pp. 53–66.

Kiernan C, Reid B (1987) The Pre-Verbal Communication Schedule. NFER-Nelson, Windsor.

Kiernan C, Reid B, Jones L (1982) Signs and Symbols: Use of non-vocal communication systems. Heinemann Educational, London.

Kiernan C, Reid B, Goldbart J (1987) Foundations of Communication and Language (FOCAL): Course manual and videotape. Manchester University Press in association with BIMH, Manchester.

Knowles W, Masidlover M (1982) Derbyshire Language Scheme. M Masidlover, Derbyshire Education Authority, Derby.

Kolb DA (1984) Experiential Learning: Experience as a source of learning and development. Prentice-Hall, Englewood Cliffs, NJ.

Kosciulek JF (1999) The consumer-directed theory of empowerment rehabilitation counselling. Rehabilitation Counselling Bulletin 42(3): 196–210.

Kot A, Law J (1995) Intervention with pre-school children with specific language impairments: A comparison of two different approaches to treatment. Child Language and Therapy 2: 144–61.

Kouri T (1989) How manual sign acquisition relates to the development of spoken language. Language, Speech and Hearing Services in Schools 20: 50–62.

Kublin K, Wetherby A, Craise E, Prizant B (1998) Prelinguistic dynamic assessment. In: Wetherby A, Warren S, Reichle J (eds) Transitions in Prelinguistic Communication. Paul H Brookes Publishing Co., Baltimore, MD.

Lacey P, Ouvry C (1998) People with Profound and Multiple LD: a collaborative approach to meeting complex needs. David Fulton Publishers, London.

Lackner J (1968) A developmental study of language behavior in retarded children. Neouropsychologia 6: 301–20.

Lahey M (1988) Language Disorders and Language Development. Macmillan Press, New York.

Lambe L (1998) Supporting families. In: Lacey P, Ouvry C (eds) People with Profound and Multiple Learning Disabilities: A collaborative approach to meeting complex needs. David Fulton Publishers, London.

Landesman-Dwyer S, Knowles M (1987) Ecological analysis of staff training in residential settings. In: Hogg J, Mittler P (eds) Staff Training in Mental Handicap. Croom Helm, London. Chapter 1.

Larcher J (1998) Leaving school – crisis or opportunity: Which is it for AAC users? In: Wilson E (ed) Augmentative Communication in Practice: An introduction. Call Centre, Edinburgh, pp. 77–81.

Latham C, Miles A (1997) Assessing Communication. David Fulton Publishers, London.

Launonen K (1996) Enhancing communication skills of children with DS: Early use of manual signs. In: von Tetzchner S, Martinsen H (eds) Augmentative and Alternative Communication: European perspectives. Whurr Publishers, London, pp. 213–30.

LaVigna GW, Willis TJ, Donnellan AM (1989) The role of positive programming in behavioural treatment. In: Cipani E (ed) The Treatment of Severe Behaviour Disorders. American Association on Mental Retardation, Washington, D.C., pp. 59–82.

Law J (1992a) The process of early intervention. In: Law J (ed) The Early Identification of Language Impairment. Chapman & Hall, London. Chapter 6.

Law J (1992b) What is language impairment. In: Law J (ed) The Early Identification of Language Impairment in Children. Chapman & Hall, London. Chapter 2.

Law J (1996) Labels and diagnosis – what happens after assessment. In: Law J, Elias J (eds) Trouble Talking: A guide for the parents of children with speech and language difficulties, Chapter 5. Jessica Kingsley Publishers, London.

Law J, Elias J (eds) (1996) Trouble Talking: A guide for the parents of children with speech and language difficulties. Jessica Kingsley Publishers, London.

Law J, Lester R (1991) Speech therapy provision in a social education centre. Mental Handicap 19: 22–8.

Law J, Brown G, Lester R (1994) Speech and language therapy provision in a S.E.C.: The value of a first step assessment. British Journal of Learning Disabilities 22: 66–9.

Le Roux A (1999) Teler Information Pack. Available from A A Le Roux, PO Box 699, Sheffield S17 3YG, UK.

Lebrun Y, Van Borsch J (1991) Final sound repetitions. Journal of Fluency Disorders 15: 107–13.

Lee M, MacWilliam L (1995) Movement, Gesture and Sign. Royal National Institute for the Blind, London.

Leeming K, Swan W, Coupe J, Mittler P (1979) Teaching language and communication to the mentally handicapped. Schools Council Curriculum Bulletin 8, Evans/Methuen Educational: London.

Lees J, Urwin S (1991) Children with Language Disorders. Whurr Publishers, London.

Lees JA, Smithies G, Chambers C (2001) Let's Talk – a community-based language promotion project for Sure Start. RCSLT National Conference – Sharing Communication, Abstracts of the College's Conference, April 2001, Birmingham, UK. Royal College of Speech and Language Therapists, London. p. 39.

Lenneberg E (1967) Biological Foundations of Language. Wiley, New York, NY.

Lenneberg E, Nichols I, Rosenberger E (1964) Primitive stages of language development in mongolism. In: McRioch D, Weinstein E (eds) Disorder of Communication. Proceedings of the Association for Research in Nervous and Mental Disease 17. Williams & Wilkins, Baltimore, MD, pp. 119–37 (cited in Rondal and Edwards, 1997).

Leonard LB (1975) Relational meaning and the facilitation of slow learning children's language. American Journal of Mental Deficency 80: 180–5.

Leonard L (1998) Chidren with Specific Language Impairment. MIT Press, Cambridge, MA.

Leudar I (1981) Strategic communication in mental retardation. In: Fraser WI, Greive R (eds) Communicating with Normal and Retarded Children. Wright, Bristol.

Leudar I (1989) Communicative environments for mentally handicapped people. In: Beveridge M, Conti-Ramsden G, Leudar I (eds) Language and Communication in Mentally Handicapped People. Chapman & Hall, London. Chapter 12.

Leudar I, Fraser WI (1985a) Behaviour disturbance and its assessment for people with learning disability. In: Hogg J, Raynes NV (eds) Assessment in Mental Handicap. Chapman & Hall, London, pp. 107–28.

Leudar I, Fraser WI (1985b) How to keep quiet: Some withdrawal strategies in mentally handicapped adults. Journal of Mental Deficiency 29: 315–30.

Lieven E, Pine J, Barnes HD (1992) Individual differences in early vocabulary development: redeveloping the referential/expressive distinction. Journal of Child Language 19: 287–310.

Lifter K, Bloom L (1989) Object knowledge and the emergence of language. Infant Behaviour and Development 12: 395–423.

Lifter K, Bloom L (1998) Intentionality and the role of play in the transition to language. In: Wetherby A, Warren S, Reichle J (eds) Transitions in Prelinguistic Communication. Paul H. Brookes, Baltimore. Chapter 8.

Light J (1988) Interaction involving individuals using augmentative and alternative communication: State of the art and future research directions. Augmentative and Alternative Communication 4: 66–82.

Light J (1989) Toward a definition of communicative competence for individuals using augmentative and alternative communication systems. Augmentative and Alternative Communication 5(2): 137–44.

Light J (1997) Communication is the essence of human life: Reflections on communicative competence. Augmentative and Alternative Communication 13(2): 61–70.

Light P, Remington B, Clarke S, Watson J (1989) Signs of language. In: Beveridge M, Conti-Ramsden G, Leudar I (eds) Language and Communication in Mentally Handicapped People. Chapman & Hall, London.

Lister Brook S, Bowler DM (1997) Intervention with children who have learning difficulties: Contributions from clinical psychology. In: Fawcus M (ed) Children with Learning

Difficulties – a collaborative approach to their educational management, Chapter 2. Whurr Publishers, London.

Lloyd LL, Quist R, Windsor J (1990) A proposed augmentative and alternative communication model. Augmentative and Alternative Communication 6(3): 172–83.

Locke J (1997) A theory of neurolinguistic development. Brain and Language 58: 265–326.

Loncke F, Clibbens J, Arvidson H, Lloyd LL (1999) Augmentative and Alternative Communication: New directions in research and practice. Whurr Publishers, London.

Lowe K, Felce D (1995) The definition of challenging behaviour in practice. British Journal of Learning Disabilities 23: 118–23.

Lowe K, Felce D, Blackman D (1995) People with learning disabilities and challenging behaviour: the characteristics of those referred and not referred to specialist teams. Psychological Medicine 25: 595–603.

Lowe M, Costello A (1988) Symbolic Play Test, 2nd edn. NFER-Nelson, Windsor.

Luckasson R, Coulter D, Polloway E, Reiss S, Schalock R, Snell M, Spitalnick D, Stark J (1992) Mental Retardation: Definition, classification and systems of supports. American Association on Mental Retardation, Washington, DC.

MacDonald A (1984) Blissymbols and manual signing: A combined approach. Communicating Together 2(4): 20–1.

MacDonald A (1998) Symbol systems. In: Wilson E (ed) Augmentative Communication in Practice: an introduction. Call Centre, Edinburgh, pp. 19–26.

MacDonald A, Rendle C (1998) Laying the foundations of communicative competence for very young children. In: Wilson E (ed) Augmentative Communication in Practice: An introduction. Call Centre, Edinburgh, pp. 51–53.

MacMillan D, Gresham F, Siperstein G (1993) Conceptual and psychometric concerns about the 1992 AAMR definition of mental retardation. American Journal on Mental Retardation 98: 325–35.

MacWhinney B (2000) The CHILDES Project: Tools for analyzing talk. Laurence Erlbaum Associates, Hillsdale, NJ.

Mahdani N (1996) The role of bilingual co-workers within speech and language therapy. Journal of the Israeli Speech, Hearing and Language Association, Part Six – Cultural, Augmentative Communication and General 19: 372–81.

Manolson HA (1992) It Takes Two to Talk. A Hanen Early Language Parent Guide Book. Hanen Resource Centre, Toronto.

Marcell MM (1995) Relationships between hearing and auditory recognition in Down's syndrome youth. Downs Syndrome Research and Practice 3: 75–91.

Martinsen H, von Tetzchner S (1996) Situating augmentative and alternative language and intervention. In: von Tetzchner S, Jensen MH (eds) Augmentative and Alternative Communication: European perspectives. Whurr Publishers, London, pp. 37–48.

Marvin C (1998) Teaching and learning for children with profound and multiple learning difficulties. In: Lacey P, Ouvry C (eds) People with Profound and Multiple Learning Disabilities: A collaborative approach to meeting complex needs. David Fulton Publishers, London.

Mattaini MA (1995) Contingency diagrams as teaching tools. Behaviour Analyst 18: 93–8.

McConkey R (1991) Community Integration. In: Fraser WI, MacGillivary RC, Green AM (eds) Hallas' Caring for People with Mental Handicaps. Butterworth-Heinemann, Oxford, pp. 285–302.

McConkey R, Jeffree D, Hewson S (1979) Involving parents in extending the language development of their young mentally handicapped children. British Journal of Disorders of Communication 14: 203–18.

McConkey R, Morris I, Purcell M (1999a) Communications between staff and adults with intellectual disabilities in naturally occurring settings. Journal of Intellectual Disability Research 43(3): 194–205.

McConkey R, Purcell M, Morris, I (1999b) Staff perceptions of communication with a partner who is intellectually disabled. Journal of Applied Research in Intellectual Disabilities 12(3): 204–10.

McCullough A (2001) Viability and effectiveness of teletherapy for pre-school children with special needs. RCSLT National Conference – Sharing Communication, April 2001, Birmingham, UK. International Journal of Language and Communication Disorders – Supplement. Royal College of Speech and Language Therapists, London, 36: pp. 321–6.

McDade H (1981) A parent child interactional model for assessing and remediating language disabilities. British Journal of Disorders of Communication 16(3): 175–83.

McEwen I, Lloyd LL (1990) Some considerations about the motor requirements of manual signs. Augmentative and Alternative Communication 6(3): 207–16.

McEwen G, Millar S (1993) Passports to Communication. In: Wilson A, Millar S (eds) Augmentative Communication in Practice: Scotland. Collected Papers: Study Day. Call Centre, Edinburgh, pp. 37–40.

McGill P (1993) Challenging behaviour, challenging environments, and challenging needs. Clinical Psychology Forum (June): 14–18.

McGill P, Clare I, Murphy G (1996) Understanding and responding to challenging behaviour: From theory to practice. Tizard Learning Disability Review 1(1): 9–17.

McGurk H (1979) Visual perception in young infants. In: Oates J (ed) Early Cognitive Development, Croom Helm: London. Chapter 7.

McLeod H, Houston M, Seyfort B (1995) Communicative interactive skills training for care-givers of non-speaking adults with severe disabilities. International Journal of Practical Approaches to Disability 19(1): 5–11.

McNaughton S (1985) Communicating with Blissymbolics. Blissymbolics Communication Institute, Toronto.

McNaughton S, Light J (1989) Teaching facilitators to support the communication skills of an adult with severe cognitive disabilities: A case study. AAC – Augmentive and Alternative Communication 5(1): 35–41.

McNaughton S, Lindsay P (1995) Approaching literacy with AAC graphics. Augmentative and Alternative Communication 11(4): 212–28.

McNeill D (1970) The Acquisition of Language. Harper & Row, New York.

McNulty B, Smith DB, Soper EW (1983) Effectiveness of Early Special Education for Handicapped Children. Colorado Department of Education, Colorado.

Meltzoff A, Moore M (1991) Cognitive foundations and social functions of imitation, and intermodal representation in infancy. In: Woodhead M, Carr R, Light P (eds) Becoming a Person Chapter 5. Routledge, London.

Menn L, Stoel-Gammon C (1995) Phonological development. In: Fletcher P, MacWhinney B (eds) The Handbook of Child Language. Blackwell Publishers, Oxford, pp. 335–9.

Mental Health Foundation (1997) Don't Forget Us: Children with learning disabilities and severe challenging behaviour. Report of a Committee set up by the Mental Health Foundation. Mental Health Foundation, London.

Mervis C, Bertrand J (1999) Developmental relations between cognition and language: Evidence from Williams syndrome. In: Adamson L, Romski M (eds) Communication and Language Acquisition: discoveries from atypical development. Paul H Brookes, Baltimore, pp. 75–106.

Miller J, Chapman R, Mackenzie H (1981) Individual differences in the language acquisition of mentally retarded children. Second Wisconsin Symposium on Research in Child Language Disorders, 1981, University of Wisconsin, pp. 130–47.

Mirenda P (1997) Supporting individuals with challenging behaviour through functional communication training and AAC: research review. Augmentative and Alternative Communication 13(4): 207–25.

Mirenda P, Iacono T, Williams R (1990) Communication options for persons with severe and profound disabilities: state of the art and future directions. Journal of the Association for Persons with Severe Handicaps 15: 3–21.

Mittler P (1987) Staff development: Changing needs and service contexts in Britain. In: Hogg J, Mittler P (eds) Staff Training in Mental Handicap. Croom Helm, London, pp. 31–65.

Mittler P, Berry P (1977) Demanding language. In: Mittler P (ed) Research to Practice in Mental Retardation, Vol. 2. University Park Press, Baltimore, MD, pp. 245–51.

Mizuko M (1987) Transparency and ease of learning of symbols represented by Blissymbols, PCS and Picsyms. Augmentative and Alternative Communication 3(3): 129–36.

Møller S, von Tetzchner S (1996) Allowing for developmental potential: A case study of intervention change. In: von Tetzchner S, Jensen MH (eds) European Perspectives on Augmentative and Alternative Communication. Whurr Publishers, London, pp. 249–69.

Money D (1997a) An evaluation of three approaches to delivering a speech and language service to people with learning disabilities. Unpublished PhD Thesis, De Montfort University, Leicester.

Money D (1997b) A comparison of three approaches to delivering a speech and language therapy service to people with learning disabilities. European Journal of Disorders of Communication 32: 449–66.

Money D (2000) Delivering quality. Bulletin of the Royal College of Speech and Language Therapists (January). 9–10.

Money D, Thurman S (1994) Talkabout communication. Bulletin of the College of Speech and Language Therapists 504: 12–13.

Montgomery JW, Windsor J, Stark RE (1991) Specific speech and language disorders. In: Obrzut JE, Wynd GW (eds) Neuropsychological Foundations of Learning Disabilities: A handbook of issues, methods and practice, Chapter 21. Academic Press, London.

Morford M, Goldin-Meadow S (1992) Comprehension and production of gesture in combination with speech in one-word speakers. Journal of Child Language 19: 559–80.

Morse JL (1988) Assessment procedures for people with mental retardation. The dilemma and suggested adaptive procedures. In: Calculator SN, Bedrosian JL (eds) Communication Assessment and Intervention with Adults with Mental Retardation. Taylor & Francis, London. Chapter 5.

Muir N, Tanner P, France J (1991) Management and treatment techniques: A practical approach. In: Gravell R, France J (eds) Speech and Communication Problems in Psychiatry. Chapman & Hall, London, pp. 244–325.

Murphy G (1994) Understanding challenging behaviour. In: Emerson E, McGill P, Mansell J (eds) Severe Learning Disabilities and Challenging Behaviours. Chapman & Hall, London, pp. 37–68.

Murphy J, Scott J (1995) Attitudes and strategies towards AAC: A training package for AAC users and carers. Department of Psychology, University of Stirling.

Musselwhite C, Ruscello D (1984) Transparency of three communication symbol systems. Journal of Speech and Hearing Research (September) 27: 436–43.

Nafstad A, Rodbroe I (1999) Co-Creating Communication. Nordic Staff Training Centre for Deafblind Services (NUD), Denmark.

Naigles L, Fowler A, Helm A (1995) Syntactic bootstrapping from start to finish with special reference to Down syndrome. In: Tomasello M, Merriman W (eds) Beyond Names For Things: young children's acquisition of verbs. Erlbaum, Hillsdale, NJ, pp. 299–330.

Natsopoulos D, Xeromeritou A (1990) Language behavior by mildly handicapped and nonretarded children on complement clauses. Research in Developmental Disabilities 11: 199–216.

Nelson K (1973) Structure and strategy in learning to talk. Monographs of the Society for Research in Child Development 38: 149.

Nelson K (1986) Event knowledge and cognitive development. In: Nelson K (ed) Event Knowledge: structure and function in development. Laurence Erlbaum Associates, Hillsdale, NJ, pp. 87–118.

Nelson NW (1990) Only relevant practices can be best. In: Secord WA (ed) Best Practices in Speech and Language Pathology. Psychological Corporation, San Antonio, TX, pp. 15–27.

Nelson N (1992) Performance is the prize: Language competence and performance among AAC users. Augmentative and Alternative Communication 8(1): 3–18.

Newell A (1987) How can we develop better communication aids? Augmentative and Alternative Communication 3(1): 36–40.

Newson E (1976) Parents as a resource in diagnosis and assessment. In: Oppé TE, Woodford YFP (eds) Early Management of Handicapping Conditions. Elsevier/Excerpta Medica, Amsterdam/New York.

NHSE (1990) NHS and Community Care Act. National Health Service Executive, Department of Health, London.

NHSE (1997) Our Healthier Nation. National Health Service Executive, Department of Health, London.

NHSE (1998a) Partnership in Action. National Health Service Executive, Department of Health, London.

NHSE (1998b) A First Class Service. National Health Service Executive, Department of Health, London.

NHSE (1998c) The New NHS: Modern and Dependable: National framework for assessing performance. National Health Service Executive, Department of Health, London.

Nichol L, Rendle C (1998) Strategies for developing pre-reading skills for nursery AAC users. In: Wilson E (ed) Augmentative Communication in Practice: An introduction. Call Centre, Edinburgh, pp. 71–3.

Nind M, Hewett D (1994) Access to Communication: Developing the basics of communication with people with severe learning difficulties. Paul H. Brookes, Oxford.

Nirje B (1969) The normalisation principle and its human management implication. In: Kugel R, Wolfensberger W (eds) Changing Patterns in Residential Services for the Mentally Retarded. President's Committee on Mental Retardation, Washington DC, pp. 179–96.

Nirje B (1976) The normalization principle. In: Kugel R, Shearer A (eds) The Principle of Normalization in Human Services. National Institute on Mental Retardation, Toronto, p. 231.

Nisbet P, Poon P (1998) Special Access Technology. Call Centre, Edinburgh.

Norwich B (1990) Special Needs in Ordinary Schools: Reappraising special needs education. Cassell Educational, London.

Norwich B (1996) Special needs education or education for all: Connective specialisation and ideological impurity. British Journal of Special Education 23(3): 100–3.

O'Brien J, Tyne A (1981) The Principle of Normalisation: A foundation for effective services. CMH, London.

O'Neill RE, Horner RH, Albin RW, Storey K, Sprague JR (1990) Functional Analysis and of Problem Behavior: A practical assessment guide. Sycamore, Sycamore, IL.

O'Neill RE, Horner RH, Albin RW, Sprague JR, Storey K, Newton JS (1997) Functional Analysis and Program Development for Problem Behavior: A practical handbook, 2nd edn. Brooks/Cole, Pacific Grove, CA.

Oakenfull S, McGregor T, Ramtin F, Stanhope J, Zinzan S (2001) Re: WILSTAAR (letter to the editor). International Journal of Language and Communication Disorders 36(1): 135–8.

Ockelford A (1994) Objects of Reference. Royal National Institute for the Blind, London.

OERI (2000) Early Intervention. Office of Educational Research and Improvement, US Department of Education; http://www.kidsource.com/kidsource/content/early.intervention.html. Accessed on 9 April 2001.

Oliver B, Buckley S (1994) The language development of children with Down syndrome: First words to sentences. Down Syndrome Research and Practice 2: 71–5.

Ostrosky M, Donegan M, Fowler S (1998) Facilitating transitions across home, community, work and school. In: Wetherby A, Warren S, Reichle J (eds) Transitions in Prelinguistic Communication. Paul H. Brookes, Baltimore. Chapter 18.

Ouvry C (1998) Making relationships. In: Lacey P, Ouvry C (eds) People with Profound and Multiple Learning Disabilities: A collaborative approach to meet complex needs, Chapter 6. David Fulton Publishers, London.

Owens RE, Rogerson BS (1988) Adults at the presymbolic level. In: Calculator SN, Bedrosian JL (eds) Communication Assessment and Intervention for Adults with Mental Retardation, Chapter 8. Taylor & Francis, London.

Owings N (1985) Communication and the mentally retarded. American Association on Mental Deficiency, Annual Convention, Boston.

Paget Gorman (1990) Paget Gorman Signed Speech. Paget Gorman Society, London.

Papagna S, Tucker E, Harrigan S, Lutman M (2001) Evaluating training courses for parents of children with cochlear implants. RCSLT National Conference – Sharing Communication, April 2001, Birmingham, UK. International Journal of Language and Communication Disorders – Supplement. Royal College of Speech and Language Therapists, London, 36: pp. 517–22.

Park K (2000) Reading objects: literacy and objects of reference. PMLD Link 12, 1 (Winter): 4–9.

Parker F, Piotrkowski CS, Peay L (1987) Head Start as a social support for mothers: the psychological benefits of involvement. American Journal of Orthopsychiatry 57: 2.

Parkes K (1997) How do objects become objects of reference. British Journal of Special Education 24(3): 108–14.

Pennington L, Jolleff N, McConachie H, Wisbeach A, Price K (1993) My Turn to Speak: A team approach to augmentative communication. Hospitals for Sick Children/Institute of Child Health, London.

Peterson K, Reichle J, Johnston S (2000) Examining preschoolers' performance in linear and row-column scanning techniques. Augmentative and Alternative Communication 16(1): 27–36.

Piaget J (1963) The Origins of Intelligence in Children. Norton, New York (originally published in 1936).

Piaget J (1973) The Child's Conception of the World. Paladin, London.

Pickstone C (2001) A sure start for a researcher. Bulletin of the Royal College of Speech and Language Therapists 587(March): 9–11.

Pine J, Lieven E (1993) Reanalysing rote learned phrases: individual differences in the transition to multi-word speech. Journal of Child Language 20: 551–74.

Plante E (1998) Criteria for SLI: The Stark and Tallal legacy and beyond. Journal of Speech, Language and Hearing Research 41: 951–7.

Plutro MA (1990) A comparative study of parental perceptions of the impact of Head Start on their lives. Dissertation Abstracts International 51.

Porter G, Kirkland J (1995) Integrating Augmentative and Alternative Communication into Group Programs: Utilising the principles of conductive education. Spastics Society of Victoria, Australia.

Premack D, Premack A (1974) Teaching visual language to apes and language-deficient persons. In: Schiefelbusch RL, Lloyd LL (eds) Language Perspectives: Acquisition, retardation and intervention. University Park Press, Baltimore, MD, pp. 347–76.

Purcell M, McConkey R, Morris I (2000) Staff communication with people with intellectual disabilities: The impact of a work-based training programme. International Journal of Language and Communication Disorders 35: 147–58.

Quist R, Blischak D (1992) Assistive communication devices: Call for specifications. Augmentative and Alternative Communication 8(4): 312–17.

Qureshi H (1994) The size of the problem. In: Emerson E, McGill P, Mansell J (eds) Severe Learning Disabilities and Challenging Behaviours. Chapman & Hall, London, pp. 17–36.

Radell U (1997) Augmentative and alternative communication assessment strategies: Seating and positioning. In: Glennen SL, DeCoste DC (eds) Handbook of Augmentative and Alternative Communication. Singular Publishing, London. Chapter 6.

Raghavan R (1996) Confusing diagnoses. Nursing Times 92(5 June): 59–62.

Raghavan R (1998) Anxiety disorders in people with learning disabilities: A review of literature. Journal of Learning Disabilities for Nursing, Health and Social Care 2(1): 3–9.

Rankin J, Harwood K, Mirenda P (1994) Influence of graphic symbol use on reading comprehension. Augmentative and Alternative Communication 10(4): 269–81.

Rasore-Quartino A (1999) The present state of medical knowledge in Down syndrome. In: Rondal J, Perera J, Nadel L (eds) Down Syndrome: A review of current knowledge. Whurr Publishers, London. Chapter 14.

Ratcliff A (1994) Comparison of relative demands implicated in direct selection and scanning: Considerations from normal children. Augmentative and Alternative Communication 10(2): 67–74.

RCSLT (1996a) Communicating Quality. Royal College of Speech and Language Therapists, London.

RCSLT (1996b) Survey of assistants in speech and language therapy. Royal College of Speech and Language Therapists Bulletin (January): 2–3.

RCSLT (2001) Sure Start: Law will evaluate language component. Bulletin of the Royal College of Speech and Language Therapists 587(March): 3.

Reason R (1993) Primary special needs and National Curriculum assessment. In: Wolfendale S (ed) Assessing Special Educational Needs. Cassell, London, Chapter 5.

Reichle J, Piché-Cragoe L, Sigafoos J, Doss S (1988) Optimising functional communication for persons with severe handicaps. In: Calculator SN, Bedrosian JL (eds) Communication Assessment and Intervention for Adults with Mental Retardation. Taylor & Francis, London. Chapter 9.

Reiss S (1994) Issues in defining mental retardation. American Journal of Mental Retardation 99: 1–7.

Reiss S, Sysko J (1993) Diagnostic overshadowing and professional experience with mentally retarded people. American Journal of Mental Deficiency 47: 415–21.

Remington B (1997) Verbal communication in people with learning difficulties: An overview. Tizard Learning Disability Review 2(4): 6–14.

Rheingold H, Adams J (1980) The significance of speech to newborns. Developmental Psychology 16: 397–403.

Richman N, Stevenson J, Graham P (1982) Pre-School to School: A behavioural study. Academic Press, London.

Rinaldi W (1992) The Social Use of Language Programme. NFER-Nelson, Windsor.

Robertson C (1997) 'I don't want to be independent.' Does human life need to be viewed in terms of potential autonomy? Issues in the education of children and young people with severe, profound and multiple learning difficulties. In: Fawcus M (ed) Children with Learning Difficulties: A collaborative approach to their education and management. Whurr Publishers, London. Chapter 12.

Robertson J, Atkinson S, Birch T, Dennet G, Kinghorne I, Lesley J, Morris D, Robertson A, Rumble G (1996) The CORE AAC Curriculum: Augmentative and alternative communication curriculum for people with little or no natural speech. SCOPE, London.

Robson B (1989) Special Needs in Ordinary Schools. Cassell Educational, London.

Romich B, Spiegel B (1999) AAC: Principles, research, and outcomes to guide in system selection. Directions: Technology in Special Education 5(8) (obtained from website http://www.prentrom.com).

Romski MA, Ruder KF (1984) The effects of speech, and speech and sign instruction on oral language learning and generalisation of Action + Object combinations by Down's syndrome children. Journal of Speech and Hearing Disorders 49: 293–302.

Romski MA, Sevcik R (1988) Augmentative and alternative communication systems: Considerations for individuals with severe intellectual disabilities. Augmentative and Alternative Communication 4(2): 83–93.

Romski MA, Sevcik R (1996) Breaking the Speech Barrier: Language development through augmented means. Paul H Brookes, Baltimore.

Rondal JA (1985) Linguistic and prelinguistic development in moderate and severe mental retardation. In: Dobbing J, Clarke ADB, Corbett JA, Hogg J, Robinson R (eds) Scientific studies in Mental Retardation. Royal Society of Medicine and Macmillan Press, London. pp. 323–45.

Rondal JA (1999) Language in Down syndrome. In: Rondal JA, Perera JA, Nadel L (eds) Down Syndrome: A review of current knowledge. Whurr Publishers, London. Chapter 13.

Rondal JA, Edwards S (1997) Language in Mental Retardation. Whurr Publishers, London.

Rondal JA, Lambert J (1983) The speech of mentally retarded adults in a dyadic communication situation: Some formal and informative aspects. Psychologica Belgica 23: 49–56.

Rondal JA, Perera J, Nadel L (eds) (1999) Down Syndrome: A review of current knowledge. Whurr Publishers, London.

Rosen N, Brock J (1998) The West Midlands Therapy Outcome Collaboration. Journal of the Association of Chartered Physiotherapists in Management 32(Winter/Spring): 15–17.

Rosen S (1997) Kinesiology and sensorimotor function. In: Blasch BB, Wiener WR, Welsh RL (eds) Foundations of Orientation and Mobility. American Foundation for the Blind. New York. pp. 170–99.

Rosenberg SA, Abbeduto L (1993) Language and Communication in Mental Retardation: Development, processes and intervention. Laurence Erlbaum Associates, Hillsdale, NJ.

Rosenberg SA, Robinson CC (1988) Interactions of parents with their young handicapped children. In: Odom SL, Karnes MB (eds) Early Intervention for Infants and Children with Handicaps – an empirical base, Paul H. Brookes, Baltimore, pp. 159–77.

Rosetti LM, Kile JE (eds) (1997) Early Intervention for Special Populations of Infants and Toddlers. Singular Publishing, London.

Rourke BP (1981) Neuropsychological assessment of children with learning disabilities. In: Filskov SB, Boll TJ (eds) Handbook of Clinical Neuropsychology. John Wiley & Sons, New York, pp. 453–78.

Rourke BP, Del Dotto DE (1994) Learning Disabilities – a neuropsychological perspective – (especially Chapter 4). Sage, London.

Rourke BP, Fisk JL, Strang JD (1986) Neuropsychological Assessment of Children: A treatment-oriented approach. Guilford, New York.

Rowland C, Schweigert P (1989) Tangible symbols: symbolic communication for individuals with multisensory impairments. Augmentative and Alternative Communication 5(4): 226–34.

Rumble G, Larcher J (1998) AAC Device Review. VOCAtion, Marlow.

Rutter M, Tizard J, Whitmore K (1970) Education, Health and Behaviour. Longman, London.

Rutter T, Buckley S (1994) The acquisition of grammatical morphemes in children with Down's syndrome. Down's Syndrome: Research and Practice 2: 76–82.

Ryan J, Thomas F (1980) The Politics of Mental Handicap. Penguin, Harmondsworth.

Savignon S (1985) Evaluation of communicative competence: The ACTFL provisional proficiency guidelines. Modern Language Journal 69: 129–34.

Schalock P (1996) Quality of life and quality assurance. In: Renwick R, Brown I, Naggler M (eds) Quality of Life in Health Promotion and Rehabilitation. Sage, Thousand Oaks, CA, pp. 105–18.

Schlosser R (1997a) Nomenclature of category levels in graphic symbols: Part I: Is a flower a flower a flower? Augmentative and Alternative Communication 13(1): 4–13.

Schlosser R (1997b) Nomenclature of category levels in graphic symbols: Part II: Role of similarity in categorisation. Augmentative and Alternative Communication 13(1): 14–29.

Schwartz IS, Anderson SR, Halle JW (1989) Training leaders to use naturalistic time delay: Effects on teacher behaviour and on the language use of students. Journal of the Association for Persons with Severe Handicaps 14: 48–57.

Schweinhart LJ, Weikart DP (1980) Young Children Grow Up: The effects of the Perry Preschool Program on youths through age 19. High/Scope Educational Research Foundation, Ypsilanti, MI.

Schweinhart LJ, Barnes HV, Weikart DP (1993) Significant Benefits: The High/Scope Perry Pre-school Study through age 17. Monographs of the High/Scope Educational Research Foundation 10. High /Scope Press, Ypsilanti, MI.

Scollon R (1979) A real early stage: An unzipped condensation of a dissertation on child language. In: Ochs EO, Schieffelin BB (eds) Developmental Pragmatics. Academic Press, New York. pp. 215–28.

Scott J (1988) Low tech methods of augmentative communication. In: Wilson E (ed) Augmentative Communication in Practice: An Introduction. Call Centre, Edinburgh, pp. 13–18.

Shonkoff JP, Hauser-Cram P (1987) Early intervention for disabled infants and their families: A quantitative analysis. Pediatrics 80: 650–8.

Siddons G, Wray N (1995) The process of change in service delivery to adults with learning disabilities. Bulletin of the College of Speech and Language Therapists 516: 12–13.

SIG (1995) Specific interest group for adults with learning disabilities and challenging behaviour, Eastern Region. Survey of United Kingdom undergraduate training in challenging behaviour for speech and language therapists. Unpublished report.

SIG (1996) Specific interest group for adults with learning disabilities and challenging behaviour, Eastern Region. Factors to consider in prioritisation. Unpublished report.

Sigafoos J, Roberts D, Kerr M, Couzens D, Baglioni AJ (1994) Opportunities for communication in classrooms seeing children with developmental disabilities. Journal of Autism and Developmental Disorders 24: 259–79.

Silverman F (1980) Communication for the Speechless. Prentice-Hill, Englewood Cliffs, NJ.

Singer N, Bellugi U, Bates E, Jones W, Rossen M (1994) Contrasting Profiles of Language Development in Children With Williams and Down Syndromes. Technical Report: Project in Cognitive and Neural Development No. 9403. University of California, San Diego.

Smith M (1992) Reading abilities of nonspeaking students: two case studies. Augmentative and Alternative Communication 8(1): 57–66.

Smith M (1996) The medium or the message: A study of speaking children using communication boards. In: von Tetzchner S, Jensen MH (eds) Augmentative and Alternative Communication: European perspectives. Whurr Publishers, London, pp. 119–36.

Smith M, Grove N (1999) The bimodal situation of children learning language using manual and graphic signs. In: von Tetzchner S (ed) 8th Research Symposium of the International Society of Augmentative and Alternative Communication, 1999. Whurr Publishers, London, pp. 8–30.

Smith N, Tsimpli I (1995) The Mind of a Savant: Language learning and modularity. Blackwell, Oxford.

Smith TEC, Polloway E, Dutton JR, Dowdy CA (1995) Teaching Children with Special Needs in Inclusive Settings. Allyn & Bacon, Boston, Mass.

Smith-Lewis M (1994) Discontinuity in the development of aided augmentative and alternative communication systems. Augmentative and Alternative Communication 10(1): 14–26.

Soto G (1999) Understanding the impact of graphic sign use on the message structure. In: von Tetzchner S (ed) 8th Research Symposium of the International Society of Augmentative and Alternative Communication, Whurr Publishers, London, pp. 40–8.

Soto G, Toro-Zambrana W (1995) Investigation of Blissymbol use from a language research paradigm. Augmentative and Alternative Communication 11(2): 118–30.

Sperber D, Wilson D (1995) Relevance: Communication and cognition, 2nd edn. Blackwell, Oxford.

Spiker D, Hopmann MR (1997) The effectiveness of early intervention for children with Down syndrome. In: Guralnick MJ (ed) The Effectiveness of Early Intervention. Paul H Brookes Publishing, London, pp. 271–305.

Stackhouse J, Wells B (1993) Psycholinguistic assessment of developmental speech disorders. European Journal of Disorders of Communication 28: 331–48.

Stackhouse J, Wells B (1997) Children's Speech and Literacy Difficulties: A psycholinguistic framework. Whurr Publishers, London.

Stamp GH, Knapp ML (1990) The construct of intent in interpersonal communication. Quarterly Journal of Speech 76(3): 282–99.

Stansfield J (1982) Current trends in mental handicap. Bulletin of the College of Speech Therapists 365: 1–2.

Stansfield J, Cheseldine S (1994) Challenging to communicate. Human Communication (May/June): 11–14.

Stansfield J, Cheseldine S (1996) Challenging Behaviour and Speech and Language Therapy: II. A comparison of the experiences of speech and language therapists. IASSID Conference, Helsinki.

Stillman R, Battle C (1985) Caller Azuza Scale (H) Programme in Communication Disorders. Callier Centre for Communication Disorders, University of Texas at Dallas.

Stoel-Gammon C (1980) Phonological analysis of four Down's syndrome children. Applied Linguistics 1: 31–48.

Stoel-Gammon C (1981) Speech development of infants and children with Down's syndrome. In: Darby J (ed) Speech Evaluation in Medicine. Grune & Straton, New York, pp. 341–60.

Stoel-Gammon C (1997) Phonological development in Down syndrome. Mental Retardation and Development Disabilities Research Reviews 3: 300–6.

Strain PS, Odom S (1986) Innovations in the education of preschool children with severe handicaps. In: Horner RH, Meyer LH, Fredericks HB (eds) Education of Learners with Severe Handicaps: Exemplary service strategies. Paul H Brookes Publishing, London. Chapter 3.

Sutton A, Morford J (1998) Constituent order in picture pointing sequences produced by speaking children using AAC. Applied Psycholinguistics 19: 525–36.

Sutton K, Thurman S (1998) Challenging communication: People with learning disabilities who challenge services. International Journal of Language and Communication Disorders 33: 415–20.

Swain I, Finklestein V, French S, Oliver M (eds) (1993) Disabling Barriers: Enabling environments. Sage, London.

Szatmari P, Bremner R, Nagy J (1989) Asperger's syndrome: A review of clinical features. Canadian Journal of Psychiatry 34: 554–60.

Tae-Kim Y, Lombardino L (1991) The efficacy of script context in language comprehension intervention with children who have mental retardation. Journal of Speech and Hearing Research 34: 845–57.

Tager-Flusberg H (1986) Constraints on the representation of word meaning: Evidence from autistic and mentally retarded children. In: Kuczaj S, Barrett M (eds) The Development of Word Meaning. Springer, New York, NY, pp. 69–81.

Tager-Flusberg H, Calkins S, Nolan T, Baum Gerger T, Anderson M, Chadwick-Dias A (1990) A longitudinal study of language acquisition in autistic and Down Syndrome children. Journal of Autism and Developmental Disorders 20: 1–21.

Tannock R, Girolametto L (1992) Reassessing parent-focused language intervention programs. In: Warren S, Reichle J (eds) Causes and Effects in Communication and Language Intervention. Paul H Brookes, Baltimore, pp. 49–79.

Tannock R, Girolametto LE, Siegel L (1992) The interactive model of language intervention: Evaluation of its effectiveness for pre-school-aged children with developmental delay. American Journal of Mental Retardation 97(2): 145–60.

Thurman S (1997) Challenging behaviour through communication. British Journal of Learning Disabilities 25: 111–16.

Thurman S, Stewart K, Jones J (1991) Talking Points: A resources file for communication workshops. Stass Publications, Ponteland, Northumberland.

Tizard B, Mortimore J, Burchell B (1981) Involving Parents in Nursery and Infants Schools. Grant McIntyre, London.

Tod J (1997) Applying the principles of the code of practice to pupils with specific learning difficulties/dyslexia. In: Fawcus M (ed) Children with Learning Difficulties: A collaborative approach to their education and management. Whurr Publishers, London. Chapter 11.

Tomasello M (1992) First Verbs: a case study of early grammatical development. Cambridge University Press, Cambridge.

Toogood S, Timlin K (1996) The functional assessment of challenging behaviour: A comparison of informant-based, experimental and descriptive methods. Journal of Applied Research in Intellectual Disabilities 9(3): 206–22.

Torgesen JK, Rashotte C, Greenstein J, Houck G, Portes P (1987) Academic difficulties of learning disabled children who perform poorly on memory span tasks. In: Swanson HL (ed) Memory and Learning Disabilities. JAI Press Inc., Greenwich, Conn.

Tyrer SP, Dunstan JA (1997) Schizophrenia. In: Read S (ed) Psychiatry and Learning Disability. W.B. Saunders, London, pp. 185–215.

Udwin O, Yule W (1990) Augmentative communication systems taught to cerebral-palsied children – a longitudinal study. I: The acquisition of signs and symbols, and syntactic aspects of their use. British Journal of Disorders of Communication 25: 295–309.

Udwin O, Yule W (1991) Augmentative communication systems taught to cerebral-palsied children – a longitudinal study. III: Teaching practices and exposure to sign and symbol use in schools and homes. British Journal of Disorders of Communication 26: 149–62.

US Department of Education (1994) 16th annual report to Congress on the implementation of the 'Individuals with Disabilities Education Act'. US Department of Education, Washington, DC.

US GPO (1991) America 2000. An Education Strategy. US Government Printing Office, Washington DC.

van Balkom H, Welle Donker-Gimbrere A (1996) A psycholinguistic approach to graphic language use. In: von Tetzchner S, Jensen MH (eds) Augmentative and Alternative Communication: European perspectives. Whurr Publishers, London, pp. 153–70.

van der Gaag A (1988) The Communication Assessment Profile (CASP). Speech Profiles, London.

van der Gaag A (1989) The view from Walter's window: Social environment and the communicative competence of adults with a mental handicap. Journal of Mental Deficiency Research 33: 221–7.

van der Gaag A (1998) Communication skills and adults with learning disabilities: Eliminating professional myopia. British Journal of Learning Disabilities 26: 88–93.

van der Gaag A, Dormandy K (1993) Communication and Adults with Learning Disabilities. Whurr Publishers, London.

van Tatenhove G (1993) What is Minspeak? Prentke Romich Company, Wooster, OH.

Vaughn S, Schumm JS (1995) Responsible inclusion for students with learning disabilities. Journal of Learning Disabilities 28(5): 264–70.

Veneziano E, Sinclair H, Berthoud I (1990) From one word to two words: Repetition patterns on the way to structured speech. Journal of Child Language 17: 633–50.

Volden J, Johnston J (1999) Cognitive Scripts and Children and Adolescents. Journal of Autism and Developmental Disorders 29(3): 203–11.

von Tetzchner S, Jensen MH (1996) Introduction. In: von Tetzchner S, Jensen MH (eds) European Perspectives on Augmentative and Alternative Communication. Whurr Publishers, London, pp. 1–18.

von Tetzchner S, Grove N, Loncke F, Barnett S, Woll B, Clibbens J (1996) Preliminaries to a comprehensive model of augmentative and alternative communication. In: von Tetzchner S, Jensen MH (eds) Augmentative and Alternative Communication: European perspectives. Whurr Publishers, London, pp. 19–36.

Vygotsky L (1978) The development of higher psychological processes. In: Cole M, John-Steiner S, Souberman E (eds) Mind in Society. Harvard University Press, Cambridge MA (originally published in 1930).

Walker C, Walker A, Ryan T (1995) What kind of future? Opportunities for older people with learning difficulties. In: Philpot T, Ward L (eds) Values and Visions, Changing Services for People with Learning Difficulties. Butterworth-Heinemann, Oxford, pp. 232–43.

Walker M (1980) Makaton Vocabulary Development Project: 31 Firwood Drive, Camberley, Surrey GU15 3QD, UK.

Ward S (1992) The predictive validity and accuracy of a screening test for language delay and auditory perceptual disorder. European Journal of Disorders of Communication 27: 55–72.

Ward S (1994) The Validation of a Treatment Method for Auditory Perceptual Disorder in Young Children. WILSTAAR, London.

Ward S (1999) An investigation into the effectiveness of an early intervention method for delayed language development in young children. International Journal of Language Communication Disorders 34(3): 243–64.

Ware J (1990) Interactions between pupils with severe learning disabilities and non-handicapped peers. Reach 4: 44–8.

Ware J (1996) Creating a Responsive Environment for People with Profound and Multiple Learning Difficulties. David Fulton Publishers, London.

Warnock M (1978) Special Educational Needs: Report of the Committee of Enquiry into the Education of Handicapped Children and Young People (DES). HMSO, London.

Warren SF (1988) A behavioural approach to language generalisation. Language Speech and Hearing Services in Schools 19: 292–303.

Wetherby A, Warren S, Reichle J (1998) Transitions in Prelinguistic Communication. Paul H. Brookes, Baltimore.

Whalley M (2001) Involving Parents in Their Children's Learning. Paul Chapman Publishers, London.

White M, Cameron RJ (eds) (1988) Portage: Problems and possibilities. NFER-Nelson, Windsor.

WHO (1997) Health for All. Alma Alta Conference, 1997. World Health Organization, Geneva.

Wicks K (1998) Equitable service provision for inclusive education and effective early intervention. International Journal of Language Communication Disorders. Supplement 33: 562–7.

Wilcox J (1992) Enhancing initial communication skills in young children with developmental disabilities through partner programming. Seminars in Speech and Language 15(3): 195–212.

Wilkinson KM, Romski MA, Sevcik R (1994) The emergence of visual-graphic symbol combinations by youth with moderate or severe mental retardation. Journal of Speech and Hearing Research 37: 883–95.

Will M (1986) Educating Students with Learning Problems: A shared responsibility. I.S. Department 2000, Washington DC (ERIC Document Reproduction Service, No, ED 279 149).

Williamson K (2000) The best things for the best reasons. Bulletin, Royal College of Speech and Language Therapists. October, pp. 17–18.

Wing L (1996) The Autism Spectrum: A guide for parents and professionals. Constable, London.

Wirz S (1995) Perceptual Approaches to Communication Disorders. Whurr Publishers, London.

Wolfendale S (1992) Primary Schools and Special Needs: Policy, planning, provision. Cassell Educational, London.

Wolfendale S (1993) Assessing Special Educational Needs. Cassell, London.

Wolfensberger W (1972) The Principle of Normalisation in Human Services. National Institute on Mental Retardation: Toronto.

Wolfensberger W (1983) A proposed term for the principle of 'normalisation'. Journal of Mental Retardation 21(3): 234–349.

Wolfensberger W (1985) Social Role Valorisation: A new insight and a new term for 'normalisation'. Australian Association for the Mentally Retarded 9(1): 4–11.

Woll B, Barnett S (1998) Towards a sociolinguistic perspective on augmentative and alternative communication. Augmentative and Alternative Communication 14: 200–11.

Woll B, Grove N (1997) On language deficits and modality in children with Down Syndrome: A case study of twins bilingual in BSL and English. Journal of Deaf Studies and Deaf Education 1: 271–8.

Woltosz W (1988) A proposed model for augmentative communication evaluation and system selection. Augmentative and Alternative Communication 4(4): 233–5.

Wong BYL (1996) The ABCs of Learning Disabilities. Academic Press, London.

Wong BYL (ed) (1998) Learning About Learning Disabilities, 2nd edn. Academic Press, London.

Wood ME (1983) Costs of intervention programs. In: Garland C, Stone NW, Swanson J, Woodruff G (eds) Early Intervention for Children with Special Needs and their Families: Findings and Recommendations. Westar Series Paper No. 11. University of Washington, Seattle, WA.

Woods P, Cullen C (1983) Determinants of staff behaviour in long-term care. Behavioural Psychotherapy 11: 4–17.

Wooton A (1989) Speech to and from a severely retarded young Down's syndrome child. In: Beveridge M, Conti-Ramsden G, Leudar I (eds) Language and Communication in Mentally Handicapped People. Chapman & Hall, London. Chapter 7.

Wright J (1993) Assessment of children with special needs. In: Beech JR, Harding L, Hilton-Jones D (eds) Assessment in Speech and Language Therapy. Routledge-NFER Assessment Library, London. Chapter 7.

Yamada J (1990) Laura: A case for the modularity of language. MIT Press, Cambridge, MA.

Yoder J, Warren S, McCathren NR, Leew S (1998) Does adult responsivity to child behaviour facilitate communication development? In: Wetherby A, Warren S, Reichle J (eds) Transitions in Prelinguistic Communication, Chapter 3. Paul H. Brookes, Baltimore.

Yorkston K, Honsinger M, Dowden P, Marriner N (1989) Vocabulary selection: A case report. Augmentative and Alternative Communication 5(2): 101–8.

Zangari C, Lloyd L, Vicker B (1994) Augmentative and alternative communication: An historic perspective. Augmentative and Alternative Communication 10(1): 27–59.

Zarkowska E, Clements J (1988) Problem Behaviour in People with Severe Learning Disability. Croom Helm, London.

Ziarnik JP, Bernstein GS (1982) A critical examination of the effect of in-service training on staff performance. Mental Retardation 20: 109–44.

Index

specialist support 250
  to early intervention (EI) 105
settings 41, 66, 68
severe learning difficulty 169
shared
  attention 158
  communication 89
  model of communication 86
sharing 59
showing 58
side effects 287
sign 158, 160
  combinations 170
  co-active use 161
  morphology 170, 178
Sign Support English 191
signal localisation 143
Signalong 191
significant others 90, 222, 263
Signs and Symbols Linkworker Network
  96
simultaneous processing 165
single word understanding 145, 159
single words 165
single-symbol messages 173
single-word to two-word utterances 180
skills
  cognitive see cognitive
  listening 43
  partner 60
  pre-linguistic 43
  social 157
  visual 43
SLT assistant (SLTA) 2, 21
SLTA competencies 2
smell and taste 141
smiling 58
Sneozelen 206
social
  benefits 110
  communication 241, 242, 285, 286
  communication skills 88, 95
  consequences 155
  constructs of disability 47
  framework 47
  functioning 282
  handicap 291
  history 70
  interaction 48, 59, 155, 240, 286

isolation 47
meanings 160
milieu 36
participation 25
policy 2
relationships 48
responsiveness 138
skills 48, 62, 76, 157, 197, 243
skills deficit 76
Social Communication Group 234
Social Communication Programme 234
social model of 47, 190
  communication 100
  disability 100, 102
Social Role Valorisation (SRV) 1, 2, 3, 4,
  18
social services 84, 91
social stories 286
social synchronisation 285
Social Use of Language Programme 77
social withdrawal 277
socialisation 77
Somerset Total Communication
  Approach 99, 100
sound discrimination 58
spatial
  relationships 143
  syntax 172
Speaking and Listening and Reading
  Package 230
special
  education needs coordinators
    (SENCO) 126
  interest groups 24
  learning difficulties 36
  needs 55
  needs co-ordinator 8
specialist role 90
specific interest group 250, 272
specific language impairment (SLI) 78
speech and language therapy assistant 20,
  233
speech and verbal language skills 64
staff
  carer interaction 84
  communication 85, 101
  initiations 85
  trainers 98
  training 93, 97